Praise for
# Radical Hope

"*Radical Hope* reveals real-world examples of how to rise to the challenges of living with cancer and to not only survive but thrive. This scientifically based and accessible book will help to transform lives, as it contains a multitude of actionable recommendations to empower people to reverse and prevent multiple diseases."

— **Lorenzo Cohen, Ph.D.**, professor and director of Integrative Medicine Program at MD Anderson Cancer Center and co-author of *Anticancer Living*

"Thanks to Kelly for so clearly presenting the 10 healing factors that constitute the holistic pillars of integrative oncology. The Action Steps will help motivate readers to begin their journey. Empowering patients with tools to take control of their own health creates hope, which, in and of itself, promotes healing."

— **Donald I. Abrams, M.D.**, Integrative Oncology, University of California San Francisco Osher Center for Integrative Medicine and co-editor of *Integrative Oncology*

"In this evolutionary and breakthrough book, Turner reveals the 10 factors that cancer patients who experience radical remission have in common and provides exercises and stories of survivors using this process. A powerful work providing tools for healing."

— **Anita Moorjani**, *New York Times* best-selling author of *Dying to Be Me* and *What If This Is Heaven?*

"Turner's revelatory research on cancer patients who survive against the odds is some of the most important work in the cancer space today. *Radical Hope* is a book that anyone who wants to survive or prevent cancer should read!"

— **Chris Wark**, best-selling author of *Chris Beats Cancer*

"*Radical Hope* is an enlivening, heart-opening, paradigm-shifting, educational, and illuminating update on Kelly Turner's extensive research into the 9 (now 10) factors that are linked to radical remission from 'incurable' cancer. It's a grounded collection of practical tools anyone who is ill can utilize to be proactive about building the foundation for better-than-expected health outcomes."

— **Lissa Rankin, M.D.**, *New York Times* best-selling author of *Mind Over Medicine* and founder of the Whole Health Medicine Institute

"Nothing—and I mean nothing—is more powerful than hope. In her latest book, Turner documents the healing power of hope and provides solid scientific evidence of the power of hope and how it is saving lives."

— **Christiane Northrup, M.D.**, *New York Times* best-selling author of *Women's Bodies, Women's Wisdom; The Wisdom of Menopause;* and *Goddesses Never Age*

"Turner is a pioneer and bright light of hope for cancer survivors. Her fierce dedication to finding and sharing practical, evidence-based healing solutions has helped countless patients thrive through a cancer diagnosis."

— **Shamini Jain, Ph.D.**, assistant professor, University of California San Diego; founder and director of Consciousness and Healing Initiative

*"Radical Hope* builds on Dr. Turner's first book, offering a deeper dive into the lives of patients who have overcome the odds, expertly woven into the latest research, tips, and revelations that takes an individual from merely surviving to thriving."

— **Nasha Winters, N.D.**, oncology naturopathic physician and best-selling co-author of *The Metabolic Approach to Cancer*

"This book is for anyone looking for the courage to heal. Don't miss out on the 10 key healing factors from survivors of cancer and other diseases! A must-read for anyone who is going through it."

— **Liana Werner-Gray**, best-selling author of *The Earth Diet* and *Cancer-Free with Food*

"The authors capture poignant stories of the human spirit and the power of being present, engaged, and proactive—and how this can positively influence even life-limiting diagnoses. *Radical Hope* brings important attention to why exceptional responders—often quickly dismissed as outliers and anecdotes—must be thoroughly studied."

— **Glen Sabin**, best-selling co-author of *N of 1*

"Turner recognizes important factors that make all the difference for people with cancer. These factors are difference-makers for people with cancer. I am one of the cancer survivors who is continually reinspired by her work."

— **Ann Fonfa**, president of The Annie Appleseed Project

"Healing completely from cancer and chronic disease is not only possible but achievable, thanks to Turner's essential insights. Her superb book serves up empowering science, inspirational stories, and proven strategies to kick cancer and chronic disease to the curb."

— **Palmer Kippola**, best-selling author of *Beat Autoimmune: The 6 Keys to Reverse Your Condition and Reclaim Your Health*

"*Radical Hope* raises fundamental questions around beliefs, and how they can trap or free us. With candor and curiosity, Turner dares us to reconsider spontaneous healings as more ordinary than extraordinary. This is a must-read for every patient and doctor."

— **Cynthia Li, M.D.**, integrative medicine doctor
and best-selling author of *Brave New Medicine*

"In these history-making pages, the impossible is made possible, and the path to the little-discussed promise land of remission is revealed for its intuitive simplicity. *Radical Hope* will uncage that small voice inside you that says, *yes*, there is a better way!"

— **Kelly Brogan, M.D.**, *New York Times* best-selling author of
*Own Your Self* and *A Mind of Your Own*

"*Radical Hope* is essential reading for anyone with a serious interest in what we can do to heal ourselves."

— **Michael Lerner, Ph.D.**, president and co-founder of
Commonweal Cancer Help Program

"If you have been diagnosed with a cancer considered 'hopeless,' read *Radical Hope* now, and then give a copy to your oncologist."

— **Dawn Lemanne, M.D., MPH**, oncologist and founder of
Oregon Integrative Oncology

"The patients described in *Radical Remission* and *Radical Hope* have important lessons to share, not only for others facing serious health challenges, but for all of us who want to live as full and vibrant a life as possible."

— **Linda L. Isaacs, M.D.**, co-author of *The Trophoblast
and the Origins of Cancer*

"If you have cancer, if you love someone who has cancer, or if you are a healthcare practitioner who cares for people with cancer, I encourage you with my whole heart to read *Radical Hope*. Allow it to fill you with hope in knowing that the 'impossible' is indeed possible."

— **Mark Bricca, N.D., MAc.**, Oncology Naturopathic Physician

## ALSO BY KELLY A. TURNER, PH.D.

*Radical Remission: Surviving Cancer Against All Odds*

# RADICAL

## *Hope*

### 10 Key Healing Factors from Exceptional Survivors of Cancer & Other Diseases

## Kelly A. Turner, Ph.D.
### with Tracy White

**HAY HOUSE, INC.**
Carlsbad, California • New York City
London • Sydney • New Delhi

*Published in the United States by:* Hay House, Inc.: www.hayhouse.com®
*Published in Australia by:* Hay House Australia Pty. Ltd.: www.hayhouse.com.au
*Published in the United Kingdom by:* Hay House UK, Ltd.: www.hayhouse.co.uk
*Published in India by:* Hay House Publishers India: www.hayhouse.co.in

*Indexer:* J S Editorial, LLC
*Cover design:* Ploy Siripant
*Interior design:* Bryn Starr Best

Cataloging-in-Publication Data is on file at the Library of Congress

Hardcover ISBN: 978-1-4019-5921-0
e-book ISBN: 978-1-4019-5923-4
Audiobook ISBN: 978-14019-5952-4

10 9 8 7 6 5 4 3 2 1
1st edition, April 2020

Printed in the United States of America

SUSTAINABLE
FORESTRY
INITIATIVE
Certified Chain of Custody
Promoting Sustainable Forestry
www.sfiprogram.org
SFI-01268

SFI label applies to the text stock

*To anyone who has ever felt fear,
when what they needed most
was hope.*

# CONTENTS

# INTRODUCTION

When a doctor says, "You have cancer," your brain stops. Your amygdala—the primal part of your brain that screamed at your caveman ancestors to "Run from that tiger *now!*"—kicks into fight or flight. You enter pure survival mode.

Most newly diagnosed cancer patients report a similar experience. Whether the prognosis is, "You need a quick surgery and then you will be fine," or "It's incurable and you should get your affairs in order," they report feeling overwhelming fear.

In that moment, what patients and their caregivers need more than anything is *hope.* They want to know that someone else has beaten their dire prognosis and they feel an instinctive need to find other survivors.

That's why we wrote this book—to provide radical hope to those affected by cancer and other diseases when they need it most.

## What Is a Radical Remission?

A radical remission is a statistically unlikely remission in which the person either:

1. heals without conventional treatment;

2. first tries conventional treatments, which do not lead to remission, so they then try alternative treatments, which do lead to remission; or

3. uses a combination of conventional and alternative treatments at the same time in order to outlive a dire prognosis (e.g., less than 25 percent five-year survival rate).

My first book, *Radical Remission: Surviving Cancer Against All Odds*, was born out of a decade of research into what the medical field terms "spontaneous remissions," and what I call radical remissions. I wanted to know how someone could be sent home to die from cancer, only to walk into their doctor's office a year later alive and well, perhaps even healthier than before their diagnosis.

Who were these miraculous survivors? Why were there more than 1,000 verified cases in medical journals, and yet no one was studying them? What had these people done to heal, and why did they think they got well?

These were the questions that fueled my dissertation research at the University of California, Berkeley. Over the course of the next decade, I went on to analyze more than 1,000 medically verified spontaneous remissions documented in medical journals and conducted in-depth interviews with hundreds more radical remission survivors from around the world. This research became my Ph.D. dissertation, and ultimately the book *Radical Remission*.

It became very clear as I interviewed people who had experienced a "spontaneous" remission that there was nothing spontaneous about it. These survivors spoke of making significant lifestyle and emotional changes in order to heal. Their so-called miracle healings occurred because they made radical shifts in their minds and spirits—not just their bodies—upending their *entire* lives in order to achieve what I came to call "radical remission."

Nine common factors emerged from my in-depth interviews with hundreds of cancer patients who had beaten the odds. The survivors didn't know they were using the same healing strategies as other survivors, and many of them tried more than just these nine healing strategies. However, all of them used all nine factors, which formed the foundation for their healing.

The nine key healing factors are listed below, in no particular order:

- radically changing your diet
- taking control of your health
- following your intuition
- using herbs and supplements
- releasing repressed emotions
- increasing positive emotions
- embracing social support
- deepening your spiritual connection
- having strong reasons for living

These nine factors are covered in depth in *Radical Remission*, and we will be expanding that discussion in this book.

## Radical Remission

Much to my surprise, *Radical Remission* hit the *New York Times* bestseller list in its first week. Numerous TV and radio programs requested interviews, and eventually the book was translated into 22 (and counting) languages. Clearly, I am not the only one fascinated by radical remissions.

As its popularity grew, *Radical Remission* became a platform for healing and support. Patients and their families continued to ask for more resources, and my small team and I did our best to answer the call. Our readers asked for in-person workshops on how to boost the immune system. We now offer them around the world, led by our wonderful group of certified Radical Remission instructors. Those who were too sick to attend workshops in person asked for an online course, which is now available on our website and can be taken from the comfort of your own home (or hospital room) at your own pace. Readers asked for one-on-one coaching after their in-person workshops ended. We now have certified Radical Remission health coaches offering in-person or virtual coaching sessions for those who need it. And, of course, we are grateful that social media allows us to join in conversation with you. We love seeing your #shelfies (photos of the book on your shelf) of #radicalremission!

Continuing radical remission research is a high priority for me, so my small staff and I actively collect new cases on RadicalRemission.com every day. Thanks to our free online database, radical remission survivors no longer need to wait for their oncologists to write up their cases and publish them in medical journals (although that remains an important task for doctors to do). Instead, a radical remission survivor can now share their remission story on our site in as little as 10 minutes. One goal of this database is to facilitate future research by building an ever-growing collection of verified cases.

We are happy to report that since *Radical Remission's* publication, our site has been flooded with new cases. Each year for the past six years, we have collected *six times* the average number of radical remission cases that are published annually in medical journals—which suggests that radical remissions occur far more often than doctors realize. The new cases reported on our website continue to support the commonality of the nine healing factors that emerged during my initial decade of research. This is exactly what a scientist hopes to see: confirmation of the original findings. I love it when someone submits their healing story to the RadicalRemission.com website and writes, "I read your book *Radical Remission* and it was like reading my own diary. Those were the exact nine things I did to heal my cancer 20 years ago!"

After *Radical Remission* was published, researchers from Harvard University approached us and asked if they could study the effects of the Radical Remission workshop on cancer patients. We are happy to report that a pilot study on this topic is currently underway, supported in part by your generous donations to our nonprofit research organization, the Radical Remission Foundation. We have also helped a biotech company that wanted to analyze the blood and genetic makeup of radical remission survivors. Thanks to many of our newsletter readers who donated blood to that study, the company is currently testing novel immunotherapy cancer treatments in its laboratory.

## The 10th Factor

During my initial decade of research, exercise was a very common healing factor among radical remission survivors, but it was not reported in *every* case. I believe this is because many of the people I interviewed were very sick when they first began to heal, and exercise was simply not possible for them at that time. For example, some of the people I interviewed were sent home on hospice care in wheelchairs and with feeding tubes before they eventually healed.

However, in reviewing our archive of radical remission cases, it has become clear that radical remission survivors make moderate to intense exercise a lifelong habit whenever they are physically able. In addition, some radical remission survivors use exercise as a direct healing method, incorporating activities such as high-intensity interval training (HIIT), rebounding on a mini-trampoline, or weight training into their healing regimen from the day they are diagnosed.

In this book, we will fully describe this new, 10th healing factor, including the latest research on why exercise is crucial when going through cancer, the ways in which radical remission survivors incorporate it into their lives, and the healing story of a woman who relied on exercise as one of her key healing factors in overcoming breast cancer.

## My Story

Cancer entered my life at a young age. My close friend was diagnosed with stomach cancer when we were both 14. Two years later, despite his trying everything conventional medicine had to offer, including surgery and chemotherapy, he died. We were both 16, and while my future still lay ahead of me, bright and full of possibility, his was gone.

It was a sad and confusing time for me, and stories provided an escape. I spent hours lost in books, movies, plays, and musicals. My love for stories, especially true and inspiring ones, followed me to Harvard University, where I balanced the analytical and creative sides of my brain by studying both psychology and screenwriting.

After graduation, I began volunteering at a local hospital on weekends, working with cancer patients. This inspired me to pursue a master's degree in clinical social work at the University of California, Berkeley, with a specialty in counseling cancer patients. It was an emotionally draining time, but I loved helping cancer patients in such a profound way. Each person's healing journey was unique, and it was an honor to listen to their stories.

One particular story that I read about during this time—a radical remission healing story—completely fascinated me. I had to know more. After some initial research, I realized there was a treasure trove of *thousands* of verified "spontaneous remission" healing stories in the medical journals that no one was investigating. At that moment, the two sides of me—researcher and storyteller—joined forces to solve an important mystery: *How had these people healed?*

To answer this question, I stayed at the University of California, Berkeley, earning my Ph.D. and later publishing *Radical Remission*. The Radical Remission Project has grown over the years, bringing more incredible healing stories to light and giving hope to those who need it. When I'm not working on the resources we offer at Radical-Remission.com, other forms of storytelling fill my time, including writing *Open-Ended Ticket*, a feature film script inspired by *Radical Remission*, and directing a 10-part docuseries on radical remissions. Most recently, writing *Radical Hope* has given me the opportunity to analyze even more amazing cases of radical remission.

## About This Book

We have structured this book in a format similar to *Radical Remission*, in that each chapter focuses on one of the key healing factors. However, you will notice that the factors are presented in a different order than they were in *Radical Remission*. This is purposeful, because we wanted to emphasize that we still do not know which of the 10 factors (if any) is more important than the others. In each chapter, we will:

- briefly review a radical remission healing factor;
- share what we and other researchers have learned over the years since *Radical Remission* was first published;
- share one in-depth healing story of a new radical remission survivor who relied on that particular factor; and
- suggest new ways you can bring that factor into your life.

It is important to remember that we, along with everyone at the Radical Remission Project, are not and have never been against conventional medicine for cancer treatment. We believe there is tremendous value in studying the thousands of anomalous cases of people who have healed without such treatment, or after that treatment has failed them. Anyone who has healed from cancer against the odds has something to teach us about cancer and the immune system.

Another important point to remember is that we are *studying* radical remissions, not *prescribing* them. We are researchers reporting on a phenomenon, as opposed to doctors telling you what you should do. As such, this book should not be used in lieu of medical advice, and we cannot promise that these 10 factors will heal your disease or anyone else's.

All we know at this point in the research process is that these 10 healing factors appear to have helped *this particular group of people* achieve remission. We will not know if these 10 factors work for other people until multiple, randomized, prospective controlled trials have been conducted. The pilot study by Harvard University researchers that is currently underway is the first step in that long process. It will take 20–50 more years and tens of millions more dollars in research funding before we have definitive answers. Nevertheless, while we wait for the research, we feel comfortable providing suggested action steps at the end of each chapter because these 10 factors have been shown in other independent clinical research trials to benefit the immune system. Whether it will strengthen your immune system enough to bring your cancer into remission is still unknown.

Please remember that, while 9 out of the 10 healing factors can be explored on your own, taking herbs or supplements should always be done under the guidance of a qualified health professional, and it is always a good idea to discuss with your doctor or other health professional any lifestyle or dietary changes you plan on making.

## Finding Hope

Despite the myriad of activities that have been happening at the Radical Remission Project, we have noticed that what patients and caregivers crave most are more real-life stories of radical remission survivors.

We understand this completely, since these healing stories are what have inspired us to continue with our research day in and day out. There is nothing more life-affirming than interviewing a real-life person who has overcome stage 4 cancer. These are not just "stories"—they are verified case reports of healing against the odds, and it is our honor and privilege to be their messengers.

A cancer coach once said to a radical remission survivor, "In your town, you seem like a 'cancer unicorn'—rare because you beat the odds by surviving so-called incurable cancer. But in my line of work, I see thousands of survivors. I wish everyone could know there are fields full of unicorns just like you."

We hope that the true stories of survival in this book will provide you with your own "field full of unicorns," and that they will inspire and empower you to take charge of your own health. Our greatest wish is that these verified case studies of real people whom we have met, spoken with, laughed with, and cried with will give you the radical hope that healing is possible at any time.

## CHAPTER 1

# EXERCISE

## Mary's Story

*If physical activity existed in pill form, it would
be the most prescribed medicine in the world.*

— GRETE WAITZ, CANCER SURVIVOR AND CO-FOUNDER
OF AKTIV AGAINST CANCER

We know exercise is good for us. It should come as no surprise that exercise provides health benefits, even for a person with cancer. However, until recently, physical activity as it relates to cancer has not captured the attention of researchers, patients, or the media. For example, a quick online search for books on "exercise and cancer" yields one-quarter the results of a search for books on "diet and cancer."

Exercise did come up as one of the healing factors that survivors used when I first researched *Radical Remission*, but it was not a factor that *all* survivors utilized, which is why it was not included in my original dissertation or my first book as one of the most common healing factors. However, I believe this is because many of the people I studied were too weak to exercise at the beginning of their healing journeys. As they grew stronger, many of them started to move their bodies, and *all* of them started to exercise or move their bodies regularly once they were physically able. At the height of their illness, they may not have been able to exercise due to the physical toll that the disease or treatment was taking on their body, but exercise was, in fact, essential to their long-term remission.

After reviewing the older radical remission cases and analyzing the new ones that have come in since the publication of *Radical Remission*, we have found that radical remission survivors added some form of movement or exercise back into their lives as soon as they were strong enough to do so. This is why we are now including exercise as the 10th common factor of radical remission cases.

It may be helpful to reframe exercise as physical activity. Many of the survivors from my early research did not think to mention exercise in our interviews because they did not consider their daily walks or movements to be exercise. Let's use Tracy (this book's co-author) as an example. As a former marathon runner, triathlete, gym buff, and yogi, Tracy used to set a high bar for what she considered exercise. She thought of the low points of her illness as a time when she was not exercising at all, because her body hurt too much to do any of her previous workouts. When she was at her weakest, she could barely walk down the street.

However, when I asked if she had moved her body *at all* during that time, she remembered doing little things to stay strong, such as walking as far as she could down the street, resting for a minute, and then turning around and walking home. She did not think of this activity as exercise, nor as a part of her treatment. It was something she did to survive.

When you are very ill, running a simple errand can count as physical activity, due to the amount of energy it can take out of you. Tracy remembers having a mini-celebration when, during her treatment, she was able to go to both the grocery store and the library on the same day without needing a two-hour nap. With this story in mind, remember that exercise does not need to be formal or intense. You do not need special clothes or a gym membership. You just need to move your body every day.

Since *Radical Remission* was published, we have heard from many more survivors via our website, RadicalRemission.com. One such person is Tremane from New Zealand. Tremane was diagnosed with stage 4 pancreatic cancer in 2012. He was very physically fit and active prior to his diagnosis—he played indoor soccer, went to the gym two to three times a week, boogie-boarded at the beach, and practiced yoga. But then his whole life changed with one sentence from his doctor.

*I was told it was terminal cancer. And they told me to stop moving because [the tumor] was pressing up against my stomach and lungs, and they didn't want it to spread. So I stopped moving, which I think—in hindsight—was a mistake. It was only a year later when, by that stage, I realized I wasn't going to die. I was in a space where I was neither recovering nor dying; I was just surviving. And one of the things that got me out of that hole was exercise. . . . I had stopped moving for a year and I thought, This is a mistake. I can't keep on doing this. It's not in my nature, anyway, to sit still. So I started walking—just walking around the block after work every day. And about a year and a half later, I started doing yoga again.*

What makes Tremane's example interesting is that he *was* exercising regularly until his doctors told him to stop after he was diagnosed. Thankfully, he followed his intuition and resumed exercise a year later, which he believes helped him to achieve his radical remission (along with practicing the other nine radical remission healing factors). Luckily, Tremane's intuition lines up with the latest scientific research, which shows that moderate to intense exercise is one of the best things cancer patients can do to support their healing.

In this chapter, we will begin by talking about why exercise is essential to anyone's health and quality of life, including during and after treatment. We will share the latest research on this topic and discuss different types of exercise for cancer patients. The heart of the chapter is an in-depth survivor story that we hope will inspire you to "jump" into this 10th factor of exercise, followed by simple action steps you can take to bring this healing factor into your life.

## Benefits for Everyone

If you are alive, you should be moving. We know exercise makes us healthier. As far back as 1996, the surgeon general was so concerned that physical inactivity was causing a national health crisis that a multiagency report was released that compiled decades of research showing the benefits of exercise for health.[1]

Any physical activity is better than none. In 2008, a second report from the surgeon general took things a step further by recommending that all Americans over the age of six engage in either 150 minutes of moderate exercise per week, or 75 minutes of vigorous exercise per week, in order to reap the substantial health benefits of exercise.[2] A third report published in 2018, the *Physical Activity Guidelines for Americans*, concluded that *everyone's* health improves with physical activity: men and women of all races and ethnicities, young children to older adults, women who are pregnant or postpartum, people living with a chronic condition or a disability, and people who want to reduce their risk of chronic disease.[3] The report goes on to say that adults with chronic conditions and disabilities (e.g., cancer) should avoid inactivity at all costs[4] and consult their physicians about what they can do.

Recent studies have also found that obesity is a global epidemic.[5] It is the number one cause of preventable deaths,[6] and it poses a direct and severe cancer risk.[7] In fact, being obese is more deadly for you than smoking or having high blood pressure, high cholesterol, or diabetes.[8] Thankfully, exercise, along with eating a healthy diet, gives us the first line of defense in combating obesity.

Here are just a few of the scientifically proven benefits of exercise.[9] Exercise can:

- reduce the risk of dying prematurely;
- reduce the risk of dying from heart disease and cancer;[10]
- reduce the risk of developing diabetes;

- reduce the risk of developing high blood pressure and reduce blood pressure in people who already have high blood pressure;

- reduce feelings of depression and anxiety;

- help you maintain a healthy weight;

- help you build and maintain healthy bones, muscles, and joints; and

- extend your life span.

That last fact is worth emphasizing: According to a recent study, regular movement or exercise can extend your life by three to eight years, depending on how much you exercise and when you start.[11] On the opposite end of the spectrum, other research has found that being a couch potato can kill you. A meta-analysis study of more than a million participants found that people who exercise with moderate intensity (a total of 60–75 minutes per day) are able to eliminate the increased risk of death that is associated with a high daily sitting time (unless that sitting time is associated with high TV viewing time, in which case the risk remains).[12] So if your job forces you to sit at a desk all day, you can overcome the negative health effects of all that sitting through exercise, but if you then choose to binge-watch TV all night, those health benefits disappear.

## Benefits for Cancer Patients

The first studies investigating the effects of exercise on cancer patients and survivors were published in the 1980s.[13] Since then, the National Cancer Institute, American Cancer Society, and American College of Sports Medicine (ACSM) have concluded decisively that exercise is not only safe and feasible during cancer treatment, but that it can improve one's physical functioning, reduce fatigue, and enhance quality of life during treatment.[14,15] In 2018, the ACSM hosted a roundtable to review the latest research and update its recommendation regarding exercise as a form of cancer prevention and control. There is a growing body of evidence to demonstrate the effectiveness of exercise in cancer prevention, treatment support, reduction in recurrence, and improvement in survival rates. The biggest challenge is spreading the word about the benefits of exercise when it comes to cancer, and educating oncologists so that they talk about exercise with their patients.[16]

As you might expect, cancer patients who exercise end up stronger than those who do not exercise. In one study of prostate cancer patients, researchers found that brief exercise significantly improved the patients' muscle mass, strength, physical function, and balance, compared to prostate cancer patients who did not exercise.[17]

In addition to making cancer patients stronger, exercise can help reduce the side effects of conventional cancer treatment. For example, one study prescribed 10,000 steps of walking per day to breast and colorectal cancer patients who were going through chemotherapy. Compared to a control group of patients who did not walk, the walkers experienced significantly fewer side effects from the treatment, had less pain and swelling, and increased their mobility.[18]

Another study looked at breast cancer patients who exercised in conjunction with their chemotherapy. Compared to a control group, the exercisers showed reduced levels of inflammatory biomarkers and were able to retain their neurocognitive function,[19] reducing their inflammation and "chemo brain," thanks to exercise.

Numerous other studies have shown that exercise improves cancer patients' quality of life during treatment, including their body image/self-esteem, sleep quality, social functioning, sexuality, fatigue and pain levels, and emotional well-being (specifically, exercise significantly reduces depression and anxiety).[20,21]

Improving one's quality of life is important, but you may be wondering, what *exactly* does exercise do to the human body, especially one that is trying to heal from cancer? Studies have shown that exercise leads to a number of specific physiological changes in cancer patients' bodies, including:

- reduced inflammation;
- reduced insulin resistance;
- increased immune cell activity and counts;
- increased lymphatic flow in the lymph system;
- improved ability of the gastrointestinal system to limit exposure to toxins;
- lowered levels of key hormones, such as insulin and estrogen;[22]
- improved oxygen delivery and utilization;
- increased mitochondrial biogenesis;[23] and
- reduced obesity.

In case you are unfamiliar with any of these terms, know that they are *very positive* physical changes for cancer patients—or anyone, for that matter—to experience. That is why the American Cancer Society recommends exercise for everyone with cancer, even those who are bedridden, in which case physical therapy is recommended.

## Exercise and Cancer Survival

Perhaps of most interest to cancer patients are the scores of studies that show exercise reduces the overall risk of cancer recurrence and mortality for certain cancers.[24] For example, exercise has been found to significantly reduce the risk of mortality from breast, colon, prostate, endometrial, ovarian, and lung cancers.[25] One of these studies concluded that a modest amount of vigorous activity, such as biking, tennis, jogging, or swimming for three or more hours per week, was found to significantly improve the survival rate of men with prostate cancer.[26]

Another study showed that women with breast cancer who walked for only one hour per week at an average pace of 2 to 3 mph had up to a 49 percent lower risk of death from breast cancer, compared with women who engaged in less physical activity.[27] In a large study of patients with colorectal cancer, those who engaged in leisure-time physical activity (e.g., tennis, golf, biking, swimming, heavy gardening, fast walking, dancing, aerobics, or jogging) had a 31 percent lower risk of death than those who did not—and this was independent of whether or not they had exercised before their diagnosis.[28] (That's inspiring news for people who do not currently exercise and may think all hope is lost. It's not!) These studies and many more like them show us that if we want to significantly reduce our chances of dying from cancer, we must—*must*—move our bodies, ideally every day.

## Exercise as Targeted Medicine

Until now, the majority of the research on exercise and cancer has focused on exercise as something that cancer survivors can do to prevent a recurrence, or something that cancer patients can do to reduce the side effects of conventional treatment. However, emerging evidence suggests that exercise may actually improve a person's direct response to conventional cancer treatment, including radiation and chemotherapy.[29]

In one such study, scientists studied mice with colon cancer over a six-week period. One group of mice was put on a running wheel for exercise, while another group of mice was not. The mice who exercised experienced unique mitochondrial changes that actually slowed the growth of their tumors, while the non-exercising group's tumors grew at a typical rate.[30]

Exercise can jump-start your body's immune system to fight tumor cells. In a different study, mice who exercised by running on a wheel reduced their tumor growth by 60 percent and increased their adrenaline, natural killer (NK) cells, and immune system function in ways that encouraged tumor healing.[31]

Just imagine if, sometime in the future, an oncologist were to tell her patient, "Due to your particular type of cancer, I recommend six weeks of targeted immunotherapy, 30 minutes per day of high-intensity interval training, and 15 minutes per day of weight training." Countries like Norway and Australia are ahead of the U.S. when it comes to studying exercise as a direct cancer therapy, rather than as a way to reduce side effects. The Exercise Medicine Research Institute in Australia works with cancer patients to add exercise to their conventional medical treatments so that patients can walk out of chemotherapy or radiation and meet with a trained physiologist who then leads them through a customized workout right there at the hospital.[32] Similarly, AKTIV Against Cancer, a nonprofit that operates 16 physical activity centers across Norway, focuses on making exercise an integrated part of cancer treatment.[33] Both organizations aim to someday "prescribe" physical activity as a targeted therapy to slow disease progression and improve survival rates for cancer patients.

Thanks in part to AKTIV's research funding, the U.S. is starting to catch up to Australia and Norway. AKTIV Against Cancer has already pledged more than $3 million to Memorial Sloan Kettering Cancer Center to fund exercise oncology research.

## Types of Exercise

There are many different types of exercise, each with its own unique benefits for cancer patients during treatment and remission. While aerobic exercise and strength training have been around for decades, there has been a recent surge of interest in high-intensity interval training (HIIT) and lymphatic training. Here is an overview of these common exercise types and the research relating to each one.

Aerobic exercise is what we think of most often when we think of exercise. The word *aerobic* means "relating to oxygen"; therefore, aerobic exercise refers to any exercise that increases our oxygen intake.[34] Any walk, run, swim, or bike ride is aerobic because these activities require us to breathe more deeply and faster in order to provide extra oxygen to our muscles. Aerobic exercise has been the most studied form of exercise, and it provides all the exercise benefits that we previously discussed.

Strength training, which is done either by lifting weights or pulling on resistance bands, is a form of physical activity that has been around for centuries but only recently has been studied with cancer patients. Don't worry, you don't have to be able to bench press 150 pounds. Studies have shown that regularly using one-, two-, or three-pound hand weights can be effective in maintaining muscle mass.[35] Two of the most debilitating side effects that cancer patients undergoing chemotherapy and radiation experience are loss of muscle mass and the corresponding loss of strength. This decline reduces their quality of life and can severely hinder their day-to-day functioning. In a large review of studies conducted on this topic, researchers concluded that strength training for cancer patients who are undergoing chemotherapy and radiation is a safe form of exercise that reduces treatment-related side effects, significantly increases muscle strength, helps to maintain a lower body mass, and reduces the overall percentage of body fat.[36]

## HIIT

HIIT has become incredibly popular in the past few years, and not just in fitness magazines or blogs, but also in the medical community. This is for good reason, since HIIT workouts have been scientifically proven to be beneficial in a variety of ways for people with and without cancer.[37]

HIIT workouts are different from traditional aerobic or continuous-intensity exercise. With the old "no-pain, no-gain" workouts, you might go for a run, take a spin class, or lift weights for 30–60 minutes straight. The goal of these workouts is to get your heart rate up into a target range and keep it there for at least 20 minutes. In contrast, a HIIT workout is designed around bursts of intense exercise (typically one to four minutes) that work your entire body, alternating with recovery periods of similar length.

HIIT can deliver the same cardiovascular benefits as aerobic exercise in less total workout time.[38]

For cancer survivors, research has shown that *any* type of exercise improves quality of life, functional capacity, and selected cardiovascular disease risk factors. However, when studying a group of cancer patients who rode a stationary bike or ran on a treadmill for 20 minutes of low-intensity training, compared to a group that exercised in HIIT intervals (seven 30-second bursts), the HIIT group members improved their overall heart, lung, and muscular fitness faster.[39]

In another study, researchers studied the effects of HIIT on colon cancer survivors, who are known to have decreased cardiorespiratory fitness and muscle mass, both of which greatly increase their risk of death. Scientists wanted to know whether there was a difference between HIIT and moderate-intensity exercise when it came to improving their chances of survival. In just a four-week period, the colon cancer survivors who engaged in HIIT saw far superior results compared to the survivors who stuck to moderate-intensity exercise. To be more specific, the HIIT group outperformed the moderate group in $VO_2$ capacity (a measure of how much oxygen you can utilize during exercise), lean mass, and decreased body fat percentage.[40]

Given these and scores of other studies that have recently been published on HIIT, it appears to be a highly efficient and effective form of exercise that can be used by cancer patients both during and after treatment.

## Lymphatic Training

The lymphatic system is a vitally important part of the immune system. Through a network of vessels and nodes, it helps to deliver illness-fighting white blood cells all over your body while collecting and disposing of unwanted viral, bacterial, and cancerous cells. In order to perform these important functions, the fluid in your lymphatic vessels needs to be flowing.[41]

However, unlike the heart, which pumps blood to your entire body with each new heartbeat, the lymphatic system does not have a pump, which means it relies on the movement of your body (read: exercise) to move lymphatic fluid through its vessels and any unwanted cancer cells out of your body.[42] During periods of exercise, lymphatic flow rate has been shown to rise to levels that are two to three times higher than when you are at rest.[43] In this way, exercise plays a critical role in supporting the lymphatic system's daily job of identifying and removing cancer cells from the body.

Rebounding (bouncing on a mini-trampoline) is one of the most popular forms of exercise that radical remission survivors report using to stimulate their lymphatic system, including Mary Rust, whose full healing story we will share next. While few research studies have been conducted on this specific type of exercise, one study found that mini-trampoline exercises led to significant and rapid increases in muscle mass,[44] while another study found that such exercise led to significant reductions in body mass and blood pressure, as well as significant improvements in glucose profiles and $VO_2$ capacity.[45] Radical remission survivors have reported being able to rebound even when they were at their weakest.

Now that we have described the myriad benefits of exercise on your physical and mental health, we would like to share with you the healing story of a radical remission survivor who used exercise, along with the other nine factors, to help heal her breast cancer. A few years after being crowned the "Fittest Woman in the World," Mary was diagnosed with invasive ductal carcinoma. Her remarkable story illustrates the importance of fitness before, during, and after a cancer diagnosis.

# Mary's Story

Cancer impacted Mary Rust's life long before her own diagnosis. When she was 18 years old, her mother was diagnosed with ovarian cancer. Ovarian cancer is often called the "silent killer" because by the time it is caught, it is often in the later stages and has already spread. Such was the case with Mary's mother. Shocked and devastated, Mary and her family struggled to understand the diagnosis. Mary's mother was healthy and active. There was no history of cancer in the family and she did not drink or smoke.

Mary remained by her mother's side during the chemotherapy, radiation, and multiple surgeries. Conventional medicine was all she had available at the time. Mary says, "She was a fighter, but I saw her go from a healthy, vibrant woman to someone who was very sick from the cancer, the chemotherapy, and the treatments." Her initial prognosis was only two years. Mary's mother made it for four.

Two days before her mother passed, sensing that the end of her mother's journey was near, Mary chose the dress she would wear to the funeral. Her mother asked Mary to sit beside her on the bed and shared what would later become a guiding light for Mary's own journey.

> She looked into my eyes and she said, "Mary, this isn't the way to cure cancer. There must be another way that the body can heal and restore itself."

Mary knew her mother had a strong will to live—to see her children grow up and have grandchildren. Unfortunately, that factor alone was not enough to save her. Only later did Mary realize that watching her mother suffer through conventional treatment would profoundly shape her own perspective on cancer treatment and healing.

Mary was raised to be a perfectionist in Loveland, Colorado, by the mother she adored so much. She internalized how happy her grade-oriented and competitive parents were when she got an A+, and their apathy when it was anything less.

This perfectionist streak drove Mary to earn the title "Fittest Woman in the World" by winning the Fitness Olympia in 1999, which has been called the "Super Bowl" of women's bodybuilding. This illustrious prize launched Mary into her dream job as a spokesperson for a major health and nutrition retailer—she and her husband were thrilled. In addition to being an inspiration for women, she was even more excited when she found out shortly after signing the contract that she was pregnant. She envisioned an idyllic future that involved starting a family and building a "fit pregnancy" nutrition program with the retailer.

Instead, she was about to enter the most tumultuous period of her life. The retailer unexpectedly terminated her contract due to her pregnancy. Professionally devastated yet still excited about motherhood, she decided to focus on her new son and immersed herself in the precious first year of his life. Soon after, she became pregnant with her second child, and for the next few years, she enjoyed being a full-time mother to two wonderful children. Her husband was enjoying a successful career as a general contractor, and things seemed to start going well for their young family.

Then the housing market began to crash in 2006 and her husband lost everything. Suddenly they found themselves facing bankruptcy, with two small children to raise, a home in foreclosure, and millions of dollars of debt. Mary and her family moved from her hometown to the isolated town of Gillette, Wyoming, to find work. She tried to stay positive about her blessings—she had a roof over her head, a beautiful family, and her health—but looking back, she realizes now that she was "barely surviving life."

Two years after the housing market crashed and her family had to move, Mary felt a lump in her breast. It didn't occur to her to have the lump checked out because other than the lump, she felt completely healthy. However, when Breast Cancer Awareness

Month rolled around in October, the lump was still there, so she decided it was finally time to get it checked out. She went in for a mammogram fully expecting a routine procedure followed by confirmation from her doctor that she was as healthy as she felt.

Instead, the mammogram identified her lump as "suspicious." Soon after, she had an ultrasound and an excisional biopsy. Despite not getting "clean margins" during the biopsy, which means not all the cancer was removed, Mary's doctors did remove as much of the lump as they could. The results came back and that December, two days after Mary's 36th birthday, it was official—Mary was diagnosed with breast cancer.

*How can the 'Fittest Woman in the World' get diagnosed with cancer nine years later?* Mary and her husband asked themselves. None of it made sense. Mary felt as good as the day she had won the Fitness Olympia championship.

Thinking back to her mother's ordeal with cancer, Mary began to panic, fearful of getting sicker and losing her hair. She desperately wanted to find a way to live a long, healthy life. She was only 36 and had one young child in second grade and one in kindergarten to raise.

> *All these voices were running around in my mind, and I was just in panic mode. Then, all of a sudden, there was this voice that just said "Stop." And in that stillness I specifically heard the words, "Mary, this is not the way to cure cancer. There's got to be another way." It was like my mother came through just at that moment, as well as this knowing that there is another way and I needed to find it.*

Mary immediately began researching everything she could: conventional treatment, holistic options, diets, and supplements. She found compelling evidence for both conventional and complementary and alternative treatments, which made her even more confused. To complicate things, she was also dealing with significant doubts and fears from her friends and family.

*It was one of those situations that I was very conflicted about whether to use conventional therapies, or to do alternative therapies, or maybe do a combination of both. And you know, unfortunately, when you're diagnosed with cancer, it's scary. It's really scary. . . . Yet there was this internal voice saying, "No, Mary. There's another way. Trust me, I'll show you. I'll lead you."*

Because there was still tissue in her body that contained cancer cells, Mary's doctors wanted to do either a full mastectomy on that breast or at least additional surgery to try to get clean margins on her biopsy. After that, they wanted her to do eight weeks of radiation, 12 weeks of chemotherapy, one year on the drug Herceptin, and then surgical removal of her ovaries.

This was a lot for Mary to process, much less accept. Thankfully, from her time as a competitive bodybuilder, Mary felt a deep connection to her body and knew how it worked in a way that few of us do. Knowing her body well is one of the main reasons she chose not to go down the conventional route her mother had chosen and instead made the personal decision to pursue alternative therapies first.

Mary's journey started at the physical level. She researched and experimented with different diet changes, vitamin supplements, and detoxification protocols, like baking soda baths, to see how her body responded best. For instance, when she tried the Gerson Therapy (a strict, plant-based diet), her hair fell out, so she stopped and added clean meat and protein back into her diet, to which she had a good response.

Although she started with alternative methods, she did not rule out the conventional treatments her doctors had recommended. She simply tried other things first. In the beginning, Mary says she felt "divinely guided . . . to the practitioners, books, and protocol plans—they all came to me." She was drawn to simple healing activities she could do at home. As time went on, she came to understand that her path might not be the right path for everyone, but that ultimately it was the right one *for her*.

In terms of her mental state, she came to believe that where her mind went, her body would follow.

> *I knew, and had an understanding, that our bodies can do incredible things. So if you can love, support, and nourish your body, it can physically change. One of the thoughts that ran through my mind was,* If my body created a condition like cancer, and I know that my body is incredibly designed to heal, why couldn't my body restore this physical illness that was presenting? *I trusted this divine knowing.*

As a lifelong athlete and competitor, Mary naturally turned to exercise in her healing process, but even that, she believed, was led by divine guidance. Mary felt a very close connection to God during this time and believed that God would lead her to the right solution each time she faced a choice. If something did not feel right, she adjusted and tried something new. Instead of returning to intensive weight lifting and bodybuilding, Mary did gentle rebounding on a mini-trampoline for lymphatic drainage and started practicing yoga. She did not go back to the gym and do heavy weights because she intuitively felt that was not the right healing path for her at that time. Nevertheless, she knew down to her bones that movement would be key for her healing.

> *Movement actually helps build your brain. We've become so sedentary in our lives, with typing on a computer and ordering out for food, that we really don't need to go out and hunt for food anymore. And yet our bodies are designed to do this! Our bodies are designed to move, so when you don't move, how are you going to take your dog for a walk? Or how are you going to play with your kids, if you don't nourish that part of your body?*

In addition to exercise, Mary intuitively brought the other nine radical remission healing factors into her healing process. Mary lived far away from her friends and family during her treatment, but she now believes this was a blessing in disguise since many of her loved ones were skeptical or fearful of the choices she was making. She started a blog to keep them up to date without having to deal with their resistance directly, and eventually found a small group of supportive friends who were an energetic match for what she was trying to do. She believes this was crucial because it allowed her to stay in a positive mind-set. Mary was also blessed to have two naturally funny young children whose antics helped keep her in the present moment and having fun.

As the months went by, she decided to track her progress with thermography scans instead of PET (positron emission tomography) or CT (computed tomography) scans, because she did not want unnecessary exposure to radiation. (Note: Thermography is a noninvasive test that uses an infrared camera to detect heat patterns in body tissue. Although it does not give off radiation like mammography, it is not as precise at detecting breast cancer as mammography.)

Much to Mary's relief, her next two follow-up thermography scans came back normal and follow-up blood work has shown no signs of cancer. It has been more than 10 years since Mary's doctor called to declare her cancer-free. However, Mary knew intuitively she was not done with her healing work.

*My mind started racing, like, Could this really be true? Am I really cancer-free? And I decided to say, "Let's accept it and just continue living each day." But then this internal voice said,* Mary, the physical part of what you did was only part of the healing process. *All I wanted to do was to spend one more day to live, to see my kids, and I was led through this beautiful healing journey that took me through the physical aspects of healing, the mental aspects of healing, and then the spiritual aspects of self-realization.*

As an athlete and nutrition enthusiast, Mary's healing journey began with the physical healing factors of exercise, diet, and supplements. Reflecting back on her journey today, she understands that the physical was only one piece of the health puzzle and that a mind-body-emotion shift was also vital to her success.

As Mary says, "Cancer can come as a wake-up call from your soul that says, 'There's so much more for you.'" Mary now believes that everything in our lives is here to serve a greater purpose. She finds relief in the fact that she can let go of the immediate crisis—whether it be physical, financial, relational, etc.—and open up her heart and mind to the bigger message that miracles can happen to anyone.

"Life happens for us, not to us," Mary says. She believes illness and healing happen for many different reasons, sometimes physical, sometimes mental or emotional, or sometimes to give a larger purpose to our lives.

Since her radical remission, Mary has pursued what she now considers to be her life's purpose of living each day to the fullest and helping other cancer patients via health coaching. Part of her ongoing learning process has been thinking about why she healed while others did not and analyzing why people who took different paths from hers survived. From the collective wisdom of herself and her many clients over the past 10 years, she has noticed some key mental transformations among people who heal.

One of these transformations is mind-set. Mary believes that the power of the mind is crucial to healing, and scientific studies on the placebo effect agree. For the past 60 years, scores of clinical trials have shown that what you believe, more than any drug you are taking, will have a significant effect on your health.[46] Over the years, Mary has experimented with supplements, diet, and mind-set to see what helps her most stay in remission. She has found that how she *thinks* a supplement or diet will work is exactly what she experiences. As a result, she has come to believe that the type of treatment a person chooses is not nearly as important as their mind-set and beliefs regarding that treatment.

When it comes to her own mind-set, over the past decade Mary has continued to work on releasing suppressed emotions. She has consulted a therapist specializing in consciousness and shadow work (a psychology practice developed by Carl Jung to understand the "dark side" of our psyche)[47] in order to talk through any repressed emotions, pains, or traumas she experienced from early childhood up to the present. In this way, Mary continues to work on letting go of old patterns, such as her perfectionistic tendencies.

Another mental transformation that Mary experienced during her healing journey relates to spirituality. She always had a strong faith in God, which helped her in her journey, but it was a different mental shift that brought this factor fully into Mary's life a couple of years after her remission.

> *While I always had faith and believed that miracles could happen, I don't know at the time if I believed miracles could happen for me. Shifting that mind-set that miracles can happen for me—that was huge. If you don't believe you can get well, then you don't believe this miracle can happen for you. It sets up a mental block for healing to happen.*

Lastly, Mary believes that no matter your course of treatment, you must be able to connect to your own inner guidance and intuition in order to heal, especially when it conflicts with the advice of people around you. Mary believes this factor of intuition has been a huge part of her own healing.

> *The miracle wasn't that my body healed from cancer, because our bodies are designed to heal. This is what they are designed to do. The miracle was that I listened to and trusted the soft, still voice—this voice that said, "I will lead you down a path." And I was able to follow that voice.*

Mary began hearing and following her intuitive voice from the moment she was first diagnosed, and for her it has led to a path of remission. When I asked Mary if she had any thoughts as to why she got cancer in the first place, she once again tapped into her intuition for the answer.

> *I was giving everything away in my life. I was doing everything for my kids, and nothing for me. I got into the messages of my body, and there was a reason why I got breast cancer as opposed to colon cancer or liver cancer. Why? The breast represents self-love and self-nourishment—it nourishes a newborn baby's life and feeds them. What was I not doing for myself? I was not feeding, not nourishing myself. I was giving everything away.*

Today, more than 11 years after her initial breast cancer diagnosis, Mary remains cancer-free and continues using the 10 radical remission healing factors, including exercise. She now adjusts her exercise regimen to whatever feels best for her body on any given day and believes that, above all, exercise should be fun. She often hikes, enjoys rollerblading outdoors, and does rebounding and gentle weight lifting. No matter what, she makes sure to move her body for at least 20 minutes each day.

Most of all, Mary hopes that sharing her story will inspire others since she believes that hope is one of the biggest things to hold on to during a cancer journey. As she puts it, "If you don't have hope, what do you have?" You can find out more about Mary at maryrust.com.

## Action Steps

It is important to always consult with your doctor to find out what type and level of activity is right for you. If you were sedentary before diagnosis, your doctors might first recommend low-intensity activities, such as stretching or brief walks. For older patients or those with bone metastases, osteoporosis, or significant impairments such as arthritis or peripheral neuropathy, doctors might recommend exercising with a fitness professional to ensure that balance is taken into account. Patients on bed rest lose their strength and lean body mass quickly, so physical therapy is usually recommended to maintain strength and range of motion while counteracting the fatigue and depression that often accompany being bedridden.[48]

Exercise is about incremental gains. If all you can do is walk around the dining room table, then make that your movement for today. See if you can build up to more and more laps around the table. Eventually, that will lead to walking outside.

A person does not get in or out of shape in a day, nor will you heal in a day. The key is consistency and making movement a lifelong habit. Here are a few tips to make exercise a regular part of your life:

1. **Set a time.**

   Research shows that people who set a specific time for exercise, instead of trying to squeeze it in, have more success. Write at least 10 minutes in your calendar and then hold yourself to it like any other commitment.

2. **Underpromise.**

   Approximately one-third of Americans make a New Year's resolution to "stay fit and get healthy,"[49] yet the vast majority of these resolutions are abandoned by February 1. We often fail at resolutions because we aim too high and do not make realistic plans. Set small goals that are achievable and that you will be proud of when you accomplish them. For instance, make a plan to walk for 10 minutes (if you are able) each day for a week. Start by walking out your front door for 5 minutes and then turning around and walking home. After a week, walk for 7.5 minutes before turning around, and eventually add time until you are walking for a total of 30 minutes.

3. **Set your clothes out the night before.**

Many people like to exercise first thing in the morning. If that is you, set out your exercise clothes and shoes the night before. This trick will get you going in the morning since you will not have the excuse of hitting the snooze because you cannot remember where your sneakers are.

4. **Find a buddy.**

Having an exercise buddy makes you accountable to someone else. If you know your buddy is coming over for a walk or waiting for you at the gym, it is more fun and you are less likely to skip the workout. (You will get extra credit for embracing social support!)

5. **Make it fun.**

If you think of exercise as a chore, you will be less likely to do it. Find creative ways to make it fun for you. For example, radical remission survivor Tremane, whom we quoted earlier, discovered that he loves doing yoga in his den while watching a comedy show. (Bonus points for increasing positive emotions!)

6. **Make it a family event.**

Chances are that everyone in the family could use a little exercise boost. Make it fun for everyone by having a family dance party before bed or going for a walk in the park. Your loved ones will feel good to be a part of your healing process, and it will give them something they can actually *do* to support you.

7. **Get outside.**

Fresh air will fill your cells with healthy oxygen, and being outside may help you tap into your spiritual connection, give you a vitamin D boost, and increase your positive emotions.

8. **Use the Internet for good.**

Are you curious about HIIT or another form of exercise but do not want to go to a gym or studio? YouTube has examples of every type of workout you can imagine. For instance, you can search YouTube for "HIIT for beginners" to find a free 20-minute workout. You'll find dance workouts, yoga practices, and pretty much anything else you can imagine. Let your curiosity open up the possibilities.

Exercise or movement is a healing factor that takes a lot of internal motivation. After all, no one can move your body except for you. Remember that basic, daily movement can add years to your life. And since many jobs today require that people sit at a desk all day long, it is more important than ever that we keep our bodies moving, standing instead of sitting, walking, and (hopefully) jumping for joy.

## CHAPTER 2

# SPIRITUAL CONNECTION

## Bailey's Story

*Do not dwell in the past; do not dream of the future;
concentrate the mind on the present moment.*

— BUDDHA

Like the various train tracks that lead to Grand Central Station, different spiritual practices act as train tracks that lead to the same important place: connection with something larger than yourself. The common healing factor of deepening your spiritual connection appears in every case of radical remission we have studied. Many radical remission survivors practice their spiritual connection once a day because they have found it leads to instantaneous, beneficial effects on both their bodies and their emotions.

For some people, spiritual connection means finding God through organized religion. Bailey O'Brien, whose full healing story we will share later in this chapter, found her spiritual connection through the church. However, this factor does not require you to participate in any particular religion or hold a particular set of beliefs. In its simplest form, spiritual practice can be a quiet walk in nature. It could also be painting, meditating, sitting on a beach, going to a temple, or walking your dog. The variations in spiritual practice are as limitless as the individuals who practice them.

Historically, people connected to God through organized religion (e.g., Christian churches, Jewish temples, Muslim mosques). For those who still regularly participate in religious services today, connection to God remains the top reason they attend.[1] In addition, an increasing number of Americans consider themselves spiritual. A recent study by the Pew Research Center found that 27 percent of Americans consider themselves "spiritual but not religious," representing an 8 percent increase over five years.[2] Another Pew study found that 72 percent of Americans who do not attend church regularly still pray regularly.[3]

Many spiritual leaders believe that this movement away from organized religions toward a more generalized spiritual practice represents a major paradigm shift in our society toward global connectedness. Supporting this belief, Janet O'Shea, a spiritual psychotherapist, healer, and metaphysical teacher, says:

> *A global shift is happening on so many different levels. I think [that] as we are progressing in time, there is an awakening [to the idea] that we're not separate beings. We're not separate from each other on the planet. We all share the same breath. An increased awareness that community is key is starting to awaken our DNA to the consciousness that we are truly all "one."*

This new view of spirituality has brought an awareness of the many ways we can connect to a spiritual state outside the traditional path of prayer. Alternative paths include meditation, mindfulness, yoga, and chanting. Along with alternative paths, we have alternative names for the spiritual state: God, soul, chi, life force, prana, the universe, or simply "energy." It is not the name that matters, but the sense of connection you feel when engaging in your daily spiritual practice and the physical and emotional changes you observe as a result of that practice.

In *Radical Remission*, I described various aspects of spiritual connection that radical remission survivors and their healers mentioned frequently. These aspects include:

- how spiritual connection is also a physical experience that is *felt* in the body;

- how spiritual connection evokes an overwhelming feeling of unconditional love;
- the theory that humans are spiritual beings in a physical body;
- the importance of a regular spiritual connection practice; and
- the significance of stopping the racing thoughts of the mind.

In our ongoing research, the new radical remission cases that we have collected continue to emphasize these five aspects of spirituality.

For example, radical remission survivor Jill Ayn Schneider embodies the essence of global spirituality because she weaves together a quilt of beliefs from around the world. In 1975, at age 29, Jill was diagnosed with class 5 cervical cancer after two positive Pap smears. Back then, doctors did not stage cervical cancer into four stages as they do now, but instead separated cases into classes—class 1 was considered healthy/normal, and class 5, the highest, was considered the most serious. Because of her two subsequent class 5 Pap smears, her doctor wanted her to have an immediate hysterectomy.

However, Jill's intuition told her that she should not jump right into surgery. Instead, she asked for a month or so to try healing herself. Her doctor was furious and stormed out of the room. Nevertheless, Jill held firm to her instincts and started taking Chinese herbs, meditating, receiving acupuncture treatments, and eating a Japanese macrobiotic diet (mostly brown rice, seasonal vegetables, miso soup, and legumes with smaller amounts of sea vegetables, nuts, and seeds). She also left her very stressful job. The results were almost immediate.

*I was studying the theory of Chinese medicine at the time and I felt so connected to the fact that they didn't call cancer anything more than an "imbalance." That resonated with me. I didn't have anxiety at all [about not doing conventional treatment]. After one month of herbs, acupuncture, and quitting a very stressful job, I just felt I was getting better. I went to a new doctor who confirmed it. [The cancer classification] went from a 5 to a 3 in one month! So then I knew that I was going to be fine. I asked myself, "Where am I going to go next to heal?" I was like a child—I trusted the universe.*

Encouraged by how much she had healed in a month, Jill felt a spiritual call to trek across Venezuela and Peru, where she consulted with local shamans, enjoyed nature, and continued her macrobiotic diet. Upon returning to the U.S. five months later, she had another Pap smear and was then classified as "class 1" (normal). Two years later, she gave birth to her son, and now she is "Nanny Jill" to two beautiful grandchildren.

Jill believes she healed herself of advanced cervical cancer in six months thanks to deep spiritual work and a diet change that was being divinely guided. By deepening her daily spiritual connection practice, she was able to tap into the deeper current of "universal love" that many radical remission survivors describe. Today, more than 40 years after her original diagnosis, Jill remains cancer-free. She spends her days leading people through healing seminars and retreats, guiding others to be more in tune with their true selves. To learn more about Jill, visit circle-of-life.net.

## Recent Developments

In recent years, there has been a surge of interest in all things spiritual and mindful. The number of people in the U.S. who meditate has increased threefold since 2012.[4] In addition, 37 million Americans now practice yoga,[5] and businesses based on wellness and organic brands are some of the fastest-growing in the world.[6]

This should not come as a surprise since, as a society, we are overstressed, overstimulated, and overworked. Practices like meditation and yoga help us to cope with these everyday pressures, and what was once considered "out there" has now become mainstream. A few years ago, simply saying the word *spirituality* would have polarized a room, but today it is often an engaging topic of conversation.

This cultural shift toward accepting mindfulness and spirituality has been supported by an increase in scientific research on meditation and prayer. Over the past 20 years, hundreds of studies have shown that when people quiet their minds and feel the state of peace brought on by a spiritual connection practice, their bodies respond with a rush of healthy hormones that flood the bloodstream, as well as an increase in oxygen in the blood, improved blood circulation, decreased blood pressure, improved digestion and detoxification, a stronger immune system, and, amazingly, the ability to turn off unhealthy genes.

Justine Laidlaw, a radical remission survivor from New Zealand, has experienced firsthand many of these physical effects from a regular spiritual connection practice. Justine was diagnosed in 2013 with stage 3c colon cancer at age 45. Because she was raised in a nonreligious family, meditation and prayer were not things that had ever been a part of Justine's life. That changed after her diagnosis.

> *It took a world-shattering cancer diagnosis to open my eyes to spirituality. I had spent years being busy, living with anxiety and depression, and didn't "have the time" to sit with my thoughts, emotions, and experiences. The more I began to indulge in daily breathwork, journaling, mindfulness, and meditation, my crippling anxiety, overwhelm, and self-criticism melted away as peaceful solitude, grounded presence, and positive perspective cascaded through my veins. . . . That's not to say that I still don't experience negative mind games from time to time. However, spirituality acted as a guiding light, a source of strength, and a powerful release that comforted me through my healing journey.*

Justine had a major surgery soon after she was diagnosed, but then made the personal decision not to do the recommended chemotherapy and radiation. Instead, she fully utilized the ten radical remission healing factors and thankfully remains cancer-free to this day. She now gives back to cancer patients by leading workshops as a certified Radical Remission workshop instructor.

In recent years, studies have demonstrated specific ways that spirituality can reduce cancer risk. For example, researchers at the Center for Mind and Brain at the University of California, Davis, compared people who went on a meditation retreat to control subjects who did not attend the retreat. Those who practiced daily meditation at the retreat showed a significant increase in telomerase activity,[7] which reduces your cancer risk by lengthening the telomeres in your DNA.[8] (Note: Telomeres are like endcaps on your DNA strands, helping to keep each strand intact—much like the stiff cap at the end of a shoelace.) Meanwhile, the people in the control group who were not meditating did not experience any increase in their telomerase activity. Therefore, meditation helps protect DNA in a way that specifically reduces cancer risk.

Another study looked at a group of experienced meditators and compared their stress and inflammatory responses to a group of non-meditators. University of Wisconsin–Madison researchers found that experienced meditators had lower levels of cortisol (the "stress hormone"), less perceived emotional stress, and a smaller inflammatory response than a control group.[9] These findings are important for cancer patients because reduced cortisol levels and lower inflammatory responses have both been associated with a significant reduction in cancer risk.[10,11]

The scientific field of epigenetics studies how lifestyle choices, such as diet and stress management, can turn a person's genes "on" or "off," or expressed or not expressed. This is one of the most important scientific discoveries of the past 50 years, because it allows us to overcome the notion that our inherited genes lead to inevitable results and instead encourages us to use daily habits to turn faulty genes off and health-promoting genes on.

Over the past several years, research has continued to show the incredible power of epigenetics. For example, a team of researchers at Massachusetts General Hospital in Boston found that a single meditation session can significantly improve a person's genetic expression. In this study, researchers first trained groups of novice and experienced meditators in an eight-week relaxation course. After the subjects were comfortable with the meditation method, the researchers evaluated both groups before, during, and after a single meditation session.

The researchers found that a significant number of genes showed increased expression after the single meditation session, including genes that improve a person's energy metabolism, insulin secretion, DNA protection, and mitochondrial function—all of which are crucial for cancer prevention. In addition, this single meditation session reduced the overall inflammatory and stress responses in their bodies, which is helpful in reducing cancer risk. Most interesting, though, is that *both* groups—the novices as well as the expert meditators—experienced positive changes in their genetic expression. However, the expert meditators experienced a much greater effect, which tells us that it is healthy to start meditating and even healthier to meditate regularly over a period of years.[12]

Finally, another team of researchers in Europe reviewed the available studies to see if mind-body practices—such as mindfulness, yoga, tai chi, qigong, the relaxation response, and breath regulation—could reverse the expression of genes that are involved in inflammatory reactions to stress. The research consistently confirmed that mind-body practices have the opposite effect of chronic stress on our genes. While chronic stress caused an *increase* in the expression of genes related to inflammation (and inflammation is a major contributor to cancer), mind-body practices significantly *decreased* the expression of these inflammation-related genes.[13] This study shows that if you want to reduce your cancer risk by decreasing your inflammation, mind-body practices are some ways to accomplish that.

Overall, society's interest in spirituality has increased along with the research supporting it. These well-designed studies, along with numerous others, conclusively show that spiritual connection practices significantly improve the health of the body and the mind, all the way down to the genetic level.

Now that we better understand the importance of developing a spiritual connection practice from the perspective of science, let's explore this healing factor on a more personal level by introducing you to radical remission survivor Bailey O'Brien. Bailey developed a deep, daily spiritual practice as part of her multifaceted healing from metastatic melanoma.

Bailey's spiritual connection comes in the form of her Christian faith and practices. To stay true to the source material, we will convey Bailey's beliefs to you in the ways she conveyed them to us. However, we want to remind you that radical remission cases have been reported by people from all major religions as well as by atheists and agnostics. Despite the disparate range of beliefs, the common thread among radical remission survivors is always the daily practice that leads to a sense of spiritual connection, which is accompanied by a deeply relaxed physical state and a deeply peaceful emotional state.

## Bailey's Story

Bailey was your typical freshman at Boston University in 2007. She came from a small town in New York, and while she was very close to her family, which included her mother, father, older sister, and younger brother, she felt excited to leave the nest and attend college, as her sister had done before her. She had been recruited for BU's Division I diving team, which added an additional layer of excitement.

The O'Briens had gone to church occasionally while Bailey was growing up, but Bailey's experience within that religious tradition had been one of rules, guilt, and rote memorization. By the time she went off to college, she did not feel a strong sense of connection to God or the divine. She says, "I felt like God was more ashamed of me for the things I was doing wrong, and that if I did something wrong, then I should be ashamed." In essence, she understood the rules and rituals of her religious tradition but had never developed a true spiritual practice. Once at college, she stopped attending church, and spirituality moved to the sidelines of her life.

All was going well until the end of her first semester. She noticed a suspicious mole on her right temple and immediately went to the doctor, who removed it and sent it off to pathology for analysis. It turned out to be the worst kind of skin cancer—melanoma.

Her doctors followed the standard protocol by making a wide excision to surgically remove the cancerous mole, followed by an injected "tracer" to see if the cancer had spread. Unfortunately, the tracer identified a cancer-filled lymph node in front of her ear, which her surgeon also surgically removed and biopsied. The lymph node came back positive for melanoma, meaning that her cancer had already spread. Suddenly Bailey went from being a typical undergrad worried about gaining the "freshman 15" to being a stage 3 melanoma cancer patient. As Bailey describes, "I was scared and shocked. How did something like this happen to someone young and healthy?"

Bailey wanted to complete the treatment as soon as possible. She followed conventional protocol to the letter, which included another more complex surgery to remove 45 lymph nodes in her neck. Thankfully, all of them tested negative for cancer.

She tried everything the doctors asked, although there was a high probability of recurrence. For five days a week for one month, she received injections of interferon, an early immunotherapy drug, because there was a chance that it might prevent her cancer from recurring. Bailey's mother prayed that her daughter would be one of the fortunate ones who did not have a recurrence. After successfully completing the surgery and the interferon injections, she returned to college and went in for regular scans to monitor her progress.

Bailey returned to school the following fall as a sophomore with hopes of staying in remission and getting back to a normal life—and, for a while, it was normal. She declared a major in nutritional sciences because she had always had an interest in reading food labels, although at this point in her healing journey, she did not really believe that food could help heal something as serious as cancer. Thankfully, her sophomore and junior years passed uneventfully, filled with diving practices, diving competitions, and classes. This blissful reprieve ended abruptly at the end of her junior year, however, when one of her routine follow-up scans showed suspicious cancer activity.

Bailey's doctors decided to monitor her closely during the summer between her junior and senior years. A follow-up scan at the end of the summer showed intensified cancer activity, which led her doctors to perform a computed tomography (CT)-guided needle biopsy of a suspicious spot behind her jaw. Unfortunately, the spot tested positive for melanoma, turning Bailey's fear of a cancer recurrence into a reality.

Frustrated and depressed, Bailey began her senior year of college by preparing for another surgery, this time to remove the new tumor. Her tight-knit family continued to pray for her, and her friends continued to rally behind her. A typical college student, Bailey just wanted to get the surgery over with so she could get back to school and finish her senior year. Unfortunately, her surgeon missed the tumor by a millimeter, and in the weeks it took to discover the mistake, a second tumor had already grown behind her ear lobe. She had yet another surgery a little over a month later to remove both tumors.

Despite being in the best physical shape of her life as a member of the diving team, this proved to be a hard surgery. The recovery took six weeks, followed immediately by radiation treatments. Bailey took another break from school to recover at home, which made her miss her friends and college life deeply. She tried to stay positive and to focus on getting well, but it was a challenge.

After completing this aggressive, one-two punch of treatments, there was still an 80 percent chance of a life-threatening recurrence. Bailey did not believe there was anything she could do to change those statistics, so she just went back to college life as usual, which is exactly what her doctors recommended. This meant eating the standard American diet, with its ample carbohydrates and animal protein and few vegetables, lots of skim milk, and the classic college add-ons: chips and alcohol.

The cancer, however, was unrelenting. In January 2011, only a few weeks after she finished radiation, Bailey felt a new, tiny lump under her chin. In an effort to confirm that such lumps were a normal part of human anatomy, she began to poll her friends at college. Discouraged that no one else had such a lump under their chin, she made an appointment with her oncologist. The lump was biopsied and, once again, Bailey was told she had melanoma. At this point, she and her family were beyond discouraged.

*I had done everything that my doctor had told me to do, and it felt like it was all for nothing. Like it was just a waste of my time.*

Her medical team followed the biopsy with a scan that revealed the cancer had definitively spread to her neck, lungs, and probably to her spine. Not even out of college yet, Bailey was now a stage 4 terminal cancer patient. She suddenly found herself praying, "Okay, God, if you're there, please heal me and give me a miracle."

There was little that conventional medicine could offer Bailey at this point. Immunotherapy drugs had not yet been approved by the Food and Drug Administration (FDA), and she did not qualify for a clinical trial because her cancer did not have the right genetic mutation. Her doctor's only recommendations were Temodar, an oral chemotherapy pill, and para-aminobenzoic acid (PABA), a vitamin B derivative—both of which Bailey agreed to try out of desperation.

It was at this point that Bailey and her mother went for a second opinion at the Cancer Treatment Centers of America (CTCA). When the first doctor she saw there recommended more surgery, radiation, and chemotherapy, Bailey had her first intuitive sense that she needed to try something radically different to save her life. She felt let down by the conventional medical system because, despite doing everything they had recommended, she was now facing a terminal prognosis.

> *I said [to the second-opinion doctor], "Okay. So if I do all of that, I get what? Two years?" And she said, "Yes." And I was like, "I'm sorry, but I'm not interested in that. I don't want to die a miserable death, and I want more than just two years." Because I believed it was possible to get more than that. When I got to the point of being terminal, all bets were off.*

While she pursued a second opinion from CTCA, Bailey's mother also leaned on her friends for support. One friend firmly believed that Bailey could and would get well, and this friend encouraged Bailey and her mom to begin researching alternative options. Through this research, Bailey's mom discovered "Coley's toxins," which had been helpful for some melanoma patients. After more digging, Bailey's mom discovered that Coley's toxins were available only in certain clinics in Mexico. Bailey and her mom told the medical oncologist in New York about the Mexico possibility.

> *When my mom mentioned Mexico, the [doctor's] assistant said, "When you're ready to follow our protocol, then you can give us a call." Basically, [they said], "We're not going to treat your daughter until she is doing what we want her to do."*

Bailey did not appreciate the oncologist's "take it or leave it" approach. It sounded like more of the same old treatments that would be very hard on her body and work for only a limited time. In addition, Bailey's sister had gotten engaged. "I really wanted to be around for my family and my sister, who I knew was getting married and going to have kids," Bailey said.

Bailey and her mother decided to go to Mexico, despite her conventional medicine team's lack of trust in the therapies offered. From the conventional medicine perspective, not enough studies had been conducted to fully assess the clinic's approach. But to Bailey, the clinic in Mexico offered "more hope than anything

I got from the medical community." This was a tough decision because it meant she would miss the upcoming springboard diving championship. However, she decided she did not want to risk even one more week of allowing her aggressive cancer to grow.

Bailey had completed just one round (five days' worth) of Temodar before she set off on her trip to Mexico. She decided not to continue with it, although she did keep taking the PABA. During her three weeks at the Mexican clinic, Bailey received intensive treatments of Coley's toxins and Gerson Therapy, both of which had treated stage 4 melanoma successfully in a handful of historical case reports. Neither treatment is FDA-approved in the United States, which means doctors in the U.S. are not legally allowed to offer them.

Coley's toxins is a mixture of bacterial toxins pioneered by William Coley, M.D., in New York in the 1890s. Dr. Coley noted that, much to his surprise, cancer patients who got infections after cancer surgery seemed to do better than patients who did not get an infection. He hypothesized that the infection must have stimulated their immune systems to fight the cancer.[14] The Gerson Therapy, in contrast, was a program designed by Max Gerson, M.D., in the late 1920s to activate the body's ability to heal itself through an organic, plant-based diet, including daily raw juices, daily coffee enemas, and natural supplements.[15]

Bailey had injections of Coley's toxins in both arms three times a week. They were so painful that sometimes she would break down and cry. In addition, she took a long list of personalized supplements, a laetrile supplement (a form of amygdalin from apricot seeds),[16] vitamin C infusions twice a week, coffee enemas three times a day, and started on a modified version of the Gerson Therapy diet.

*It was a radical change in my diet—and that was not fun! I was drinking 13 juices per day. I had one [freshly squeezed] orange juice and [a bowl of] oatmeal for breakfast. Then half an hour later I had my first fresh vegetable juice. I did about six carrot-apple juices and six green juices throughout the day, every hour. I had a Hippocrates soup [a vegetable soup from Gerson Therapy] for lunch and dinner, and fruit for snacks, and nuts and seeds. I did have a little bit of animal protein that they gave me in the [Mexican] hospital. It was not like a strict Gerson hospital. It was like a more modified Gerson [diet] for each individual patient.*

Bailey felt she was very blessed to have a lot of support during this time. Her mother was by her side the entire three weeks at the clinic. In addition, friends, family, teammates, and even rival teammates rallied around her to show their support, including hosting a fund-raiser for her trip to Mexico. Bailey said, "Having the encouragement of friends and people to talk to meant a lot. People were praying for me, and I was trying to stay more positive."

Bailey returned to the U.S. hopeful that her time in the Mexican clinic had slowed down the aggressive growth of her cancer. She decided to take the rest of the school year off while her mother helped her integrate the dietary and lifestyle changes from Mexico into her life in New York. Bailey lived at home with her parents for the next five months, while friends of the family would come over in shifts to help Bailey and her mother make Bailey's daily regimen of Hippocrates soup, organic coffee (for the coffee enemas), and six fresh vegetable juices per day. Bailey continued to do three injections per week of the Coley's toxins.

Three weeks after she returned from Mexico, after a total of six weeks on the new treatment program, Bailey met her original oncologist for a follow-up PET scan, a few days before her 21st birthday. Bailey was thrilled that she could no longer feel the cancer lump under her chin and prayed hard for a miracle. As she sat in the office awaiting the verdict, the doctor and his team seemed flustered while looking over the scans. They kept asking her questions about Mexico. Worried that all the hemming and hawing meant it was bad news, Bailey finally asked, "So, what are the results?"

Her doctor replied, "It would appear from your scan that you have no sign of active disease." Bailey was relieved, elated, and most of all, grateful to God for the grace she believed He had just shown her. She celebrated that night with lots of hugs and tears from her family and planned a trip to Boston the following weekend to share the news with her friends.

During that summer, Bailey started attending local church services occasionally. She wanted to make a conscious effort to increase her positive emotions and let go of any negative thoughts and emotions that might come up, and she thought that going to church might support her in achieving these goals. However, while she found the church to be a more pleasant experience than it had been in years past, she still did not feel a deep connection to God.

That August, Bailey's parents packed up the family car once again to drive her up to Boston University, this time for a "redo" of her senior year. Bailey was very diligent about continuing her new treatment regimen while back at college, which was no easy feat. She feels blessed that she continued to have help from friends and her dedicated mother. Her roommates helped with the Coley's injections, which she now received once per week. She continued taking her supplements and doing coffee enemas twice a day—not exactly a simple thing to do when you are sharing a bathroom with roommates.

And while her fellow college students feasted on the all-you-can-eat meal plan, Bailey stayed true to her restrictive Gerson-based diet. Her experience in Mexico had proven to her that diet can significantly impact your health, and her major in nutritional sciences gave her a powerful new career direction.

*It was by the grace of God that I believed in the nutritional aspect [of healing], because it just came naturally to me, whereas other people might never think during their whole lives that nutrition matters.*

Miraculously, Bailey's mother was able to convince the BU dining hall staff to make Bailey's Gerson therapy juices and soups, including buying the fresh produce that was required for them (approximately 17–20 pounds of organic produce a day!). Bailey just had to bring two sets of empty bottles to the kitchen every morning instead of spending two and a half hours a day prepping the juices herself.

It was around this time that spirituality took a front seat in Bailey's healing journey. When she returned to college that fall, she stumbled upon a "Christian Fellowship for Athletes" table at an athletic barbecue.

> The girls who were at the table were really nice and normal, and just like me. I went to a [fellowship] meeting, and I felt from the first time that I went there like I'd found what I was looking for—because there were other people there like me, who were looking for answers and who had doubts, and yet they still had faith.

When she was wrestling through her doubts about what she believed, Bailey spoke with the leader of the fellowship, who challenged her to think about God as a spiritual force who works through people, instead of a tangible being. Bailey recalls:

> I could see God whispering to someone, not audibly, but putting it in their heart to go over and talk to someone who's going through a hard time, and [yet] they have no idea the other person is struggling. . . . So on my own, I was thinking about how Jesus was kind of like my cancer treatment.

Bailey came to realize that following Jesus blindly as she had done growing up—following the "rules"—was no different from the way she had blindly followed her doctors' recommendations during her cancer treatment.

With her doctors, Bailey had kept an open mind, willing to try the conventional treatments her doctors prescribed both because scientific evidence suggested they would work and because her doctors believed they would work. To be fair, the treatments *had* worked, at least temporarily. However, when the treatments stopped working, Bailey realized she needed to stop following blindly and instead to ask questions—lots of questions. She needed to share her doubts, press for answers, and seek healing wherever she could find it.

Bailey applied the same logic to her newfound faith. Growing up, she had reasoned that because there was so much historical evidence of Jesus's life, death, and resurrection, and so many people who believe in Him, who was she to have doubts? She assumed she would just have to fake faith in order to fit in. But in her new faith community, she learned that doubts and questions are normal and that they can lead to deeper understanding. Her life had hit a pivotal point of either believing or not believing, and she chose to believe.

*I remember I was in my college dorm, sitting at my computer, and I looked out my window on the Boston skyline. I was like, okay, here we go. And I decided, I'm going to walk by faith, not by sight anymore. And then things in my life that I believe contributed to my cancer, like stress . . . they started to change. I had more positive thoughts. I felt more peace in my heart, rather than such overwhelming anxiety and fear. I still struggle with those things, but to a lesser degree.*

Unwittingly, Bailey had added the 10 radical remission healing factors into her life. Already an active athlete, she rediscovered the importance of increasing positive emotions, empowered herself in her medical decisions and followed her intuition, worked to release stressful emotions and embrace the support of her friends and family, found a new reason to live with her sister's upcoming wedding, and undertook a radical and new diet and supplement protocol—and all of it felt divinely inspired to Bailey.

*God can heal a person with the snap of a finger. . . . I did take big steps in trying to physically restore my body, but it was God's gift of healing. And ultimately all good things come from Him. By the grace of God, I was able to finish school and stick with my [healing] regimen.*

Bailey has wound down some of the Mexican clinic protocols but continues with some to this day. She has reduced the coffee enemas to once a day and continues with a mostly plant-based diet. She drinks about two fresh vegetable juices per day and eats a raw mix of colorful veggies with a dressing of apple cider vinegar, olive oil, and spices. She eats animal protein, such as fish or chicken, from time to time, but still avoids eggs and dairy products. She discontinued the Coley's injections after five years.

In addition, Bailey evaluated why she may have gotten cancer in the first place. She believes many factors caused her cancer, including many epigenetic and lifestyle factors, such as spending a lot of time in a chemical-laden pool as a lifelong competitive diver; eating "comfort" junk food in high school and college; being exposed to toxic chemicals in carpets, new cars, and everyday products; consuming pesticides in the nonorganic food she ate for most of her life; and possibly from the vaccines she received as a child. As she considered these potential sources of toxins, she worked to clean up her life as much as possible in order to stay healthy and toxin-free.

A big part of Bailey's ongoing spiritual journey has been to remain positive and grateful. When her doctors first shared her clear scan results three weeks after she returned from Mexico, Bailey said to herself, "Oh my gosh, I'm set for life! Anything else is a bonus." However, as time passed, she found herself slipping back into old patterns of unhappiness, fear, and ingratitude, which surprised her.

> *I was like,* What's wrong with me? Why am I acting and thinking this way when I have so much to be grateful for? *It would be even worse for me to have this second chance at life and to waste it by feeling the way that I feel right now.*

It was her spiritual community and faith that helped her get back to a better mental state. Bailey did deep spiritual work to understand her purpose in life and why she had been given a second chance.

*I believed that I must have a purpose, because I knew that so many people didn't get well [from cancer]. And I didn't take that lightly. . . . I believe that everyone has a purpose and I wanted to know what mine was. If I had a purpose, it had to come from somewhere or someone. . . . For that reason, I'm so grateful for the cancer I had, and for how my story unfolded. . . . Like with the treatments—so that I could try out conventional medicine and realize that it's not everything, it's not all that's out there.*

Bailey channeled the gratitude she felt for her radical remission into providing service to others as a cancer advocate and spiritually minded health coach. She feels strongly that it is possible to heal from cancer and that God wants a relationship with us. As a cancer coach, Bailey interacts with many people aspiring for a radical remission like hers. When asked what she says to new coaching clients, she replied:

*I would tell [a newly diagnosed cancer patient] to wait and pray before doing anything. Gather as much information as you can. Seek counsel from multiple advisers, as many as you feel like you need, both conventional and alternative and integrative. Pray for wisdom. . . . I won't tell someone, "Don't do chemotherapy," because maybe that's what they need to do. Praying is important, because everyone is an individual, and God works in mysterious ways.*

Today, more than eight years after she received her first "all-clear" scan in 2011, Bailey still has no evidence of disease. Along with continuing to practice the other nine healing factors, she continues her spiritual connection practice by starting each day with Bible reading and prayer. You can find more about Bailey at baileyobrien.com.

# Action Steps

A spiritual connection practice improves not only your emotional well-being, but also your physical health. The most important part of developing a spiritual connection practice is that during the practice, you feel a deep sense of peace, love, and calm—both in your body *and* your emotions.

In *Radical Remission*, I identified the following action steps to help increase your spiritual connection: deep breathing, walking outside, guided imagery, guided meditation, daily prayer, spiritual groups, and online groups. All remain excellent ways to practice finding a spiritual connection, and here are some additional ideas for you to try along your healing path.

- *Meditation Apps*

    App stores are full of tools to help increase mindfulness, wellness, and build a meditation practice. The three most well-reviewed apps at the time of this writing are Calm, Headspace (started by a monk), and 10% Happier.

- *Energy Healers and Energy Groups*

    Finding a local energy healer may not be as hard as you suspect. Ask for recommendations at your local yoga studio, wellness center, or community center. You can step out of your comfort zone by asking friends and family if they know of anyone. In addition, the Internet is a great resource. Search engines and review sites will have a listing of local providers near you.

- *"Worship Shop"*

    If the structure and community of a traditional church, temple, mosque, or other place of worship sound appealing to you, ask around for recommendations, or "shop around" until you find one that feels right for you.

- ***YouTube and Internet Videos***

  If you are more comfortable flying solo, the Internet may offer a starting point. More than 400 hours of content are streamed on YouTube every minute.[17] With this abundance of content, you will be able to find free yoga classes, healing frequency music, prayers, chants, affirmations, guided meditations, and even shamanic rituals. In addition, well-known spirituality pioneers like Deepak Chopra and Oprah, as well as spirituality leaders like Gabby Bernstein and Eckhart Tolle, offer vast video and online content to help you in your spiritual journey.

We hope you now understand more fully the power of developing a spiritual connection practice. Whether it be prayer, meditation, or a walk in nature, finding a way to radically shift your physiology in such a way that your breathing slows down, your heart rate slows, and most important, your "thinking" mind quiets down, is one of the most powerful things you can do to recharge your immune system.

---

## CHAPTER 3

# EMPOWERING YOURSELF

---

## Bob's Story

*The most successful people who heal cancer do everything they can to create conditions for healing to occur.*

— MARK BRICCA, N.D.

Most of us grew up believing that the "doctor knows best." After all, medical doctors are trained for a long time: four years of prerequisite courses during college, four years of medical school, two to three years of residency, and, for many, two additional years spent in a fellowship. On average, most medical doctors have been training for 12 years by the time they hang out their shingles and begin practicing medicine.

Such extensive education can be intimidating. Most patients feel that their doctors must be much smarter than they are—and in so many ways, they are. Doctors are true experts in their field, having mastered complicated subjects such as organic chemistry, molecular biology, and human anatomy and physiology. In addition, they keep abreast of the latest cancer statistics, evolving standards of medical care, and the latest pharmaceutical drugs and medical treatments. However, doctors are not experts in *you*. Only you can be the expert in you.

Don't get us wrong; the expertise of doctors and their medical technologies are incredibly valuable. They have eradicated diseases like polio and smallpox and provided successful treatments for diseases such as strep throat and tuberculosis. In addition, modern medical technology allows doctors to fully map your heart, brain, and even your DNA. If you break a leg, have a heart attack, or get a nasty infection, you will want a doctor to give you the correct pharmaceutical drug or perform the appropriate surgery. But in this context, it's easy to forget that doctors do not yet have all the answers, especially when it comes to chronic conditions like cancer, Lyme disease, Alzheimer's disease, and multiple sclerosis.

Another problem is the influence of money in modern medicine. Pharmaceutical companies can easily fund multimillion-dollar clinical trials on new drug treatments, spend millions to market new drugs, and create financial incentives for doctors to prescribe their drugs. As a result, over the past few generations, patients and doctors alike have become accustomed to the notion that there must be a pill to solve any problem. If you have an issue with your body, the assumption is that there should be a drug or surgery to fix it.

However, we still have not been able to "cure" cancer in the same way we have cured polio, most likely because cancer is so individualized. For example, two women with breast cancer standing side by side may *appear* to have the same type of cancer, yet, on a molecular level, they may be dealing with completely different diseases that require drastically different treatments.

In addition to any differences in the molecular properties of their cancers, these hypothetical women would have different underlying genetic profiles and immune systems and would have been exposed to different cancer-causing factors during their lifetimes, including environmental, lifestyle, and psychological factors. Thus it should come as no surprise that these two cancer patients would likely need radically different treatments. This is one reason why a single cancer "cure" remains elusive, and why radical remission survivors require multiple healing strategies. And in order to research and implement these healing strategies, radical remission survivors need to be empowered when it comes to their health.

In *Radical Remission*, I called this healing factor "taking control of your health." However, as my research has continued, the radical remission survivors I speak to have fine-tuned my language around this factor. Since having complete control over your cancer, or your life in general, is a technically impossible task, I have learned that a more accurate term for this healing factor is *empowering yourself.* Radical remission survivors empower themselves by strengthening the following traits:

- an active (versus passive) role in their health
- the willingness to make (sometimes drastic) changes in their lives
- the ability to deal with resistance from friends, family, and doctors

Think of your health as a business and imagine yourself as the CEO. You want to understand how every part of the business functions and surround yourself with a loyal and trusted team of talented employees. You want to ask questions, challenge assumptions, research your options, seek second and third opinions, and then determine the next steps in your healing strategy in collaboration with the talented health professionals on your team.

As a good CEO, you must be willing to make changes to your business strategy at times. Radical remission survivors are always willing to analyze their lives and make changes, even when those changes are time-consuming or emotionally difficult. Since there is no quick-fix pill or surgery that can magically cure cancer, they instead invest time and emotional resources to heal their whole body-mind-spirit systems. This could include replacing their personal care and cleaning products, overhauling their diets, leaving a stressful job, or moving to a new house.

Lastly, radical remission survivors report needing a strong backbone to deal with the criticism and resistance of many well-intentioned people surrounding them, including medical doctors who may refuse to treat them if they do not follow an exact protocol, loved ones who are scared of their choices, and friends who are unwilling to accept their decisions. Swimming upstream can be challenging, especially when you fear for your life, but it is this resolve that every radical remission survivor has found to be a key factor to their survival.

Put bluntly, radical remission survivors are not afraid to be labeled "bad patients." As radical remission survivor Jane McLelland puts it, "Passive patients die. Noisy ones survive."

In 1994, Jane McLelland was diagnosed with stage 3 cervical cancer at the early age of 30, but it took five years for her to become a "noisy" patient. At first she followed her doctors' recommendation for a radical hysterectomy, which meant a devastating loss of her fertility. Initially too depressed to look beyond conventional care, she allowed her medical team to attack her cancer aggressively and she obediently followed their conventional medicine protocol of surgery, radiation, and chemotherapy, which was considered the best practice at that time.

A physical therapist by trade, Jane was naturally inclined to look for additional healing resources. When her mother died of breast cancer two years later, in 1996, Jane realized conventional care was not enough. She took matters into her own hands. Using herself as a guinea pig, she began exploring the healing factors of diet, exercise, and supplements, which for her included using medicines for conditions other than their original purpose (known as "off-label" use). Thankfully she remained in remission for five years while continuing to be vigilant with her diet, exercise, supplements, intravenous vitamin C, and ultraviolet (UV) blood irradiation (a procedure that exposes a small amount of your blood to UV light to improve your body's immune response and to kill infections).[1]

Unfortunately, in late 1999 Jane's cervical cancer returned, this time spreading to her lungs and therefore classified as stage 4. Survival at this stage is ordinarily measured in weeks, and Jane was told she was terminal. Once again, Jane attacked her cancer aggressively through conventional medicine (more surgery and chemotherapy), along with her growing list of complementary treatments. Becoming her own "Sherlock Holmes," Jane added new off-label drugs to her supplement regimen, such as using aspirin as both an anti-inflammatory and COX-2/VEGF inhibitor (note: COX-2 and VEGF are enzymes that stimulate blood growth around a tumor). She also used berberine to lower her blood glucose (the simple sugar found in carbohydrates), promote healthy fat metabolism, and fight off intestinal infections.

Amazingly, Jane was back in remission by early 2000, only three months after her stage 4 recurrence. But three years later, Jane was diagnosed with terminal leukemia, which can be a side effect of receiving strong radiation and chemotherapy treatments. Jane was only 39 years old and she was devastated.

At this point, Jane was convinced that the medical industry was missing opportunities by disregarding off-label drugs. She ignored advice to undergo yet more chemotherapy and instead worked with trusted integrative doctors to create her own off-label drug "cocktails." These cocktails included medicines that were either long forgotten by conventional medicine or were being used for purposes other than treating cancer (e.g., lovastatin, usually used for high cholesterol, and metformin, normally used for controlling diabetes). Having worked in the medical industry herself, Jane believed that the field was so focused on patenting new drugs that doctors were overlooking the potential of older (and more affordable) drugs that could help "starve her cancer." The time had come to take control of her own treatment.

*I have come to realize that many patients die of politeness to their oncologist and fear of upsetting their loved ones. But I'd already found my integrative doctors and my complementary treatments. I was also empowered with knowledge. I didn't wait around in limbo. There was so much more I could do. I felt it was good to be proactive, to be taking control, not waiting for the ax to fall, knowing each time the cancer would become more and more difficult to treat. No, I was going to be obstinate!*

Jane's tireless sleuthing led to a third remission, but this one didn't last long, as her markers once again soared the following year after she admits she "fell off the wagon" of her normally super strict diet and supplement regime. Again she took her cocktail of off-label drugs and key cancer-starving supplements; however, this time she took them for longer than three months. Today she still occasionally takes some of the drugs when she has moments of "quiet panic."

To her joy, Jane's remission has lasted 15 years and counting. She has had no evidence of disease since 2004. Now she educates cancer patients around the world on how to use off-label drugs and natural approaches to starve cancer cells and has written the best-selling book, *How to Starve Cancer*, which describes her journey in detail.

## Recent Developments

Since *Radical Remission* was published, many radical remission survivors, including Jane, have mentioned the intense fear they felt upon first hearing their diagnosis, often in the form of an urgent desire to "just get the cancer out as soon as possible." Doctors inadvertently increase this fear by rushing their patients into quick decisions regarding their medical treatment. Radical remission survivors feel this panic and pressure to make quick decisions, but they also feel empowered enough to ask their doctors for some time to think—even if it is just for a few days. Radical remission survivors use this critical window of time to seek out second or third medical opinions, begin researching complementary and alternative therapies, and make sure they feel fully informed when it comes to deciding their first step of treatment.

Another mental shift that radical remission survivors tend to make is to trust the diagnosis, but not the prognosis. They believe that their cancer diagnosis is accurate, but they often refuse to believe the dire statistics—especially when they know that those statistics are based on people who have only tried one way to heal their cancer, as opposed to using a multipronged strategy to address a multifaceted disease.

In order to expand their options beyond conventional treatment, many radical remission survivors begin with online research, which can be both a blessing and a curse. On the positive side, the Internet empowers patients with a vast array of medical and wellness resources, and they no longer need to rely solely on their doctors for health information. Many long-term radical remission survivors remember a time 20-plus years ago when they had to go to an actual library to do their research, one book at a time. Now we have information from every encyclopedia and medical journal right at our fingertips, available within seconds.

One online resource that remains an absolute must for radical remission survivors is PubMed.gov. The U.S. government lists nearly all medical studies conducted around the globe on this single, comprehensive website (which is funded by your tax dollars). On this site, you can look up the most current studies by cancer type or modality. For example, you can search for "breast cancer" or "acupuncture and cancer," and have access to the scientific studies conducted on that topic since the 1970s within seconds. You have an opportunity to increase your knowledge while improving your chances of being taken seriously by your medical doctors.

In recent years, we have seen a sharp increase in the number of advocates teaching online about body-mind-spirit approaches to cancer. People everywhere are sharing their healing stories and methods online, including at our own database at RadicalRemission.com as well as on the online platforms and social media groups of radical remission survivors such as Kris Carr, Anita Moorjani, and Chris Wark. Online summits and webinars have surged in popularity, with views numbering in the millions. This technological advancement has provided an important resource for cancer patients because it allows inexpensive access to the latest research and theories from experts in the conventional, integrative, and alternative medicine fields. This is something we at the Radical Remission Project celebrate.

One recent study showed that technology allows patients to be more proactive with their health,[2] and there is no doubt that the Internet has made it easier for cancer patients to learn about different approaches to wellness, especially integrative and com-plementary approaches about which their oncologists were not trained and therefore may not know. Mark Bricca, a naturopathic doctor specializing in integrative cancer care who trained under Dwight McKee, M.D. (one of the pioneers of integrative oncology), has seen such a huge increase in demand for integrative cancer care that he is rarely able to take on new patients.

While Dr. Bricca is encouraged by this increase in empow-erment among patients and by the general shift away from a reductionist view of health (when doctors are trained in only one specialty or area of the body, as opposed to doctors who are trained to treat the body as an interconnected whole), he has noticed a concerning trend.

> *Given the great amount of information that the Internet has made available, I am seeing people who are quite well-informed regarding their health care choices. Unfortunately, I also see too many people draw black-and-white lines and make "good/bad" distinctions between all-conventional therapeutic approaches to cancer treatment versus all-alternative ones. This is unfortunate, because there are no "good" or "bad" cancer treatments, only treatments that are more or less supportive for a given individual facing a unique set of circumstances.*

Radical remission survivors acknowledge how challenging it can be to wade through the confusing and sometimes conflict-ing information they find online, regarding both conventional and alternative treatments. Most radical remission survivors say they felt like they were forced to take a crash course in cancer, going from "Cancer 101" to "Cancer Graduate School" in a matter of months.

One thing that can help reduce the feeling of being over-whelmed is to expand the number of experts on your healing team. For radical remission survivors, conventional doctors fre-quently represent only one part of their healing teams and are not the sole members. Because conventional medicine doctors are trained to treat diseases in a reductionist manner, as opposed to looking at the person as a whole, radical remission survivors often choose to bring additional experts and healers onto their healing teams, such as psychotherapists, naturopaths, herbalists, and bodyworkers.

## Empowerment Research

Scientists have long debated whether your thoughts and behaviors, including those related to empowerment, have any relation to your physical health and immune system. In the past few years, some groundbreaking studies have made a direct correlation between these psychosocial factors and cancer.

For example, stress is a very disempowering emotion. When we feel stressed, we feel out of control—that certain aspects of our lives are not manageable. A University College of London meta-analysis of several hundred studies investigated the association between stress and cancer outcomes; it found that cancer patients with a stress-prone personality, poor coping styles, negative emotional responses, or poor quality of life were associated with higher cancer incidence, poorer cancer survival, and higher cancer mortality. In addition, the researchers found that stressful life experiences were related to decreased cancer survival and increased mortality,[3] meaning that stressful situations that make us feel powerless may contribute to our getting cancer in the first place or not healing from it after being diagnosed.

Researchers at the Wake Forest School of Medicine followed more than 500 breast cancer patients over a period of 18 months and similarly found that those with negative coping skills, such as not taking any action and blaming oneself, led to a significantly poorer quality of life. On the other hand, having positive coping skills—such as taking action, receiving help and support, and reframing things positively—led to a significantly higher quality of life.[4]

Along the same lines, breast cancer patients who had an "adaptive" coping style—meaning they had low levels of helplessness and high levels of action—experienced less anxiety and depression and enjoyed a higher quality of life than breast cancer patients who had "maladaptive" coping styles.[5] Yet another study showed that cancer patients who reported high levels of self-efficacy (belief in their ability to succeed) in regard to managing their disease symptoms enjoyed a significantly higher quality of life and significantly lower levels of distress as compared to cancer patients who self-reported lower levels of self-efficacy. These studies show us that finding a sense of control over a cancer diagnosis can lead cancer patients to have a better quality of life.[6]

Unfortunately, the stress of a diagnosis and the fear of the unknown can quickly cause cancer patients to fall into a state of "learned helplessness" by perceiving their lives to be out of control and therefore losing the ability to cope with future stressors, which in turn leads to more anxiety, inaction, and depression. One recent study set out to understand exactly what happens in the brain when an unpredictable stressor, such as a cancer diagnosis, occurs. Researchers found that the key parts of the brain that control depression and stress response (the habenula and septum) are overactive when people feel helpless.[7] This means that the helplessness brought on by a cancer diagnosis can quickly lead to depression, stress, and feeling like a "deer in the headlights," which is why it is so important for cancer patients to feel like they are in the driver's seat.

Luckily, there are scientifically proven things you can do to shake off helplessness and gain a sense of control. Empowerment can be taught in a relatively short period of time. For example, in only eight weeks, cancer patients with low levels of optimism who participated in a support group that taught them problem-solving and stress-management skills showed higher levels of positivity and lower levels of helplessness than patients who joined a support group that was strictly psychological in nature.[8]

A similar study on psychoeducational workshops that aimed to empower cancer patients found that 85 percent of participants reported increased confidence in discussing treatment options with their doctors and in making treatment-related decisions with their health care team.[9] Yet another study showed that using the Internet to conduct health research left 73 percent of the study's participants feeling more in control of their health and with a better outlook.[10] These studies show there are concrete things you can do to feel more empowered.

What we find most exciting is how empowerment may help cancer patients enjoy a higher quality of life while living longer. In one recent study of women with invasive ovarian cancer, those who started off their medical treatment with higher levels of optimism and lower helplessness scores ended up living significantly longer than the patients who had lower optimism levels and higher helplessness scores.[11] Feeling empowered from the get-go *can* help to lengthen your life.

Scientific studies continue to demonstrate what radical remission survivors have long believed, namely that feeling empowered when it comes to your health is a key factor in healing. Radical remission survivors empower themselves by taking an active role in their decision-making, asking questions, doing their own research, refusing to be passive patients, and being willing to make whatever changes are needed. One such radical remission survivor is Robert Granata, a man who continues to defy the odds each day with his sheer willpower.

## Bob's Story

Bob Granata is a no-nonsense Midwesterner who in 2014 was enjoying a satisfying career as the founder and managing partner of several businesses and family time spent with his loving wife of 17 years and their three wonderful daughters, then ages 14, 15, and 17. After experiencing sudden abdominal pain, Bob thought he was going to have an easy appendectomy (surgical removal of his appendix) before quickly getting on with his life.

However, during what was supposed to be a simple operation, Bob's doctors discovered that his appendix was severely inflamed. In addition, they found an abscess around his appendix, which meant there was fluid leaking from somewhere, although they were unsure of the source.

As the surgery progressed, Bob's doctors found cancer cells in both his appendix and in his omentum (a sheet of fatty tissue that stretches over the inside of the abdomen), in 11 out of 72 abdominal lymph nodes, on his peritoneal wall, and in his colon. As a result, his surgical team had to remove one-third of his ascending colon, one-third of his omentum, and his entire appendix via a full open-incision surgery, as opposed to a laparoscopic surgery. Bob awoke from surgery with a much larger incision than he had anticipated—and missing many more of his internal organs. A few hours later, his doctors delivered the shocking news: He had a very rare cancer of the appendix known as appendiceal cancer.

Based on the large amount of cancer discovered throughout his abdomen, Bob was given a stage 4 diagnosis and a survival prognosis of a mere six months. Bob immediately told his doctor he was not prepared to accept that prognosis. While his doctors urged him to quickly "get his affairs in order," he instead moved every resource he could think of into high gear. He did not plan on going anywhere anytime soon.

> *Having teenage daughters at that time, all a year and a half apart, I wasn't quite prepared to throw in the towel. I'm fortunate that I had the wherewithal to look at all different types of solutions and become my own advocate to understand what people have done internationally, domestically, medically, naturopathically, and mentally to harness this disease.*

Like many people diagnosed with cancer, initially Bob was shocked. More surprising was the news that his cancer was incredibly rare. Only nine in a million people are diagnosed with appendiceal cancer,[12] so there was very little existing research he could study. Faced with grim statistics based on so few people, he decided he was not going to believe them and instead intended to use his own skills and determination to fill in the gaps that research had not filled yet.

He put his efforts into healing his cancer, immediately beginning the aggressive conventional treatment that was recommended by his doctors. Following his surgery, Bob started a five-round chemotherapy protocol that was originally designed to treat colon cancer. Because appendiceal cancer is so rare, there was not a specific protocol for his doctors to follow, so they decided to treat it like colon cancer. For about 15 weeks, Bob did the CAPOX protocol, which uses a combination of oral capecitabine and intravenous oxaliplatin chemotherapies, and then he continued a portion of that protocol by taking six capecitabine pills a day for the next year and a half.

During this time, Bob started working with a naturopathic clinic in Ann Arbor, Michigan, to explore more holistic approaches. He did extensive research on the Internet and at libraries and came to believe that his cancer, which was present on his peritoneal wall, would be better treated with a peritoneal cancer protocol, rather than with a colon cancer protocol. (The peritoneum is the cavity and lining surrounding your abdominal organs.)

Bob's research convinced him that traditional intravenous chemotherapies may not work as well on peritoneal cancers, because there is not enough blood flow to the peritoneum. In addition, once a patient with peritoneal cancer progresses to stage 3 or 4, the lining becomes covered with mucus and the cancer spreads quickly within the peritoneum. Peritoneal cancer is very serious, and there is little that can be done for the patient. Bob started to question his oncology team and specifically their decision to treat his cancer like colon cancer.

*So, I lost a little confidence in the medical field and started looking elsewhere. I had an oncologist in the Detroit area that discouraged what I thought was the direction to go [treating it like peritoneal cancer]. Patients need an advocate. I think if you can't be your own advocate, you need to find an advocate. You have to do a lot of reading and a lot of research on your own. A lot of the doctors don't like you doing your own [research], but I tell you, many people along the way have asked me if I were a doctor, because I'm so apprised of my situation. Some doctors have even asked if I were a doctor! . . . Knowledge is power.*

Through his tireless research, Bob learned of Paul Sugarbaker, a doctor in Maryland who had established a new protocol in the 1980s aptly named the "Sugarbaker Technique." Instead of treating peritoneal cancer systemically with intravenous chemotherapy, as doctors had been doing for years, Dr. Sugarbaker's technique perfused hot chemotherapy directly into the peritoneum. This method is now known as HIPEC (hyperthermic intraperitoneal chemotherapy).[13] Bob describes the procedure as follows:

*A midline incision is made from your belly button to your chest to open the cavity up and do what's called a "debulk-ing." If there's any type of tumor activity, they "debulk" the tumors [by surgically removing them], and they also take out any organs that you can spare [live without]. Then they perfuse [spray] hot chemotherapy into the belly and let it circulate for about 90 minutes in your abdomen. And it is that hot chemo-therapy that actually kills the microscopic cells that are floating around in your peritoneum.*

As soon as he read about it, Bob felt a strong, intuitive know-ing that this HIPEC procedure was the right next step in his heal-ing journey, so he took matters into his own hands and scheduled the procedure on his own. He had to schedule it in Pittsburgh, though, as that was the nearest location that offered HIPEC. At first Bob's oncologist was decidedly against him having the HIPEC procedure. However, once the oncologist saw that Bob was not responding to traditional intravenous chemotherapy, he began to see how valuable the HIPEC procedure might be. Bob recalls:

*My original oncologist said, "No, don't do it. There is no data to support that a HIPEC procedure is going to be helpful. They couldn't do a blind study on it, so they couldn't really document it as a true clinical trial." I said, "Well, I'm going to do it." And interestingly, some time into my fourth systemic chemo, he changed his tune. He said, "You need to get down there right away and do your HIPEC." I said, "Well, how did you change your tune so quickly?"*

This wavering continued to degrade Bob's confidence in his oncologist and more broadly in the medical system's approach to cancer.

*I lost confidence in him because he was also in academics and I thought, He's teaching it. Why doesn't he know about [HIPEC] or its effectiveness? Doctors aren't God. Part of the problem in the whole medical field is that there's just not enough time. There are too many patients and not enough doctors, which means not enough time for the doctors to really understand their patients and also to stay on top of the latest and greatest technology and developments.*

Bob finished his five rounds of traditional intravenous chemotherapy before he was ready for the HIPEC procedure. Then he went down to the University of Pittsburgh Medical Center (UPMC), led by Dr. David Bartlett, for his first HIPEC. During the procedure, Dr. Bartlett took out the rest of Bob's omentum and stripped his peritoneal wall. Going into it, Bob did not realize how arduous the surgery was going to be for his surgeon. In retrospect, Bob feels that this naivete helped him to go into the surgery with a more positive mind-set, which he believes led to a quicker recovery.

*I found out later that [my medical team] considered the HIPEC [to be] the "mother" of all surgeries. But I went in with a clear mind-set. I wasn't looking at it as being the "mother of all surgeries." I thought it was going to be very standard. I think that goes back to the mind, and how strong your mind is going forward. If I had gone in saying, "Oh, no, this is a tough surgery. Can I make it through it?" then chances are it may have turned out differently.*

After Bob's HIPEC surgery, nine months after his initial surgery and diagnosis, he was declared in full remission with no evidence of disease (NED) based on the results of PET scans, CAT scans, and blood tumor marker levels. Although he was in remission, Bob refused to take a "watch and wait" approach to see if the cancer would come back. Instead, he actively continued to work on improving his health and immune system using as many methods as possible.

During this time of remission, Bob continued to work with his naturopathic doctors by making changes to his diet, taking supplements, and taking steps to reduce his stress levels. In addition, Bob traveled to Kliniken Essen-Mitte, a health clinic in Germany, 15 months after his initial diagnosis. There, he started taking subcutaneous shots of mistletoe into his abdomen. (Note: Extract of the mistletoe plant is a well-known immune-boosting therapy in Europe that is now gaining traction in the United States. We talk more about mistletoe therapy in our chapter on herbs and supplements.) Mistletoe injections have been shown to "wake up" a patient's immune response. As Bob describes it:

> *We all know of mistletoe as something we ought to kiss under at Christmastime. Jokingly, I said, "If I take this, will it mean I'll have a lot of women wanting to kiss me?" That didn't happen, but it would have been a nice add-on to taking shots every other day! [laughs] Mistletoe works much like a flu shot. Your immune system basically becomes familiar with that flu virus so when you get the real flu, your immune system knows how to respond to it. This is the same as it is with mistletoe. Every time I took a subcutaneous shot [of mistletoe], it made my immune system wake up, recognizing there was some type of a foreign substance going on. So the theory behind the mistletoe is*

*that it would wake up [my immune system] every other day, so
that eventually my immune system could help fight my cancer.*

Bob continued taking mistletoe injections every other day for
nearly two years, from April 2014 until March 2016. Mistletoe is
not yet FDA-approved, so it cannot currently be prescribed by U.S.
medical doctors, but it can be prescribed by naturopathic doctors,
since it is considered a supplement. Bob was able to work with his
naturopathic clinic in Ann Arbor to receive his mistletoe supply.

Simultaneously, Bob worked with his naturopathic team to
fine-tune his overall supplement regimen. He says, "I had cabi-
nets for my supplements, and taking them on time and regularly
was quite arduous." Bob's long list of customized supplements that
were appropriate for his body at that particular time included his
main fallbacks of turmeric; CBD oil; mushroom supplements such
as turkey tail; vitamin D; a cayenne pepper mixture; and various
herbal teas.

In summer 2015, Bob flew from Michigan to California to
attend one of the first Radical Remission workshops ever offered.
At the two-day workshop, he learned about the nine radical remission healing factors and decided to embrace them as enthusias-
tically as he had the conventional and naturopathic medicine
protocols.

The Radical Remission workshop reinforced his gut instinct
about needing to play an active role in his healing process, which
is why when Bob got a recommendation from a fellow workshop-
goer to check out a naturopathic clinic nearby in California, he
quickly made an appointment for the next day. By the time he
was on the plane back home to Michigan, he had secured another
naturopathic team in California, which helped him participate
in RGCC (Research Genetic Cancer Centre) testing being done in
Greece, in order to identify which chemotherapies would work
well on his particular cancer cells.

Like many radical remission survivors, Bob discovered he
needed to build an extensive healing team around his medical oncologists. The naturopathic teams that Bob found first in

Michigan and then in California were an important part of his healing process, especially when it came to determining the right supplements for his body.

In addition to taking numerous herbs and supplements, Bob changed his diet drastically. Like many Americans, Bob loved a good steak and was a big beef eater. However, as part of his healing, he eliminated red meat from his diet and began replacing it with fish that was high in vitamin E. Since one-third of his colon and other digestive organs were removed during his first surgery, he could not eat a lot of fruits, vegetables, or other high-fiber foods because they are hard to digest without a full colon. He also started to limit his sugar intake. However, unlike most radical remission survivors, Bob *increased* his intake of refined flours and white bread while decreasing his intake of what he calls "fibering bread," meaning those from whole grains.

> *I always knew if you eat a high-fiber, whole-grain bread, it's much better for you, right? Well, in my case, my digestive problems after the hemicolectomy [partial, surgical removal of the large intestine] made that much more difficult.*

The rest of the radical remission factors played a big role in Bob's recovery. He relied heavily on his wife and three daughters for social support and to help keep up his positive emotions, and Bob's sister—who works in the health field—played a key role in supporting him during his treatment. She served as his primary advocate, acting as a sounding board to discuss his treatment and speaking on his behalf when he was in surgery or could not communicate well for whatever reason (e.g., when he was groggy post-surgery). For Bob, it was essential to find someone like his sister whom he could trust to advocate for him during his most vulnerable times.

Although Bob never sought out any professional counseling or therapy, he found a way to process his emotions on his own, especially the fears and "what-ifs" he felt surrounding the possibility of leaving his family before he was ready.

*I'm always thinking through things, and I just never really surrendered to the disease. I look at it and say, "I am blessed enough to still be here and, you know, it could have been worse." So I just kind of deal with it that way.*

Bob's international business provided an unexpected source of support during his cancer journey. Friends and colleagues from his hometown and all over the world offered social support through friendship and spiritual support through prayer, helping to deepen his spiritual connection and give him additional reasons for living. He believes that prayer, in particular, contributed greatly to his remission.

*I think the power of prayer was really evident in my case. I had people from my international business praying. And people from China who were typically atheists praying for me, and praying to Buddha. People in Europe and people in America and Canada were praying to other gods. So I have a lot of great friends globally. And I really felt that the power of prayer had a lot to do with where I'm at.*

Exercise was more difficult for Bob, since his core muscles were radically affected by his abdominal surgeries. Nevertheless, he was still able to engage in walking and low-impact exercise daily to stay fit and strong.

In Bob's opinion, his multifaceted healing efforts helped to keep him alive far past his six-month "expiration date." Unfortunately, though, his cancer came back in April 2016, a little more than two years after his initial diagnosis, and 19 months after his HIPEC surgery. During his HIPEC surgery, there had been a seemingly benign and very small nodule on his transverse colon that his doctors had not touched, but since then that nodule had grown into a cancerous tumor. Knowing there was probably more cancer surrounding this tumor, Bob opted to do a second HIPEC surgery, despite the inevitable challenges it would bring. He remembers how he felt during this difficult time.

*I believe in the whole concept of peritoneal disease. Most doctors are really anxious to give you [intravenous] chemotherapy at $14,000 a hit that isn't getting to the space you need it to. So logically [a second HIPEC] made a lot of sense. That's really the premise behind my doing the second one. I thought,* Well, if in fact I have a tumor, *which I did and they removed it,* then it has probably left some seeding back in the peritoneal cavity that needs to be addressed through the HIPEC procedure. *However, if the first HIPEC was the "mother of all surgeries," then this was the mother, the grandmother, and the great-grandmother of all surgeries!*

Bob's second HIPEC procedure was tougher than the first. Due to scar tissue from Bob's prior two surgeries, it was "like cutting through cement" for his doctors. All they could see was one big mass, because his colon was completely pulled together by scar tissue. As a result, Bob experienced many perforations of his colon and intestines as they tried to cut away the scar tissue to get to the tumor. He ended up coming out of this second HIPEC surgery with one-third of his colon and an ileostomy instead of the expected colostomy.

Bob's surgeons were forced to give him an ileostomy because they had to remove his transverse colon. With an ileostomy, the final section of your small intestine is diverted to an artificial hole in your abdomen, which then connects to a plastic pouch so that your fecal matter can leave your body without needing to travel through the colon. This meant his doctors recommended that Bob no longer receive his nutrition through food, but through a daily intravenous infusion of total parenteral nutrition (TPN). Bob remembers it this way:

*They said, "You'll probably never eat again. You'll be on TPN the rest of your life." It was devastating. You know, my travels would be affected. My life revolves around entertainment and food. You go out to dinner, you go out to lunch. An ileostomy is an extra bag that mounts above your colon. Any food or liquid [you consume] goes into the bag versus through your [digestive] system. Basically, every night I took two to three liters of TPN intravenously for nearly 18 months. I didn't eat any solid foods for nearly 18 months! I went from 220 pounds at the onset of my disease to about 145. It was a big life-changing moment. I had to have a strong enough mind to wrap around how my life would really change.*

Bob's medical oncology team at UPMC then took his treatment into "breakthrough" territory by creating a custom immunotherapy vaccine from Bob's own tumor. UPMC is an academic hospital that was leading an immunotherapy trial specifically for peritoneal cancer. The team took a part of the tumor that they removed during Bob's second HIPEC surgery and froze it. Nearly a year later, in April 2017, they unfroze that tumor in order to develop a personalized vaccine that they combined with cytokine proteins. These cytokine proteins were there to help Bob's body identify and "notice" the cancerous cells to which they were attached. Bob was reinjected with his original tumor, now in the form of a vaccine, with the goal of ensuring that his body's immune system would eliminate any remaining cancer cells.

*They took my tumor and developed my own custom vaccine. They actually reinjected my body back with the original cancer that they salvaged, which was strange because I'm thinking,* I don't want the cancer back. Why are you doing that? *But it goes back to that same principle behind flu shots and mistletoe, where it trains your immune system to recognize the cancer. It seems reasonable to assume that [the vaccine] had some positive effects.*

Soon after receiving four cancer immunotherapy injections, Bob achieved a major healing milestone in that he was able to reverse his ileostomy after having it for about a year. He was unwilling to accept that he would have an ileostomy for the rest of his life and attributes this milestone to having a positive, determined attitude. While he has since used TPN off and on during bowel obstructions, Bob is proud to have returned to eating solid food and to have defied the doctors who said he would need to be fed through an IV for the rest of his life.

Bob has shown no evidence of disease (NED) since his second HIPEC surgery, and, to the surprise of many of his doctors, was still NED in January 2020. That's six and a half years after his diagnosis, when his doctors gave him only six months to live.

*It's been a big journey of both surgical and naturopathic solutions. We're not really sure why I'm doing as well as I'm doing with such a dire prognosis. I have no complaints, of course. I'm convinced the takeaways from that Radical Remission workshop that have stuck with me over the years, and the different medical things that we did have had positive effects on my health.*

Bob embodies and consciously practices the 10 radical remission factors, yet he feels that taking control of his health is the most important one for him.

*I don't think I would have taken the different courses of naturopathic, mental, and medical procedures if I weren't my own advocate. And knowing what to expect going in [to the surgeries] was also important. I could understand what my expectations should be and what my recoveries would be like. And although there were a lot of challenges along the way, and there were many times I could have gotten down, I kept in mind that in reality, I was very blessed that I was still here considering my original prognosis was only six months.*

When asked about what made him push so hard to take control of his health, Bob says:

*I find some people innately will take charge [of their health] and others will just sit back and depend on their doctor to lead the way. It's just the personality of the person. But I do believe you have to be prepared to fight, and the day you start giving up is the day you probably start going down the wrong path. I do believe that.*

While Bob's efforts have resulted in a full NED remission, Bob has not been content with just saving his own life. Instead, he has made it his life's purpose to help save other cancer patients' lives, especially those with appendiceal or peritoneal cancers. Beating the odds inspired Bob to offer a grant to William Beaumont Hospital in Royal Oak, Michigan, to bring the HIPEC procedure to his local community. Since Bob helped to launch the program in October of 2016, doctors in Royal Oak have performed more than 60 HIPEC procedures for Michigan cancer patients, many with excellent results.

*I was fortunate because I had my own business and had a partner who could help run the business while I was sick. It provided me the wherewithal financially to fly to Germany and California, to do some of the things that unfortunately some people can't do. I knew when I went down for the HIPEC in Pittsburgh that we were there from three weeks to a month at a time, which is quite cost-prohibitive for most people. You have the cost of the hotel, the travel, and if you have children, it's difficult. How do you take care of your family and also your loved one who's fighting a disease?*

Bob's biggest challenge is staying hydrated, as well as the potential for bowel obstructions. Since most water is absorbed in the body's colon and Bob has only one-third of his colon left, he is not able to absorb fluids well. At least once every other day, he used to self-administer his hydration therapy intravenously to keep his body properly hydrated, but recently he has been able to rely solely on orally ingested water and fluids.

Bob now eats solid foods, but without a properly working colon, most fruits and vegetables—which are inherently high in fiber—are still a "no-no." However, he still eats a lot of fish. Bob and his doctors have yet to uncover what causes his bowel obstructions, which seem to occur with no rhyme or reason, and which land him in the hospital for 7 to 10 days at a time until the obstruction clears. At first, Bob thought his food choices were causing the obstructions, but now he thinks they are more related to scar tissue moving around internally.

Bob currently takes no medication or supplements (with only one-third of his colon, he has trouble absorbing oral supplements), but he continues to work with his naturopath to determine when supplements, perhaps intravenous ones, might be brought back into his health maintenance plan. He spends his winters in Florida, so he gets his vitamin D naturally from the sun. Now that he is in a warm climate year-round, he is able to walk and continue with his low-impact exercise daily.

Regarding what may have caused his cancer, Bob believes his international business travel created a perfect storm. He spent a lot of time in China (approximately 150 days a year) and thinks the cause of his cancer may have been environmental pollution and bacteria that he was constantly exposed to while traveling, exacerbated by the subsequent antibiotic treatments.

He noticed every time he came back from a trip, he had some type of respiratory infection. He was always coughing and the infection would take months to resolve. Each time, his doctors would prescribe a slew of antibiotics. At one point, Bob was on six different antibiotics in six months. As he describes it, his immune system was "getting beat down pretty bad." In his opinion, the combination of the continuous exposure to bacteria, plus all the travel and changes in time zones, not to mention the repeated rounds of antibiotics, came together to weaken his immune system and make him susceptible to cancer growth.

Looking back on his experience, Bob says:

> *I think we all have a purpose, and for me, it was funding the HIPEC program in Royal Oak, Michigan, to help more than 60 people so far. Maybe at some point [the HIPEC program] will help a thousand or more people. There's a higher purpose and a higher reasoning for why things happen.*

Bob exemplifies how hard radical remission survivors are willing to work toward their own recovery. The day after his diagnosis, he began researching every conventional, complementary, and alternative treatment method available to him. He pushed back with his doctors when needed and ultimately changed his traditional oncologist's mind about the usefulness of the HIPEC procedure. He sought out naturopathic clinics in the U.S. and in Europe to find the best solutions for himself, and he participated in a clinical trial with state-of-the-art immunotherapy.

It has been six years since Bob was given a terminal prognosis, and he is grateful to be alive and to be seeing his three daughters through college (his eldest graduated in 2019). He has bought a retirement home in Northern Michigan and a condominium in Florida, where he vacationed for many years and now spends the winters as a "snowbird." However, Bob shows no signs of actually retiring. In fact, he just acquired more divisions for his company and is actively growing his business. Like so many other radical remission survivors before him, Bob applied his "take charge" attitude from his life and business and applied it to his healing—with odds-defying results.

# Action Steps

In *Radical Remission*, we recommended some simple ways to empower yourself when it comes to your health, including finding a general practitioner who welcomes your questions; expanding your healing team to include naturopaths, energy healers, acupuncturists, etc.; learning how to do your own research using tools like PubMed.gov; evaluating which areas of your life could use some improvement; and finding an accountability partner. These remain great first steps to take for empowerment, and here are some additional steps you can take to feel more empowered about your health.

- **Find an advocate.**
  If you have a friend or family member who knows medical jargon, they can help you translate what the doctors are saying and conversely can express your concerns to the doctors. If possible, bring your advocate with you to medical appointments and hospital visits. Having someone familiar with the medical world is like having a translator in a foreign country. Less will get lost in translation and you will get the care you need.

- **Be thoughtful online.**
  Many online sites, including PubMed.gov, are trustworthy sources of information, while other crowdsourced websites can sometimes provide false information or send you down rabbit holes of confusion. Look for therapies that have clinical trials behind them that have been published in peer-reviewed medical journals and include a control group. However, also keep in mind that many complementary and alternative therapies do not have clinical trials supporting them due to a lack of research funding.

  In that case, look for multiple, verified case reports on the outcomes of a particular therapy from a variety of different sources (i.e., not all from the same clinic or practitioner). Also, be aware of how your online research is making you feel. Notice if the site you are on is making you feel empowered and energized or deflated and hopeless. If you need a pick-me-up, browse through and learn from the hundreds of case studies in our free online healing story database at RadicalRemission.com.

- **Get additional opinions.**
  As you evaluate whether your doctor and team are the right fit for you, be sure to get a second, third, or

even fourth opinion until you feel like you have your healing dream team in place. Ask yourself, *Do I trust this person with my life?* If the answer is not a firm yes, then keep searching. Note: Many health insurance plans automatically cover second opinions.

- **Consider a coach.**
  Lifestyle coaching has been around for decades, but it has recently gained momentum in the cancer world. This is due, in part, to an increase in cancer survivors—like Bob and Jane from this chapter—who are so transformed by their own radical remissions that they feel inspired to help others work toward remission as well. Due to high demand, we recently launched a Radical Remission coaching program to help people implement the 10 healing factors into their own lives in a customized manner. You can learn more at RadicalRemission.com/health-coach-program.

We hope this chapter has inspired you to feel more empowered when it comes to your health. For radical remission survivors, becoming empowered and taking an active role in their healing process has given them something to do in between doctor visits and has helped them feel more in control at a time when so much of their life feels out of control. We wish that this sense of empowerment will give you the same kind of radical hope that it gave to Bob, Jane, and hundreds of other radical remission survivors like them.

## CHAPTER 4

# INCREASING POSITIVE EMOTIONS

## Di's Story

*Folks are usually about as happy
as they make their minds up to be.*

— ABRAHAM LINCOLN

Look no further than the immense popularity of cat videos on the Internet for proof that humans today are in desperate need of quick joy fixes. (Googling "cat videos" produces 3.7 billion results alone!) Humans want to feel happy because it is our natural state. We love to laugh and feel joy, and children playing embody this natural state of human happiness. However, as adults, many of us have lost touch with these feelings of joy and ease. Life and all its responsibilities, deadlines, pressures, and bills can weigh us down and distract us. Add in something like a cancer diagnosis, and you begin to wonder what there is to be happy about in life.

In fact, adults today are more unhappy than ever. The incidence of depression and suicide continues to rise at an alarming rate,[1] and the World Health Organization notes that more than 300 million people around the world suffer from depression, which is the leading cause of disability.[2] Sadly, cancer patients are more vulnerable to depression and suicide, with rates almost double that of the general population.[3]

While depression is an understandable side effect of a cancer diagnosis, radical remission survivors report that the act of purposely increasing their positive emotions for at least five minutes a day helped them to counteract their diagnosis-induced depression. Radical remission survivors believe that returning to their natural state of joy, if only for a brief moment, was essential to their physical recovery. This theory is backed up by decades of scientific research, which we will explore later in this chapter.

For radical remission survivors, positive emotions include feelings of joy, happiness, contentment, peace, gratitude, laughter, and love. They often start out feeling more short-term positive emotions, such as a few seconds of laughter while watching a comedic TV show, and then develop a more constant feeling of peace and contentment from practicing happiness on a daily basis.

In *Radical Remission*, I wrote that "positive emotions are like rocket fuel for the immune system." When your body feels stress or fear, it goes into "fight-or-flight" mode, and therefore cannot heal itself. This is a well-established, scientific fact, and the opposite is also true. Positive emotions help you get out of this frame of mind and into a "rest and repair" state, which significantly improves your immune system's ability to heal. Here is a recap of what happens inside your body when you experience emotions such as love, joy, or happiness.

The first thing that happens when you feel positive emotions is that your brain instantly releases healing hormones, including serotonin, relaxin, oxytocin, dopamine, and endorphins into your bloodstream.[4] These so-called happy hormones could just as easily be called "healing hormones," because they tell the cells in your body to start performing healing activities, such as:

- lowering your blood pressure, heart rate, and cortisol (the "stress hormone") level
- improving blood circulation
- deepening your breathing in order to increase oxygenation levels in your blood
- slowing digestion in order to absorb more nutrients

- strengthening your immune system by increasing the number and activity level of white and red blood cells and natural killer cells, clearing out infections, and looking for and destroying cancer cells (via apoptosis)[5]

These physiological changes help you both in the short term and over the long term. Numerous studies have revealed what many healers have long known: Happy people live longer, period. In one recent study, elderly people were up to 35 percent less likely to die over the course of five years if they self-reported feeling happy on an average day.[6] The top 10 happiest nations in the world, as ranked in the 2019 World Happiness Report survey by the United Nations, are among the top 20 percent for life expectancy.[7]

Many radical remission survivors believe that cancer cells are simply healthy cells that have been damaged and now need to be repaired and healed. While conventional medicine agrees that cancer cells are damaged cells, the conventional medicine perspective is that cancer cells are beyond repair. Since the cancer cells have been damaged by either a toxin, virus, bacteria, mitochondrial failure, or genetic mutation, conventional medicine believes that cancer cells must be destroyed by chemotherapy, radiation, or surgery. This perspective assumes cancer cells are separate from the body and worthy of attack, whereas many healers and radical remission survivors believe that cancer cells were once healthy cells and therefore should be healed, not destroyed.

It is important to note that radical remission survivors are not Pollyannas with their heads stuck in the sand, feeling happy all the time. It would be impossible to feel happy all the time, especially while going through a health crisis. Instead, radical remission survivors make a conscious effort to incorporate a few minutes of happiness into their daily routine, just like the habit of brushing their teeth. Radical remission survivors view happiness not as a personality trait you are born with or a mood that comes and goes, but as a skill that must be practiced every day. That is why radical remission survivors set aside at least five minutes daily to increase their positive emotions in some way.

By giving themselves permission to feel happy for at least five minutes each day, radical remission survivors sidestep the misguided notion that a person who is trying to heal from a physical illness should try to feel happy all the time, which can cause many patients to feel guilty and fearful of making their cancer grow if they do not feel happy every second of every day. Some may "put on a happy face" and try to suppress their negative emotions. Embracing the reality that it is impossible to feel happy all the time helps radical remission survivors accept when they need to express fear, sadness, or frustration. (Note: We will discuss this idea further in the chapter on releasing suppressed emotions.) The goal here is emotional freedom, allowing yourself to feel and then release uncomfortable emotions like fear and anger while experiencing more authentic moments of joy and love.

Finally, for radical remission survivors, increasing positive emotions means focusing on a special type of love: love for oneself. Radical remission survivors develop a love and respect for themselves that frees them up to accept themselves as they are, faults and all, instead of trying to change or hide their true selves in order to please others. It is only after they find a way to love themselves fully and truly that radical remission survivors have been able to extend that love to others.

## Recent Developments

The good news is that happiness and mental health have finally gained the global attention of lawmakers and society at large. The not-so-good news is that this attention is being driven by an increase in depression, anxiety, and suicide that has been linked to our fast-paced, technology-driven lifestyles. Here are a couple of recent trends we have noticed regarding positive emotions.

## Happiness as Public Policy

Happiness has become a government matter in several countries around the world. Given the rising rates of depression and suicide, countries like the United Kingdom, Bhutan, the United Arab Emirates (UAE), Ecuador, and Australia are now making their citizens' happiness a central part of their government policy.[8] For instance, the U.K. has appointed a ministerial lead on loneliness, while the UAE has appointed a minister of state for happiness.[9] Despite the "pursuit of happiness" being a central theme in the United States' Declaration of Independence, unfortunately the U.S. government has not yet done anything to incorporate happiness into public health policy.

As governments become increasingly concerned about the mental health of their citizens, more government-funded programs will become available to cancer patients to help combat depression and anxiety, thereby increasing their positive emotions. And while the United States has not officially adopted any substantial new mental health policies, a number of high-profile suicides in the past few years, including those of Robin Williams, Kate Spade, and Anthony Bourdain, have brought mental health to the forefront, leading to an increase in public awareness and private funding for mental health programs. We hope that the U.S. government and health insurance companies alike will begin to understand the crucial importance of mental health on both the physical health and work productivity of its citizens.

## Daily Gratitude

Over the past few years, gratitude has become a pop-culture phenomenon. Every bookshop, app store, and retailer now carries gratitude journals, books, and products—even gratitude T-shirts. The hashtag #blessed going viral on social media shows just how mainstream the practice of expressing gratitude has become. Cultivating gratitude as a healing strategy means being grateful for both the big and little things in your life. For instance, radical remission survivors share that they strive to feel grateful for almost every part of their lives, including big things like their medical treatment and little things like wildflowers along a highway or a smile from a stranger.

One radical remission survivor who developed a daily gratitude practice to increase her positive emotions is Kristi Cromwell, who was diagnosed in 2013 with a primary, low-grade glioma (brain tumor). Because the tumor was in the brain stem area of her brain, her doctors told her that surgery was not an option. Instead, they suggested radiation and possibly chemotherapy, which came with no guarantee and the possibility of severe side effects. Understandably, this was shocking and unsettling news. Kristi opted not to do the recommended treatment and decided to explore alternative strategies for healing. Eventually she found a way to be at peace with her situation.

> *With a diagnosis of an inoperable brain tumor, I couldn't have surgery to remove it so I needed to learn to just "sit with it" and make peace with it. This was not an easy task at first, especially with being told to "watch and wait." I wanted to take part in my healing. One of my favorite quotes is "Where the mind goes, the body follows." So I sought out activities that made me happy, brought more joy into my life, and raised my internal positivity. I became certified as a Laughter Yoga leader, began watching funny videos with my daughter, spent more time with my photography creating images that evoked a sense of happiness and peace, expanded my gratitude practice, and now start each day with a "Thank you" for wherever I am in life. Staying positive in the midst of uncertainty isn't an easy task, but finding joy can help alleviate stress and has the added benefit of improving your immune system!*

Instead of watching and waiting, Kristi decided to bring the 10 radical remission healing factors into her life. Today, she gives back to other cancer patients as a certified Radical Remission instructor leading workshops in Massachusetts, and thankfully her tumor has been stable over the past six years.

But how does gratitude relate to healing? First, numerous research studies support the premise that gratitude is healing to both the psyche and the body. For example, a recent clinical trial found that an intervention designed to elicit gratitude by keeping a daily gratitude journal for two weeks increased the subjects' positive feelings, happiness, and life satisfaction, while at the same time reducing negativity and depressive symptoms.[10] One of the most commonly researched interventions is a "gratitude list," where individuals list three to five things they felt grateful for at the end of each day.[11] This daily act of purposeful gratitude has been scientifically proven to improve physical health symptoms and sleep quality.[12] A similar study showed that people who have a tendency to feel grateful have better physical health and participate in more healthy activities (e.g., exercise) compared to people who do not tend to feel grateful.[13]

## Technology Addiction

Technology, the Internet, and smartphones have improved health care in so many ways. You can now access doctors and nurses via video conferencing; pay medical bills and view test results instantly via apps; use remote health monitors at home to reduce your number of hospital visits; and track your symptoms, food intake, and vital signs via sophisticated phone apps.

However, technology has a dark side: It is eroding our happiness by damaging our social connections, making us addicted to our devices, bombarding us with negative news, interrupting our sleep patterns, and lowering our self-esteem. This technology negatively affects our brains, and therefore our physical health. Apps are designed to be addictive. Studies have shown that technology addictions are caused by the brief spurts of dopamine that are released whenever someone "likes" your social media post or when you win a silly game, which then demands an increase in technological stimulation in order to produce another dopamine "high."[14]

This leads us to *always* being on our phones. One-third of global consumers say they check their phones within five minutes of waking up in the morning,[15] and roughly 20 percent of smartphone users report checking their phones more than 50 times per day—that's once every 20 minutes while we are awake.[16]

To be clear, this is not a healthy habit. A recent review of the research showed that Internet addiction leads to neurological complications, psychological disturbances, and social problems.[17] Multiple studies have shown a strong correlation between escalating smartphone use and increased levels of depression, anxiety, and impulsivity.[18] Finally, a recent study of smartphone users in China found that excessive use of social media and messenger apps impaired the subjects' motor, cognitive, and behavioral functions within the brain.[19] In summary, smartphone use is certainly not helping us to increase our positive emotions in any lasting way.

In addition to these psychological effects, smartphones and Bluetooth usage may contribute to cancer and other physical health problems. Studies have shown that smartphone use is associated with an increased risk of brain and salivary gland tumors, and at least nine studies (and counting) have reported an increased risk of malignant brain cancer due to smartphone use.[20] There is preliminary evidence to suggest that smartphone use may increase the risk of leukemia and breast, testicular, and thyroid cancers.[21] Furthermore, a recent study showed that radiofrequency radiation from mobile phones is associated with an increase in DNA damage.[22] After reviewing the research available on this topic, a group of epidemiologists from around the world urged the International Agency for Research on Cancer to recategorize radiofrequency radiation from mobile phones and other wireless devices as being officially "carcinogenic to humans," as opposed to just a "possible human carcinogen."[23]

## Psychoneuroimmunology

Researchers continue to study happiness in order to understand its connection to physical health. One growing field of study is psychoneuroimmunology (PNI), which focuses on the links between one's thoughts and emotions ("psych"), brain activity ("neuro"), and immune system.[24] Over the past 50 years, this fascinating field of study has demonstrated that the mind and body are tightly interconnected.

A recent review of many studies related to PNI-based interventions, such as meditation, mindfulness, and cognitive behavioral therapy, found that PNI interventions have led to reductions in inflammatory markers for cancer and HIV, as well as in depression, anxiety, and other symptoms.[25] For instance, a recent study of pediatric leukemia patients found that a PNI intervention—which included guiding the children through an exercise where they imagined their immune cells removing their cancer cells—increased multiple immune markers in the children, while improving their quality of life, shortening the duration of their fevers, and reducing their use of therapeutic drugs.[26] As a bonus, this PNI intervention reduced hospital costs.

Scientists are beginning to figure out exactly how—on a cellular level—positive emotions can remove cancer cells from the body. One promising study showed that when mice who had cancer were injected with "happy hormones," their cancerous tumors shrank significantly.[27]

Dr. Henning Saupe, an integrative oncologist from Germany known for prolonging the lives of end-stage cancer patients through his various healing modalities, understands the power of psychoneuroimmunology, especially when it comes to positive emotions.

*Feelings and emotions are interconnected with our immune system on a molecular basis. They are like two sides of a coin that cannot be separated. The study of PNI has revealed that our brain produces immunoactive transmitters parallel to every feeling or emotion we experience. That is why feelings of guilt, fear, and shame block the effectiveness of our immune system. Conversely, feelings of love, forgiveness, and gratitude empower our immune system and support the chances for healing.*

## Psychobiotics

Another fascinating area of research that is gaining momentum is "psychobiotics"—the study of improving one's mental health by ingesting "good" bacteria (e.g., probiotics and prebiotics). Good bacteria can positively alter your digestive microbiome,[28] which in turn will have a positive impact on your serotonin, dopamine, and endorphin levels. The digestive microbiome refers to the trillions of microorganisms that live in the approximately 18 feet of your intestines. These microorganisms help to break down and absorb your food, remove bad bacteria, viruses, and toxins from your body, and have serious implications on your psychological state and immune system. Scientists' understanding of how much the gut microbiome affects your physical and mental health is a rapidly evolving and highly promising area of study for many diseases that affect the immune system, including cancer,[29] and we will cover more on this topic in both the diet and supplements chapters.

When it comes to the microbiome's effect on mental health, a recent study found that giving psychobiotics to mice lowered their anxiety and depression, improved their nervous and immune systems, and produced positive changes in their emotional, cognitive, and neural markers.[30] In a similar study, human patients who underwent fecal microbiota transplantation (FMT) for gastrointestinal problems such as irritable bowel syndrome (IBS) experienced an improvement in their irritable bowel symptoms, as well as their depression and anxiety, which suggests that an increase of microbiota diversity may help to improve a patient's mental health.[31]

Both the fields of psychoneuroimmunology and psychobiotics show great promise when it comes to better understanding the physiological benefits of happiness.

## Oxytocin

A third interesting area of research is oxytocin. It was once believed that happiness was a result of being born with a "cheery" disposition or living a "good life" of economic means, a strong social network, and access to higher education. Recent studies, however, have found that happiness is actually a result of multiple internal and external factors. One of the most important biological factors that influences your happiness is the body's regulation of oxytocin—perhaps the most famous "happy hormone."

Recently, researchers at Hunter College in New York reviewed current studies and found that oxytocin slowed down the growth and spread of both breast and ovarian cancers.[32] Additional studies indicate that oxytocin reverses the cancer-causing effects of cortisol (the "stress hormone") by increasing autophagy (cancer cell death),[33] suggesting we need to raise our oxytocin levels in order to reduce cortisol, which, in excess, is harmful to the immune system and hinders cancer recovery. The good news is that it is relatively easy to increase your oxytocin—it happens automatically and instantaneously any time you feel positive emotions.[34] Oxytocin helps us to be more social and trusting and reduces fear, anxiety, post-traumatic stress disorder, and stress.[35] It truly is a healing hormone on so many levels.

One specific thing that leads to an increase in oxytocin is laughter. Interestingly, the laughter does not have to be real in order to work—you can fake it. Laughter continues to be scientifically proven to be one of the best natural medicines. In 1979, Norman Cousins rocked the medical world when he published *Anatomy of an Illness,* outlining his own radical remission journey about healing a life-threatening autoimmune disease using laughter and high-dose vitamin C. Recent studies on laughter have found that when patients are exposed to a one-hour comedy video, their cortisol levels decrease, natural killer cell activity increases (which helps attack cancer cells), pain tolerance increases, anxiety and stress levels decrease, and blood pressure improves.[36]

It is unclear from the research whether increasing positive emotions kills cancer cells or rehabilitates them back into healthy cells, which then die "on time" as they are supposed to. Nevertheless, what is crystal clear is that increasing positive emotions significantly strengthens the immune system, which in turn can help the body remove cancer cells.

The life-affirming message of this chapter is that joy is essential to physical health and healing. When your body is under constant stress, it cannot heal itself. However, making happiness a high priority with a daily practice—as with exercising or taking vitamins—can play a major part in your healing journey. Even if it is only five minutes a day, a daily dose of joy is just as important as any medicine you take. Our next featured radical remission survivor, Di Foster, exemplifies the importance of practicing positive emotions on a daily basis.

# Di's Story

Di Foster is a radical remission survivor from New Zealand with a strong Kiwi accent, ready smile, and hearty laugh. While many of her friends describe her as the most positive person they know, she is quick to correct this notion. She does not think of herself as a positive person but "an absolute realist who believes in miracles." Her radical remission from stage 4 breast cancer shows us the power of increasing one's positive emotions when it comes to healing.

As a teenager, Di had experienced recurrent chest infections, which led to the discovery that she has IgA deficiency, a hereditary condition in which your body does not make enough immunoglobulin A (an antibody protein). People with this condition have compromised immune systems and are more prone to sinus, lung, and digestive infections.

During Di's teenage years, her doctors gave her numerous broad-spectrum antibiotics to get over her stubborn and mysterious chest infections. At that time, the doctors still did not know about her IgA deficiency, so they thought antibiotics would help to knock out whatever the infection was. Di eventually asked them to stop prescribing the ineffective antibiotics, but not before they had damaged her digestive microbiome so much that she had developed autoimmune conditions, including chronic digestive issues and alopecia (a condition in which you temporarily lose your hair). This early experience with the medical system—and learning firsthand how it does not always have the answers—turned out to be good preparation for Di's cancer journey nearly two decades later.

Di was first diagnosed in August 2003, when she was just 31 years old. At the time, she was living in Napier, having moved from her hometown of Dunedin to do contract work. It was an exciting and challenging time as she explored life on her own instead of working for her family's business. Although she lived far away from her family, she was very close with her parents, three siblings, and adorable niece and nephews. She dreamt of someday getting her black belt in karate, finding a life partner who would love her just as she was, and having children with that person. Unfortunately, those dreams disappeared when she was diagnosed via a biopsy with an aggressive form of breast cancer in her right breast (stage 3, infiltrating ductal carcinoma, HER2 positive). With classic Di humor, she remembers:

> My surgeon said, "Di, we've got a bit of a problem. We've got quite a large tumor in a very small breast." I thought, That's not exactly what you want to hear from a cute doctor every day! Can we just talk about some of my best features, rather than how small my breasts are and how big this tumor is?

Her doctor recommended an immediate radical mastectomy of her right breast, followed by aggressive chemotherapy and radiation.

A few weeks before her diagnosis, Di had serendipitously taken a weekend self-help course led by Dr. John Demartini that focused on gaining mastery over your mind, emotions, and personal issues. This unwitting preparation helped Di understand that she was deeply connected with her body. It also taught her that she had the power to think positively and could work on changing things herself as opposed to waiting for outside people or situations to change. Already a longtime meditator, Di recalls:

> When they explained to me what they wanted to do, I said, "Give me a couple of days and I'll think about it." And they said to me, "You don't understand! You don't have a couple of days. You need to decide now! Di, you really don't have a choice." And I said, "No, this is my body. I have a choice. I will take two days to decide if that's what I need." My gut feeling told me that anybody who feels in control over their own health is going to have a far better survival rate. So two days were not going to make any difference. And every time I meditated [during those two days], I heard a ticking time bomb. I thought, I don't have time to figure out how to do this naturally. There was an overwhelming sense that I needed to follow the traditional path. But I didn't sign up for all three things at once. I signed up to have the surgery first. I meditated and felt certain that it was the right thing for me at that point in time.

Di's deep trust in her ability to make her own decisions is an excellent example of the radical remission healing factor of empowering yourself. Di stood up to her doctors by insisting that she needed time to consider her treatment decision. Today, more than 16 years later, she continues to be happy with the decision she made during those two days and is glad she did not rush into things. The extra time allowed her to adjust to the sudden change in her life, from being a "normal" person to a "cancer patient."

> I totally believe that was the right choice for me. I accepted that my life had changed because of these events. I wasn't responsible for everything that was happening, but I was definitely 100 percent responsible for my reaction to what was

*happening. I took control of how I felt about the situation, and I went to my happy place before I went in for the surgery.*

Di showed an enormous amount of self-awareness and positivity as she continued to take responsibility for her reactions as events unfolded. For example, when she woke up the morning after surgery, the first thing she did was shower and put on a beautiful silk robe, with striped pajamas underneath. She had never been overly feminine, but rather a good balance of both masculine and feminine. However, at that moment, she wanted to feel "incredibly feminine and in my own right."

As Di remembers, she was "swanning around" in her pajamas and robe when her father arrived at the hospital at 7 A.M. He was the first of 46 people to visit Di at the hospital that day. This was the first time many of her friends had seen her since her move to Napier the year before. By 8:30 that night, eight friends still lingered in her hospital room, catching up on that lost time. As much as she loved her friends, an exhausted Di quietly asked her sister to play "bad cop" by asking the friends to leave.

While the many visitors provided great social support, Di realized that the extra energy she needed to entertain so many people was not helping her healing process.

*I knew I needed privacy and some healing time, so that's what I did. I just left the hospital. By 7:30 [the following morning], I was at home, recovering alone. I knew in my heart that I would recover far better that way than being in the hospital on show for everybody else.*

By listening to her intuition and empowering herself by speaking up, Di was able to fine-tune the level of social support she needed. She learned an important lesson.

*I learned that first day that of those 46 people who came to visit me at the hospital after my surgery, 30 of them I would call "cancer friends"—and I didn't need them in my life. Some people are drawn to suffering and only turn up because there's a drama. Those 30 people were coming to make themselves feel better, not to make me feel better. They came in like I was some sort of zoo animal that they needed to look it. That may sound harsh, but when you're talking about energy and wellness, let's just get down to the nuts and bolts.*

After Di healed from the surgery, she agreed to follow up with the six rounds of chemotherapy her doctors recommended. She had three nieces and nephews she desperately wanted to see grow up, so she was very motivated to do whatever her doctors suggested.

Because Di was only 31, her doctors decided to treat her cancer aggressively. Their theory was, "The younger you are, the more you can handle." The chemotherapy they gave her was so hard on her body and its side effects so brutal that there were times when Di did not think she would live through it. After she finished the six difficult rounds of chemotherapy, her doctor admitted that he, too, had been unsure if she would survive the treatment.

While the chemotherapy was extremely difficult, the radiation Di received a few weeks after finishing chemo was harder. Because the chemotherapy treatments had been spaced out every few weeks, she had always had someone with her during treatment. However, her radiation treatments were scheduled every day for six weeks straight, so she was alone during most of those treatments.

Her hardest moment was when she received two, pinhead-sized tattoos—one on her chest and the other under her arm—at the beginning of the radiation treatment so that the radiologist would know where to direct the laser. The radiologist was so flippant about these tattoos that it pushed Di over her emotional edge. Never one to shy away from difficult emotions, though, she remembers that she "cried and cried over these two pinhead tattoos. It was the straw that broke the camel's back."

Di's mood continued to decline during the course of the radiation treatments, and she grew increasingly tired in the weeks following the radiation. Her radiology team warned her that during this posttreatment time, there was a high likelihood of depression, which Di decided to face head-on.

> *Each morning I'd wake up and say, "I'm going to get depressed today. Can I just do it now? Just bring it on!" But I never did get depressed, and I just slowly got back to normal. To stay positive, I actually dove into the negative emotions to find out what they were about, and I chose to let go of the outcome of things. I didn't say, "Why me?"* I thought, Why not me? What can I learn from this? *I reviewed my life and decided that I had a few things that I wanted to do, like travel, so I made some changes to do them.*

Di believes that finding this pathway to positivity is what helped her heal the most out of all the radical remission healing factors.

> *It's a paradox in life that I think people miss. If my goal were to be happy, then I might think that I couldn't dive into sadness. But if my goal is to be present and to grow, then I get to dive into sadness—and then I get more happiness! Then there was the paradox of death. I embraced death. In embracing death, I get life. I know with every cell in my body that I want to live today. We put so much pressure on ourselves to be positive, but the answer is in the balance of embracing the sadness and anger and working through it. We need to let negative emotions go, so the positivity can just shine out of us. It is not having to put on a "happy face."*

This positivity, along with utilizing several of the other radical remission healing factors and, of course, conventional medical treatment, led to a seven-year remission. This was no small feat, given that her oncologist had strong doubts that Di would live that long.

> *I had a small celebration when I hit that five-year mark because my oncologist told me that it wasn't entirely likely that I'd see five years. I explained to him that I understood statistics,*

*that statistics were based on averages, and that I wasn't average, so they didn't count for me. I wasn't trying to be arrogant—I was just claiming my own space and my own life.*

During the years after her diagnosis and subsequent treatment, Di traveled extensively, broke up with her boyfriend—who, as it turned out, was not "Mr. Right"—bought her first house on her own, and prepared for her black belt test in karate. It was an incredible time of personal growth and physical healing, during which Di came to the realization that she loved living on her own, and that if a partner were to ever come into her life, he would have to significantly add to her already full and blessed existence.

As fate would have it, six years into her remission, Di met the man who would later become her husband. She recalls, "It wasn't until I met my now-husband that I felt I could have it all. Love, be loved, and love someone—be supported, be challenged, and be a better person. He accepts me just as I am, regardless of who I choose to be each morning." As their relationship grew more serious, Di went with her boyfriend to visit his father on the North Island, traveling from Christchurch on the South Island.

Di had always been hyper-allergic to pets, and therefore asked her boyfriend to double-check with his dad that he did not have any dogs or cats. As fate would have it, two days before Di and her boyfriend arrived, his dad took in a rescue cat. Di did not want to make a scene, so she stayed in the family's home the first night, but had to leave the next day because of her allergies.

Unfortunately, this allergy attack was the start of a series of severe chest infections—something she was very familiar with from her teenage years. In 2009, Christchurch was a new city for Di, so she did not have her usual medical support team near her, and she struggled to find a good general practitioner to help her resolve the worsening chest infections. She says she felt like she was hitting her head against a brick wall when each doctor she tried told her to take broad-spectrum antibiotics.

She knew how much antibiotics had damaged her health as a teenager and how ineffective they had been at that time, so she only agreed to take them now if her doctors first ordered a sputum test to determine whether her chest infection was bacterial. As she predicted, none of her sputum samples produced any bacterial growth, which meant they would not respond to antibiotics. However, her doctors offered no further solutions, although Di insisted that her chest infection was not normal for her body and that something was wrong.

A few months later, after making no major changes, she began to feel slightly better, so she decided to start sparring in her martial arts karate practice. Di had been practicing karate since she was 24 years old, but sparring took the discipline to a new level. In her first sparring class, she took a very hard hit to the left of her chest that dropped her to her knees. She felt "off" immediately after the hit, and she continued to get worse over the next eight days. Di knew that something was very wrong, and yet she still struggled to get taken seriously by any doctor. Out of desperation, she turned to her good friend, a mental skills coach and karate instructor, for advice. He sent her to an acupuncturist and a sports doctor, who—after examining her—ordered some tests and then sent her to a respiratory specialist. That led to further tests, a scan, and finally a needle biopsy.

Di's cancer recurrence in February 2010, at age 38, was devastating. The biopsy confirmed that her breast cancer had metastasized to her lungs, meaning she now had stage 4 breast cancer. There was cancerous activity in her left lung, a significant tumor and other active spots in her right lung, and her entire left lung had collapsed. After the needle biopsy by the respiratory specialist confirmed the diagnosis, he immediately referred her to an oncologist.

While at the oncologist's office, Di once again trusted her intuition and her intense need for positivity.

> *I was quite unwell and fragile. When the doctor and I were getting down to the pointy end of the conversation [about my prognosis], I asked my fiancé to leave and he just quietly got up and left the room. I turned to the oncologist and I said, "You*

*won't repeat this, but I want to know how long you think I've got." He told me I had 12 months [to live] with a 0 percent chance of [living for] 18 months. I had asked my fiancé to leave the room because I didn't want the prognosis repeated—I didn't want it to get an energy of its own. I was very clear that it was just a piece of information that I wanted so I could feel the urgency (or not) and know what I was about to embark on. . . . He said 12 months. I decided five years.*

Di left the hospital that day with her secret prognosis, and the following week her doctors offered her palliative chemotherapy since her cancer was too far advanced for any other conventional treatment. The doctors told her, "There is nothing we can do for you. There is too much of a mess to take the lung out [surgically]." Di felt grateful that she did not have to argue with them about not wanting to do more conventional treatment since they were not offering it anyway.

*The doctors offered me palliative care chemo. It was my right to refuse it. I'd done traditional treatment and it was my right to say, "I've done chemo before. Thank you very much, but no thank you. You're offering me candy and I'm looking for fruit and vegetables. I'm in the wrong store." It was the easiest decision in the world for me because at that moment, I thought, If I've only got 365 days [to live], what am I going to do with them? I only had 365 days to learn all the lessons I'm meant to learn before I die. I'd better listen because it is going to be a journey and a half!*

This does not mean Di took her diagnosis lightly. In fact, she was devastated by the cancer's return. Di's sister came with her to the appointment in which the respiratory specialist had unexpectedly told her she had recurrent, now terminal cancer. When they heard the news, both of them started sobbing. In addition to the thought of leaving her fiancé behind, Di was devastated at the thought of leaving her family and their families—as well as the thought of them having to deal with her death.

Now that conventional medicine had no further treatment to offer, Di once again turned inward via her spiritual connection practice of meditation to listen for intuitive guidance on her next steps. One night while meditating at home, she had a particularly insightful meditation session.

*I had got a whisper at the oncology appointment. The quietest of whispers within me said, "If you've got 365 days left, be happy, go natural, and be grateful." I chose to listen to it. At that point, however, I had an entire collapsed lung and I couldn't do a lot. I thought,* What the hell do I have to be grateful for? *And then I thought,* Don't worry about it. You've got 365 days to figure it out. *I left the hospital with those three things on my mind, and each day I honed them. Being happy for 365 days very quickly turned into being present for 365 days. That meant if I was angry, or if I wanted to cry, or if I wanted to hide under the duvet covers and tell the world to leave me alone, then that's what I did. I was just really present in it.*

Di initially did not know what that intuitive whisper of "go natural" meant, but she came to understand that for her it meant doing whatever felt right for as long as it felt right, and then either stopping it or switching to something else. For instance, she had decided early on in her healing journey not to search on the Internet for anything, but instead to trust her spirituality and intuition. At the start of each meditation session, she would pose a question to herself: *What do I need to do?* After that, she would meditate and listen for any answers that popped into her mind. She trusted that a higher force would guide her toward the people who could help her.

One person who helped Di tremendously along her healing journey was her chiropractor. After reading her medical records, her chiropractor looked at her and said, "Everyone is going to say, 'You're toast. You're done. You're dead already.' I just want you to know that you're not. I don't know how we're going to do it, but you are not 'toast.'"

Hearing this gave Di a glimmer of much-needed hope, which she says was crucial in her recovery. In addition, Di did not allow her healing to become a stressful to-do list. She decided she would schedule one wellness appointment per week, and the rest of the time she was going to immerse herself in living fully and learning about wellness and miracle healing, instead of dwelling on being ill.

*I actually opened my life up for the space of living. I worked out that what you're grateful for you get more of. And what you focus on is where your energy goes. So instead of researching terminal cancer and how I was going to die, or what I could do to prevent it, I decided to embrace exactly where I was at. So I read books about innate healing, energy healers, and miracles—not books about cancer. I just quietly read, and with every cell in my body, I knew that my body could heal.*

Di made a conscious decision to not pressure herself to heal. She read miraculous healing stories and thought that if such incredible turnarounds could happen, she could at least reduce her symptoms a bit. Instead of putting pressure on herself to become the next miracle, she focused on improving her wellness a little bit every day.

*I let go of the pressure of having to heal. People get so attached to healing. Instead of focusing on the 75 percent of my lungs that weren't working well, I focused on the 25 percent that was un-bloody believable! I got grateful for that 25 percent and said to my lungs, "Breathing is really important to my living, so can you just move up just a little bit and get to 26 percent? That's okay with me." I remember one day looking at my feet and thinking, There is nothing wrong with them. Those are some beautiful feet. And my legs are quite sturdy. I thought, You guys have carried me through this journey and you just stay right where you are. You are just doing a great job! And my eyes were working fantastically. So many parts of me were unbelievable. I said, "Come on, guys, this is awesome!*

*You've done a great job so far. You're doing well for almost 40 years and I'm really proud of you!"*

This gratitude and positivity toward her body led Di to a common perspective held among radical remission survivors, which is respecting or loving your cancer, as opposed to fighting it. We often hear about the "battle against cancer." The confrontational language from the "war" on cancer in the 1970s continues to dominate the public discourse on cancer today. In contrast, many radical remission survivors have come to believe that cancer is a part of their body, and they credit this shift in perspective with helping them to heal. Di says:

*I don't have a fight with my body. When people say they "battle" cancer, I don't even understand the language they're using. It's like they're on a different planet. I connected with my cancer and I said, "I'm not evicting you. I'm not asking you to leave. You can stay because you are part of my body. I created you. I can uncreate you. But if you're meant to be here, then I am happy to live with you. I know that you've got something to teach me and I'm prepared to listen."*

Although Di had never been one to suppress her emotions, she realized that she was suppressing her fear. She decided to face the dark cloud of fear that had crept over her self-described "peachy" nature. So, taking a rare day off from work, Di decided to face her deepest fear head-on as a way of releasing the suppressed emotion of fear from her mind-body-spirit.

*I very calmly slipped my hand around this dark cloud and said, "Hello, death. It's time we had a chat." I can't remember exactly what we said, but I remember that when death and I finished that conversation, I felt like a different person. I knew in my heart that one day I will die, and on that day I will go with ease, grace, and flow because it's my day to go. Death comes with me every day, not as a reminder that it's going to be dark and sad, but as a reminder of the joy that I get to have today. Death is my very best friend to remind me that one day I won't be here, and every single day it's my job not to worry about the days that I will never see.*

Di views her positivity as a garden in which no beautiful flowers will grow unless she deals with her suppressed emotions, which she views as weeds.

> *I pulled the biggest "weeds" and dealt with those. Then I picked up every single stone in my garden and said, "Do I have any stuff to deal with here, or can I put you back down? Do I need to polish you?" I looked at every situation in my life that I might've had some emotion about. I didn't get into the drama of what may or may not have happened. I just looked at my reaction to it and how I felt about it. . . . I wrote letters to the people who had hurt me. I did not send them, because this wasn't about making peace with them. This was about making peace with myself, my life, and my past."*

This type of forgiveness is echoed by numerous other radical remission survivors who attest to how such a practice has helped them forgive and heal. In Di's view, releasing suppressed emotions is a necessary precursor to increasing positive emotions.

> *I think that we're going for the wrong goal in trying to be happy and trying to be positive. I wouldn't know what joy felt like unless I had some bad times to tell me what sadness felt like. I can't have one without the other. We're actually missing the whole balance of life, which is to love as much as you can. Grief is a result of great love. That doesn't mean I get stuck in it, though. And that's the point.*

In order to release suppressed emotions and increase positive emotions, Di practices a daily breathing meditation. For her, a big part of that entails facing her fears instead of running away from them.

*We must be aware of the stories we tell ourselves. We can grab on to a single, negative thought as it runs past us and turn it into a paragraph in our mind. Then we take that one negative thought and turn it into a full story, and then into a film because we get really attached to it. Then we might even make it a 3-D, surround-sound, high-definition film! That is a good way for our whole body to think that this negative thought is now true, rather than taking a step back and asking ourselves, "Is that thought even true?" We get mixed up with the fact that we're not supposed to have any negative thoughts, rather than acknowledging that they might be there. Being positive doesn't mean not thinking about something bad that might happen to you. For me, it's about having a plan so that I know I can cope with [something bad], and then the fear goes away, so I get to be more positive.*

Spirituality was key in Di's healing, especially in terms of her spiritual practice of meditation. Di considers herself an "old soul born to seek growth," as opposed to someone who is "religious." By the time she was diagnosed with stage 4 breast cancer, she had had more than 15 years of martial arts training, which included physical combat training, mental focusing exercises, meditation training, and learning how to harness the body's energy. As a result of the latter practices, she developed a spiritual understanding that she drew on to help with her healing.

*I am a mind, a body, and a spirit. That's me. I can't separate it. I spoke to the big guy upstairs a couple of times, but that's different from my spirituality. I might've thought about spirituality a bit more [after my diagnosis], and polished it some, but it wasn't some light-bulb moment where I thought,* I need to open myself up to spirituality, *because I'd done that my whole life.*

Given her autoimmune issues, Di had always been health-conscious when it came to her diet, but she changed her diet and increased her use of supplements after the cancer spread to her lungs.

In general, she tried to ensure that everything she put in her body was nutritious and helped to increase her lung capacity. She added a morning green juice, switched to eating mostly vegetables and smaller amounts of "clean" fish, chicken, and meat while cutting out *all* processed foods. Meanwhile, her personalized supplements, which were chosen and overseen by her medical herbalist, included high doses of vitamin C, fenugreek, reishi mushrooms, and apricot kernels. Whenever someone told Di that she should enjoy life by eating a sweet dessert, she would respond, "Honestly, the best treat I can think of is being here tomorrow."

During this period of lifestyle changes and daily gratitude, Di never missed a day of work or exercise. She believes that exercise and movement help connect her to her body, which is why she practiced karate twice a week after her stage 4 diagnosis. However, she purposely switched to kata, which is a form of karate that involves no physical contact and is focused on a specific pattern of movements. She took these classes at her own pace. For instance, she would do one series of kata movements and sit out the next series if she needed to. In addition, an important part of Di's healing was continuing to live her life as close to normal as possible, which meant she never stopped working at her husband's business or as a part-time contractor at an energy company.

After her first diagnosis of cancer, Di learned that she needed a smaller, closer support group. When her cancer recurred, she hand-selected a small group of friends with whom she shared her full emotional experience, while choosing to project only positivity to those who were outside of that group. Di was acutely aware that she had a tendency to take on other people's energy, so she made sure to hang out only with positive people.

*I learned after the first cancer that I didn't need many people, and that it was better for me to hold my own energy than to get everyone else's stuff. So the second time, I locked down five people, and they were the only people that I spoke to about my cancer. In fact, if I had a superpower, it would be that I can push people's energy back to them. So if someone comes at me with sympathetic eyes after seeing me sit out half of a karate class, I just push it back. I just didn't want or need the sympathy.*

Di's husband provided "rock-solid and steadfast" support after her recurrence, and he never questioned her choice not to have the palliative chemotherapy treatment. One day, when Di and her husband were having a loving and comical exchange, her husband told her "the nicest thing anyone has ever said" to her. Di remembers it this way:

*I said to him, "Do you understand that I am the love of your life? If I die, there is no point in you dating anybody else." And he said, "Darling, I do understand this about our relationship, but if you want to have a say in who I date, you have to be here."*

As if there wasn't enough going on in their lives, Di and her husband went through the massive earthquakes in Christchurch six months after her recurrence diagnosis. They lived at Di's sister's house after the second devastating earthquake because their own home was in an area so unstable that they couldn't visit to see if it was still standing.

Despite this turmoil, over the next 14 months Di cherished each day she had with her husband. They hardly talked about her illness and instead got on with putting their lives and businesses back together post-earthquakes. They were not ignoring her illness—they simply did not allow it to take over their lives. Privately, Di knew she was approaching her 18-month, "100 percent guaranteed" expiration date—at least according to her doctor. However, she also knew that she was feeling better than ever.

In the fall of 2011, Di's husband was the first to notice her significant improvement, as her characteristic spunkiness had returned. She recalls:

*My husband and I had an amazing 14 months after being diagnosed [with the recurrence]. We got married, took an extended family holiday in Fiji (which my sister hijacked to get married), and worked on healing. It was intense and calm and amazing. At the end of it he said to me, "You are seriously a pain in the ass again. I think you're well. What are we going to do with the rest of our lives?" I agreed that I was well, and I said, "I'm not having children after I'm 40. I've done the math. You've got six weeks to impregnate me." Nothing phases him, but he said, "Sweetheart, we've been through five-and-a-half-thousand earthquakes in Christchurch. We've relocated two businesses. We're about to relocate one of them again. We don't even know if we're going to have the house to get back to. We're living at your sister's [house] with six people. Do you think having a child at this point in time is a particularly good idea?" And I said, "Yeah."*

Given the crowded, unromantic living situation, she booked them a weekend getaway in a beautiful location. According to Di, her husband "performs well under pressure," and as a result, Di gave birth to a beautiful baby boy nine months later in December 2011—three weeks before her 40th birthday, and almost two years after she had been diagnosed with "terminal" stage 4 cancer.

Because conventional medicine had given up on her long before, Di trusted her intuition and the way her body felt to decide she was well enough to have a baby—and it turned out she was right. Because her husband was prepared to raise their child alone should Di's cancer ever overtake her, she never checked in with her medical team to determine the status of her cancer. Instead, she stayed in the present and enjoyed every moment of her pregnancy, the birth, and the daily bliss of seeing her baby boy slowly transform into a walking, talking toddler.

Over the next few years, Di continued to tweak her personal wellness plan, especially whenever she felt the occasional flare-up in her lungs. By early 2012, she wanted to test for a second black belt in karate but did not think it was wise to take the test without first confirming with her doctors that she was well. So she got a computed tomography (CT) scan, which—to her oncologist's utter bafflement—showed no evidence of disease. Three years after being given only 12 months to live, with a 0 percent chance of making it to 18 months, Di was conclusively cancer-free with no sign of disease in her lungs or breasts.

Ever since Di first heard her intuition whisper "go natural," she has not taken any conventional medicine or treatment. She remembers taking a few paracetamol (acetaminophen) tablets for a headache she had while visiting family, and she received pain medication during the birth of her son, but those are the only medications she has had since her stage 4 recurrence was diagnosed more than nine years ago. She has successfully given up the asthma inhalers she had relied on for more than 30 years for her exercise-induced asthma, thanks to the lifestyle changes she has made.

When asked about her reasons for living, Di explains that she is her own reason for living—both now and nine years ago when she got her stage 4 diagnosis. She feels that women should have permission to be their own reason for living, instead of living for other people, such as their children or partners.

> *I wake up every morning passionate about being the best version of myself. I do not wake up to live for my son. That, to me, is a second-rate reason. Being a mum is so inherent in me that I don't even think about it. I'm very intentional about having my son fill his [own] cup, but not needing to fill mine. Of course, I get to share [my life] with other people, and I'm so incredibly grateful for that, but they are never my reason to live.*

In addition, as is typical with radical remission survivors, Di has found a higher calling to help other cancer patients who are at the beginning or in the middle of their healing journeys.

> *If I was "only" a mother, then I wouldn't spend every other hour of the day communicating my [healing] story, connecting with people, giving them hope, shifting the way they think, and spending hour after hour coaching people.*

The book *Radical Remission* was not released until after Di had her own radical remission, but when she heard about it, she bought it immediately to make sure she had "all [her] bases covered." As she read the book, she was elated to find out she had intuitively found all the healing factors on her own.

Di empowered herself to make decisions on her own time line and followed her intuition, which she accessed through the spiritual connection practice of meditation. She found strong reasons to live with both diagnoses, first in her niece and two nephews, and then in her own self-worth. She fine-tuned her social support with each diagnosis so that her friends and family could give her the support she needed, and she adjusted her diet and supplements to support her body's changing needs. With regard to exercise, Di continued to practice karate, and while she already had a deep connection to spirituality before her diagnosis, she deepened her spirituality during her illness. Last but not least, she actively worked to release any suppressed emotions in order to increase the amount of positive emotions she felt each day, and she views this emotional work as an absolutely vital factor in her recovery.

Today, Di continues to practice the 10 radical remission healing factors and tries to lead a balanced life, which means she is constantly making small adjustments. For example, she recently had her DNA analyzed to determine the best foods for her body. After receiving the results, she changed her diet slightly. In general, Di believes that people should personalize their diets to their own bodies and not just follow whatever everyone else is doing.

Di continues her daily meditation practice and does a guided meditation from her hypnotherapist first thing each morning, which allows her to continue to tap into her spirituality and intuition. She continues to do karate twice a week and moves her body regularly, and she got her third-degree black belt in 2016. Di focuses on helping others and being the best person she can be as her reasons for living. She draws social support from her husband, son, family, and close friends. Di has started a beautiful tradition with her beloved niece and nephews in which she travels with each of them on their 16th birthday. So far, she has taken them to Melbourne, Australia, and Vietnam. Next year she and her youngest nephew will travel to Japan. Finally, as a self-proclaimed "realist who believes in miracles," Di focuses on maintaining her positivity and naturally "peachy" disposition, while consciously feeling and then releasing any suppressed emotions she uncovers in her emotional "garden."

It has been more than nine years since Di's doctors told her there was nothing else they could do to treat her stage 4 cancer and gave her just 12 months to live. Today, you can find her savoring each new day in New Zealand, helping others on their journeys, and experiencing all that life has to offer. To learn more about Di, visit DiFoster.com.

---

## Action Steps

---

As you can see from Di's story, making an effort to bring joy into your life, even in the middle of a traumatic cancer journey, can support the healing process. In *Radical Remission*, we noted the following activities as ways to increase your positive emotions: starting every day with a feeling of gratitude; monitoring your media to avoid being bombarded with negative information; examining your entertainment choices to ensure that the shows and movies you watch bring you joy; finding friends who energize instead of drain you; finding a physical or social activity that brings you joy (watching TV does not count); and doing a nightly check-in to recall a moment that brought you happiness or joy during the day. These remain wonderful ways to increase your positive emotions, and here are a few additional ideas to boost your oxytocin levels:

- **Fake it 'til you make it**
Laughter Yoga is a combination of laughing exercises and yoga breathing based on the principle that your body does not know if you are "faking" laughter. In Laughter Yoga, group exercises that involve faking laughter quickly lead to real laughter. Because laughter can be as contagious as a cough or sneeze, being in a group setting that induces laughter is thought to provide the same physiological and psychological benefits as spontaneous laughter.[37] Search online for a class or workshop in your area.

- **Try a digital detox.**
Given the amount of research reflecting the negative effects of technology on our mental health, one way to increase your positive emotions while on a cancer journey is to consider a technology detox—a voluntary reduction of screen time. Try starting small: Give up social media for 24 hours (perhaps every Saturday or Sunday) and see if you feel lighter and happier. Or the next time you reach for your phone for a distraction, try a non-digital form of entertainment like a book, game, exercise, magazine, nature, music, or phone call to a friend to make a real-life social connection.

- **Reconnect with what brings you joy.**
It is not uncommon for radical remission survivors to admit that before their diagnosis, they had either forgotten what brought them joy and/or could not remember the last time they had fun. If this applies to you, and you have forgotten what brings you joy, try to reconnect with your favorite things from when you were younger, say 10 or 11 years old. At that age, what was so fun that you would lose track of time? Maybe you would lose yourself in ice skating,

reading, watching the clouds, or riding your bike. Whatever that thing was, try it again and see if you can rekindle that youthful joy.

- **Find a furry friend.**
  Contact with animals has been shown to lower blood pressure, reduce anxiety, decrease depression, and reduce pain perception.[38] In addition, visits with a therapy dog, specifically, have been shown to increase the social and emotional well-being of cancer patients undergoing radiation and chemotherapy.[39] You might consider temporarily fostering or permanently adopting a pet, volunteering at your local animal shelter, or finding an organization that provides cancer patients with free animal therapy. There are many hypoallergenic breeds of dogs these days if allergies are an issue.

- **Build a joy squad.**
  Sometimes it is hard to make yourself laugh and feel joy, so consider building your own "joy squad." Caregivers, family members, and friends often feel helpless and are unsure of how to help their loved ones heal. Enlisting others to help increase your happiness and lighten your mood creates a win-win scenario for everyone. You and the other person share the positive endorphins of a good laugh or happy experience, and the other person feels like they are contributing to your healing (which, in fact, they are!). Consider asking your friends and family— children, too—to send you daily memes, gifs, videos, or jokes to make you laugh or smile. Ask the jokester in your life to call you once a week to lighten your mood or ask members of your joy squad to plan a surprise event once a month that will make you feel happy.

This chapter illustrates the old saying, "Laughter is the best medicine," while the latest research from the field of psychoneuroimmunology highlights the scientifically proven connection between happiness and longevity. We hope Di's story and the latest trends and research inspire you to boost your own healing by increasing the amount of positive emotions in your life.

## CHAPTER 5

# FOLLOWING YOUR INTUITION

## Palmer's Story

*The only real valuable thing is intuition.*

— ALBERT EINSTEIN

Have you ever walked into a room and felt the hairs on the back of your neck stand up, making you want to leave immediately? Or have you ever met someone for the first time, looked into their eyes, and trusted them right away? Have you ever thought of a friend you haven't seen in a long time, only to have that person call or text you later that day? These are examples of your intuition communicating with you.

Intuition is rooted in a particular area of your brain that communicates almost instantly with the millions of neurons in your gut and with your sweat glands, heart rate, and hair follicles. It operates out of the basal ganglia area of your brain, known colloquially as the "reptilian brain" because these brain structures are also present in reptiles' brains. The basal ganglia is quite different from the prefrontal cortex (the front part of the brain), which is in charge of planning, reasoning, and decision-making.

Intuition is our natural-born instinct. As humans, we were once very connected to this instinct. Our survival depended on it. If we sensed danger from a predatory animal, our intuition would send us running. If we sensed a storm coming, our intuition would urge us to seek shelter. Intuition is the ability to know something without analytic reasoning, and it helps us bridge the gap between the conscious and unconscious parts of our brains.

However, beginning with the Age of Reason in the 1600s, and increasingly over the past few centuries, society has valued logic over instinct to the point where we have now lost touch with our sense of intuition. Today, we are overloaded with outside data and have forgotten that we have a deep, intuitive sense at the back of our brains that was designed to guide us away from danger. We have learned to disregard our intuitive impulses because society deems it "crazy" to follow an intuitive impulse that may be difficult to explain or defies rational logic.

But while saying that you have a strong gut feeling about something may not be received positively in this day and age, radical remission survivors report hearing or feeling intuitive guidance at some point during their healing journeys, and they have taken that guidance into consideration. This does not mean that they act upon every intuitive impulse, but that they stop and at least listen to what it has to say.

In this chapter, we will explore how radical remission survivors learned to tap into their intuition and inner guidance system. Interest in intuition has exploded over the last few years, both culturally and in research communities, so there is much progress to report. We will also share the healing story of Palmer, a woman who used her intuition to heal from the autoimmune disease multiple sclerosis, and will end with action steps to help you start following your own intuition.

When I first began the research that led to *Radical Remission*, I was not expecting "following your intuition" to be one of the most common healing factors among the survivors I studied. To my surprise, I found some fascinating research studies showing that our intuition knows what is best for our bodies even when the thinking part of our brains does not yet understand what's happening.

Radical remission survivors describe three aspects of intuition that they believe were key to their recovery:

- Our bodies innately know how to heal.
- There are many ways to access intuition.
- Everyone has a different change they need to make.

Regarding the first point, radical remission survivors either always believed or grew to believe that the body has an innate, intuitive knowledge about what it needs to heal, and often about why it got sick in the first place. While this belief clashes with conventional medicine—which often removes the patient entirely from the decision-making process—radical remission survivors nevertheless came to believe that it was vital to check in with their intuition when making healing decisions.

Elizabeth Gould is a breast cancer survivor from Australia who enjoyed a successful legal and corporate career before cancer abruptly changed her life path. She decided to trust her intuitive voice from the very beginning, and it led her to receive medical treatment in the nick of time, guiding her to each next step in her healing journey.

*I remember being advised to have a lump checked in my breast. I'd had benign cysts in my breasts before, and I was so sure the doctors would tell me there was nothing to worry about. Then I heard a quiet voice inside say, "Perhaps you should be worried." Now, 13 years later, I still remember the exact stretch of road I was driving when I heard those words spoken deep inside me. Within two weeks, I had been diagnosed with aggressive breast cancer, undergone a mastectomy, a lymph node clearance, and was preparing for chemo.*

Although that was the first time Elizabeth heard her intuitive voice, it certainly was not the last. She spent the next few years developing a variety of imagery, emotional, and meditative practices that would help her to access that inner wisdom.

*I wish I could conjure up that quiet voice whenever I want. But intuition is very different from thoughts or feelings. Intuition speaks rarely, softly, and often takes us unaware. We cannot demand our intuition to appear in times of crisis—it speaks only when we are ready to listen. With focus, I've achieved an understanding about the mental space I need to create before that voice will speak. Many times, my intuition tells me what I don't want to hear. I now understand that my intuition is a guide, a compass pointing toward my own personal truth.*

Thanks to her surgeries and chemotherapy, along with utilizing her intuition and the other radical remission healing factors, Elizabeth has been cancer-free for more than 13 years. Today, she is a best-selling author and speaker focused on personal reinvention and overcoming life's challenges.

In addition to trusting that the body knows what it needs in order to heal, radical remission survivors report that there is no single "right way" to access your intuition. For instance, some people hear an internal voice, while others get a physical feeling in their bodies, and still others experience vivid dreams, have insights during meditation, or are able to access their intuition while journaling. Some highly intuitive people experience all of the above. These methods are valid ways to access the instinctual, intuitive part of your brain. Like a muscle, this connection will grow stronger the more you use it.

For many radical remission survivors, especially at first, it can be hard to determine which thoughts come from intuition and which come from the panicked, thinking area of their brains. Gabby Bernstein, a renowned spiritual teacher, author, and speaker, advises the following when it comes to identifying your intuition over your logical mind (what she calls the "ego"):

*When you're being led from your inner guidance system, you're not questioning it. You feel a sense you're on the right path. Maybe you can't explain it. It's more of a visceral feeling than an intellectual idea. If you're feeling anxious, insecure, tense, nauseous, or sick over the idea or the thought, it's likely you're being guided by your ego. If you're feeling at peace, then that's definitely your inner guidance system.*

The third common belief among radical remission survivors is the idea that everyone has a different change, or set of changes, that they need to make in order to heal. For example, some people may need to change their diets, while others with the exact same diagnosis may need to change their marriages, while still others may need to leave their jobs. This notion clashes with conventional medicine, which strives to find a single cure for a single disease. However, finding a single cure for cancer is unrealistic, given that cancer is a multifaceted disease with multiple potential causes. Perhaps this is why radical remission survivors find intuition to be so helpful when trying to figure out the particular change that *their* body-mind-spirit needs in order to heal.

# Recent Developments

## Meditation Goes Mainstream

For centuries, meditation has been a primary method for monks, yogis, and seasoned meditators to access and activate the intuitive part of their brains. Fortunately, as mindfulness and meditation have exploded in popular culture over the past few years, people who are new to meditation now have many ways to use and practice it as a way of connecting with their intuition. For example, you can find a wide variety of meditation classes, workshops, apps, and online videos dedicated specifically to using meditation to access your intuition.

Meditation helps connect you to your intuition because a busy mind that is constantly thinking about to-do lists, responsibilities, and deadlines cannot access the brain's deeper intuitive areas. The brain has two "systems"—the front part of your brain, which handles logical thought processing, and the back part of your brain, which handles survival instincts. These two systems are mutually exclusive, which means when one system is "on," the other is "off." Meditation helps turn the front system off, so that the back system can turn on and start providing intuitive guidance.

Christian Kurmann, a radical remission survivor from Switzerland, followed his intuitive insight that meditation would aid his healing. Christian was diagnosed in 2007 with a very aggressive brain tumor (grade 4 anaplastic meningioma) at age 41. Although his doctors gave him only a few months to live, they still recommended high doses of chemotherapy. When he asked his doctors about the potential side effects, they told him he would lose his ability to think clearly, that the treatment would decrease his quality of life, and that he could potentially lose his eyesight. While he was shocked at the diagnosis, he was more rattled that his medical team would recommend treatment with such severe side effects, especially when there was no guarantee of lengthened survival time. If he chose to do chemo, he would essentially lose what little time he had left.

Soon after his diagnosis, Christian heard a clear and calm inner voice that told him this was not the path for him—although his logical mind did not know what the right path would be. He decided to listen to that intuitive voice and left the hospital, heading straight to the Swiss mountains to think about his next steps. Serendipitously, while he was in the mountains for those few days, his best friend gave him a book on meditation by Thich Nhat Hanh, a Buddhist Zen Master, which led Christian to sign up for an upcoming Buddhist retreat in France.

As a businessman leading a high-flying corporate lifestyle, Christian had never meditated before the retreat. However, he was so moved by the way he felt in meditation that he decided to move to a Buddhist monastery in the Himalayan mountains for several months. Being single at that time, he felt that he had nothing to lose and perhaps much to gain by immersing himself in this new (to him) meditative experience.

He spent the next few months meditating for several hours a day, and eventually in complete isolation for 100 days, living a simple monastic lifestyle in a tiny wooden hut. During this time, his fears came up, especially his fear of death. Nevertheless, his intuition told him to stick with the meditation practices.

> It took me many weeks and months to actually understand [how] not to think, but to feel, contemplate, accept, and be insightful. It's a feeling. It was in meditation and during these calm moments that I absorbed that. There were moments that were beyond thinking. Feelings and emotions are much stronger than thoughts or knowledge or experience. Meditation helped me to detach from this illness, this tumor, this fear, from this incredible anxiety. . . . You don't always need the answer. The answer will come to you when you're in this calm state.

After four months at the Buddhist monastery, Christian returned to Switzerland and went back to his doctors. They ran a scan on his brain and found that his tumor was gone; it had completely disappeared. It has been more than 10 years since his diagnosis, and the tumor has not returned. Meanwhile, Christian has continued to listen to his intuitive voice, which he hears most clearly during meditation.

## The Rise of Energy Healing

Energy healing is a form of complementary and alternative medicine based on the flow of energy through the human body. Energy medicine practitioners believe that when this vital energy is off-balance or stagnant, the body becomes ill, and therefore realigning one's energy can help the body to heal. The goal of energy healing is to balance energy flow in the patient, making sure it is neither too weak nor too strong and that it is flowing smoothly throughout the body without blockage or stagnation.

Energy healing has been used for thousands of years across many cultures. In Chinese and Japanese cultures, this energy flow is referred to as ki, chi, or qi (most often pronounced "chee"). In India, the energy is referred to as prana, and Indian ayurvedic medicine practitioners describe seven energy centers called chakras, located in the body from the base of the spine up to the top of the head.

Today, more and more people are returning to these energy healing practices that have been around since ancient times. As energy healing grows in popularity, people in the mainstream culture are trying a number of practices, such as:

1. acupuncture

2. ayurveda

3. chakra clearing

4. healing touch

5. qigong

6. Reiki

7. Sat Nam Rasayan (the healing practice of Kundalini yoga)

8. tapping/EFT (emotional freedom technique)

Along with the public's increased interest in energy healing, we have seen an uptick in the number of research studies on the subject. Preliminary research studies have demonstrated that energy does indeed exist and can be measured.[1,2,3] In one study, researchers were able to see and measure acupuncture points (compared to areas without any acupuncture points) by using a specialized form of computed tomography (CT) imaging.[4]

With regard to cancer, energy healing is currently being studied in patients receiving cancer therapy to find out if it can improve quality of life, boost immune systems, or reduce side effects. Hospitals around the country are beginning to offer acupuncture, Reiki, healing touch, and therapeutic touch to cancer patients. So far, studies have shown that these energy healing modalities are safe and side effect–free, and can help ease patients' chemotherapy-related side effects,[5] as well as strengthen their immune systems.[6] In one study, an energy healer performed energy healing over a petri dish of lung cancer cells. Afterward, his energy healing was shown to significantly slow tumor growth and produce twice as many immune-boosting cells compared to a control group of petri dishes that were not exposed to energy healing.[7]

If you are skeptical about this new area of scientific study, rest assured that these energy healing modalities fall under the heading of "Can't hurt, might help."

## Interest in Energy Kinesiology

In the last few years, there has been an increasing interest in energy kinesiology, a healing modality that purportedly allows practitioners to communicate with your body's intuition. The term *energy kinesiology* was first used by Donna Eden, a pioneer in the field of energy medicine back in the early 1970s. Energy kinesiologists use muscle testing, a biofeedback method (also known as muscle monitoring, muscle checking, or applied kinesiology) to uncover areas of imbalance in your body and therefore identify ways to bring your energy back into a healthy balance. Healers across many disciplines use muscle testing as a biofeedback tool for assessing a patient's health.

In muscle testing, a patient holds her arm straight out from her body, parallel to the floor. Then the practitioner places their hand gently on the patient's forearm and asks a question, either out loud or silently, such as, "How is your gut health?" The practitioner then gently presses down on the patient's forearm. If the patient's gut health is strong, the theory is that her arm will remain steady and in place; if her gut health is weak, the theory is that her arm will lower toward the ground. Although the patient could just answer the question verbally—by thinking about it and speaking her answer—practitioners who use muscle testing prefer to ask the intuitive part of their patients' brains for answers, which they believe is connected to the arm's muscles via energy flow (or lack of flow) in the body.

Some muscle testing practitioners do not ask verbal questions but instead ask you to hold a glass vial containing a vitamin supplement or substance (e.g., gluten or cat dander) in the palm of your hand before they press down on your forearm. With this method, the patient does not know what is in each vial, and in fact, sometimes it is just a placebo vial of water. This allows the practitioner to do muscle testing without worrying about the patient's logical mind getting in the way.

You can learn to muscle test yourself to access your body's intuition and help inform your decisions. For instance, some radical remission survivors—like Palmer, whom we will feature later in the chapter—use self muscle testing to determine which vitamin supplements are good for their bodies at that particular time. There are several ways to test yourself, but two common methods are the swaying method and the balancing method. In the swaying method, you first ask your body a question, and perhaps hold something in your hand (like a certain vitamin supplement). If the answer is that it is good for your body, the theory is that you will naturally sway forward. If it is not good for your body, the theory is that you will sway backward slightly or just stay neutral. In the balancing method, while balancing on one foot, it is believed that you will stay solidly balanced if the answer to your question is "this is good for your body" but will fall off balance if the answer is "not good for your body." It is important to note that muscle testing is still in the very earliest stages of being researched scientifically; however, the initial studies indicate that it is safe and potentially helpful for reducing pain and other uncomfortable symptoms.[8,9,10,11]

One popular form of energy kinesiology is BodyTalk, a fast-growing healing modality founded by John Veltheim, an Australian chiropractor and acupuncturist who now has more than 200 instructors in more than 50 countries around the world. Like most energy healing systems, BodyTalk addresses the emotional, physical, and spiritual well-being of the entire person, instead of one specific issue. It is believed that this whole-person focus helps the practitioner and the patient find the underlying causes of illness and communicate with the body's innate wisdom to heal itself. To accomplish this, BodyTalk therapists use noninvasive techniques to establish what is wrong in the body, find out what communication in the body needs to be improved, and then align the body's energy for optimal healing.

More specifically, BodyTalk practitioners and patients believe that illness and pain are signs of your body trying to communicate with you about deeper underlying issues. In a BodyTalk session, a trained practitioner will first use muscle testing to identify the areas of your body that are not communicating/functioning well. Typically, you will lie down flat on a table, fully clothed. The practitioner will place their hands on your arm or body and ask your body questions, either out loud or silently. They may stretch your body gently to see where energy is trapped. They are trained to understand subtle physical responses in the body that may be imperceptible to you.

These body cues tell the practitioner where both physical and emotional past traumas may be stuck in the body, which may be contributing to current physical problems. The idea that emotional trauma can lead to physical problems, especially physical pain, is one that is supported by many top neurologists, physicians, and psychiatrists.[12] Once a BodyTalk practitioner understands the body's underlying issues and energy blockages, they will use gentle tapping on various acupressure points to get the nervous system to "talk" to the areas that need better communication with other parts of the body. This tapping is thought to use the body's acupressure points to address the underlying physical or emotional issues. Relief may be instant if the trauma is not too deep, or it may take days or months if it is a deep emotional issue buried in the body.

As a culture, we are slowly beginning to appreciate the importance of using our intuition during a healing journey, and consequently, the resources for accessing intuition are becoming more readily available. For instance, while meditation has always been a long-standing tradition for accessing your intuition, you can now take a multitude of meditation classes online or in apps, or attend live classes at a local yoga or meditation studio. Likewise, energy healers such as Reiki masters, acupuncturists, or qigong masters are now readily available to help you tap into your body's intuition and clear any energetic blockages, so you do not have to do all the work. And these days, it is not difficult to find a skilled energy kinesiologist or BodyTalk practitioner to help you tap into the deeper parts of your body's intuitive wisdom.

If this is brand-new to you, it may sound a little far-fetched. Fortunately, there is increasing scientific evidence to support the idea that accessing your inborn intuition is a safe practice that will enhance your decision-making and may improve your physical health.

## Intuition Research

Although most people agree that intuition (a rapid, unconscious decision-making process) exists, it has largely gone unstudied because it is so hard to demonstrate empirically and researchers were not sure how to quantify it. However, in recent years, an increasing number of studies have validated intuition as an inherent trait of the brain and illustrated the existence of both your thinking brain and intuitive brain.

First, as I mentioned in *Radical Remission*, researchers have discovered that the gut has millions of neurons—the same type of cells found in the brain—that can actually think and feel just like the brain can. When these gut neurons get fired up, you might start feeling "butterflies" in your stomach or have a strong "gut feeling" about something. Scientists have known for decades that the cells in your gut can communicate with your brain by releasing hormones into your bloodstream, a process that takes anywhere from 3 to 10 minutes. However, a recent study revealed that the gut's neurons communicate with the brain nearly instantaneously via a newly discovered "neural circuit," which bypasses the bloodstream altogether.[13] This new discovery (of something that has been in our bodies all along) explains why we experience "gut feelings" so quickly when faced with a new situation or person.

Another study from a team of researchers at the University of New South Wales purports to have measured intuition for the first time, as opposed to relying on questionnaire answers, as many prior studies on intuition have done. To measure intuition, these researchers designed an experiment in which participants were exposed to brief, emotionally charged subliminal images as the subjects attempted to make accurate decisions on a computer screen. The results demonstrated that although the subjects were not consciously aware of the emotionally charged images, their brains were still able to process the subliminal information from the images to make more accurate decisions. What's more, the study found that the subjects' intuition improved over time, which suggests that intuition can be strengthened with practice.[14]

Another study explored whether our bodies can respond to an event physically before experiencing it. Researchers at the HeartMath Institute conducted an experiment using roulette. Study participants were told that they were participating in a gambling experiment. They were given an initial starting fund and told they could keep any winnings. Researchers then monitored participants at three points during the experiment: 4 seconds before the bet was placed, 12 seconds after the bet was placed, and 6 seconds after the result of the bet was revealed. The subjects were monitored via an electrocardiogram (ECG) to record their heart rate variability (HRV) and via skin conductance to record changes in their nervous systems and sweat glands.

Amazingly, the subjects' bodies accurately "knew," via HRV and sweat gland opening, whether they had won or lost 18 seconds (on average) *before* the roulette ball fell into its final slot, meaning their bodies knew what the outcome would be—a win or a loss—before the outcome had occurred. Studies like these suggest that our bodies—through our heart rates and sweat glands, at least—may be able to predict the future.[15]

A team of researchers in Hamburg, Germany, recently set out to better understand what determines the dominance of intuition over deliberation by studying whether hormones could shift the brain from deliberate thinking into intuitive thinking. To do this, researchers performed a cognitive reflection test (CRT) on healthy participants after they were given either a placebo pill or cortisol (hydrocortisone), which increases the flight-or-fight response. The study found that taking cortisol caused a shift from deliberate, reflective decision-making toward automatic, intuitive information processing. In essence, participants who were given a "stress pill" relied more on intuitive thinking, while their cognitive thinking capabilities were impaired.[16] This study provides a possible explanation for why patients who have just been delivered a stressful cancer diagnosis tend to suddenly hear—often out of nowhere—an inner intuitive voice.

Another recent study found that high-level executives from several countries across various industries believed that intuition was an important component of their decision-making process, despite the data and computer analytics they had at their disposal.[17] Only one-third of CEOs trusted their data and resulting analytics over their gut instincts,[18] while 59 percent of business decision-makers said their decisions required human judgment (i.e., intuition) instead of relying on machine algorithms alone.[19] If the world's business leaders are using their intuition, along with data, to assist in their decision-making, it seems logical that cancer patients may want to check in with their intuition while making life-altering health decisions.

Medical doctors also report relying on their intuition to do their work. A team of researchers set out to understand the role intuition plays with family physicians, and found that intuition acted as a compass for these doctors when faced with uncertain or complex situations. Family physicians reported that gut feelings (either a "sense of reassurance" or a "sense of alarm") played a substantial role in their diagnostic reasoning.[20] If doctors are using their intuition to guide their diagnoses, patients should also be given the freedom to check in with their intuition when it comes to making health-related decisions.

Taken together, these provocative research studies indicate that intuition is an inherent ability based in our brains, and that this ability can be strengthened with practice.

Cancer inspired my original radical remission research. The project grew out of my curiosity about people who had healed from advanced cancer after conventional medicine had given up on them, or after they had declined conventional treatment altogether. Much to my delight and surprise, ever since the release of *Radical Remission*, people have been reaching out to share how they used the radical remission healing factors to heal from diseases *other* than cancer. One such radical remission survivor who has strengthened her intuition over time to achieve a radical recovery is Palmer Kippola. As you read her story, we hope you are inspired by her courage to rely on her gut instinct, despite her doctors' insistence that there was nothing she could do to improve her condition.

## Palmer's Story

Palmer Kippola, from Santa Monica, California, was diagnosed with multiple sclerosis (MS) when she was just 19 years old. MS is a chronic and debilitating disease that affects the central nervous system, including the brain and spinal cord, and predominantly strikes women of childbearing years.[21] MS is considered an autoimmune disease in which your body mistakenly attacks itself because your immune system—which is doing its protective job of destroying invaders like toxins or infections—misfires, cross-fires, or overreacts. In the case of MS, the body's immune system mistakenly attacks and damages myelin, the fatty material surrounding nerve cells. When myelin is damaged and destroyed during an MS autoimmune attack, patches of nerve cells become exposed and then scarred. This scarring is known as sclerosis.

In the summer of 1984, Palmer was a happy, healthy, and well-adjusted 19-year-old, home for summer break after her freshman year at Middlebury College in Vermont. Out of the blue, she woke up one morning with the "feeling you get when you've slept on a limb or sat on it too long, and when the blood flows back, you have a tingly, pins-and-needles sensation." However, no matter how hard she shook her feet and legs, nothing happened. They remained numb. Figuring it would go away on its own, she headed to her summer job as a restaurant hostess, as she did not want to be late for work.

Over the course of the morning, the tingling sensation continued up her calves. By noon, the tingling had reached her knees. At this point, Palmer knew something was very wrong. She called her parents, who called their family doctor, who advised that Palmer see a neurologist as soon as possible.

Later that same afternoon, Palmer and her mother and father were in a neurologist's office at the University of California, Los Angeles. The doctor asked her to walk across the floor—heel, toe, heel, toe—and to touch her finger to her nose with her eyes closed. She tested Palmer's reflexes. Only five or so minutes had passed when the neurologist abruptly announced, "I'm 99 percent certain that you have multiple sclerosis. And if I'm right, there's nothing you can do except take medication and prepare for life in a wheelchair."

In that one moment, Palmer's entire life changed. Neither she nor her parents had ever heard of MS before, and this was long before the Internet.

> *We left that office with very little information and even less hope. It was dizzying and disorienting. I didn't even know what to do with the information. It seemed like I got hit by a Mack truck. One day I'm a happy-go-lucky girl hanging out with her friends, doing well in school, and the next day, all of a sudden, I'm flattened. We didn't know what to expect and were told to just go home and rest.*

But first, the doctor sent Palmer for nuclear magnetic resonance (NMR) imaging, which confirmed the diagnosis of MS. Palmer refused the doctor's recommended medication, because the potential side effects truly scared her, and also because there was no guarantee that the medication would help. Her neurologist reluctantly agreed to a "wait and see" approach, which meant that Palmer went home and waited for the flare-up to retreat, if only it would. By nightfall, the tingling had crept up her body to her collarbone. By the time she got in bed that night, her mother held her and they both cried. Her entire body had gone completely numb and would stay numb for the next six weeks. With no guidance other than the doctor's advice to rest, Palmer laid on her living room couch for most of those six weeks. Her father would hold her steady as she grabbed on to furniture each morning to make it from her bedroom to the couch.

Palmer is an only child, and during this time her parents were her rocks of support. Her mom empathized and cried with Palmer when she needed it, and helped her envision an uncertain future. Meanwhile, her dad took a more motivational approach, encouraging her that they would somehow find a way to beat this illness. She had many friends stop by to support her with flowers or cookies, or to watch movies or bring books. These visits provided social support and helped increase her positive emotions during this fraught time.

One friend brought Norman Cousins's book *Anatomy of an Illness*, in which Cousins famously recounts his own experience of reversing a mysterious autoimmune condition with laughter therapy. As Palmer remembers:

> *We really made it our mission to watch more funny things [on TV]. There was* I Love Lucy, M*A*S*H, America's Funniest Home Videos. *Laughing is absolutely one of my favorite things to do in life. I see the humor in things because it's uplifting and brings you joy. You connect with other people through laughter.*

Another family friend who was into metaphysical topics changed Palmer's entire perspective when she visited Palmer that summer. This friend asked Palmer why she thought she got MS in the first place. Palmer was initially offended by the question. She held her tongue, but thought to herself, *Are you implying that I caused this?*

While stuck on the couch, however, she had plenty of time to ponder this provocative challenge. It would not leave her alone.

After much contemplation, Palmer recalled a pivotal moment that had happened when she was a little girl. She had been adopted as a baby by her loving parents, but they weren't perfect. Her dad—a former fighter pilot—was opinionated and liked things to be a certain way. One night when Palmer was about four years old, her mother had shut herself in her bedroom, crying. In the memory, Palmer's father was standing in the hallway yelling at her mother through the closed door.

*I stood up to my dad, and with my little dukes up, I yelled, "You call my mom names and I'll sock your lights out!" In that instant lying on the couch, I could see myself as a child warrior. After that, I became hypervigilant and experienced periods of insomnia. I didn't close my eyes to go to sleep, because what if something happened? What if my mom needed help? I think my body got stuck in that fight-or-flight pattern. In that moment on the couch [in 1984], I thought to myself, maybe my immune system is acting as a proxy for that hypervigilance. And maybe, even though it's supposed to be fighting viruses and parasites and bacteria, when it doesn't have something to fight, it fights me. That's the autoimmune attack.*

As soon as the thought came to her, Palmer intuitively knew there was truth to it and that part of her healing journey would entail learning how to turn off the constant fight-or-flight pattern in her body. She later found a therapist to help release her suppressed emotions of stress, hypervigilance, and fear, which she now realized had started at a very young age.

*A big part of my healing journey was releasing stored emotions. It started with traditional talk therapy, by letting go of suppressed anger that I felt for my dad around having to protect my mom, and eventually realizing there was some anger toward [my mom] in that triad as well. At the same time, I worked on practicing forgiveness and feeling more gratitude. So it's both letting out suppressed emotions as well as cultivating the positive. I discovered that you can't supplement your way out of a bad diet, and you can't exercise your way out of emotional trauma—you just need to address it and find peace.*

Palmer notes that her dad sometimes comes off as a villain when she shares this part of her healing story, when in fact he became her biggest motivator, teacher, and ultimately the hero. Palmer has come to believe that everyone, no matter how loving and pleasant their childhood may have been, likely has some suppressed emotions they have to deal with and release. She references the now-famous CDC-Kaiser Permanente Adverse Childhood Experiences (ACE) study from 1997, which found that two-thirds of 17,000 people surveyed had at least one adverse childhood trauma, and one-fifth of them had three or more traumas.[22] More incredible is the connection the researchers found between adverse childhood traumas and the emergence of chronic illnesses like autoimmune conditions decades later.[23]

When it came to her own emotional healing and release, Palmer realized that it was about understanding and honoring how she, at age four, had felt in that moment and in the years that followed. How could she, at age 19, give herself what that little girl had needed back then?

*I needed to support that little girl who didn't feel safe at the time. It doesn't matter that she may have been completely protected. It's the perception of not feeling safe or having the support, and the meaning we associate with that, that ends up coloring our lives and our belief systems. We feel, "I'm not good enough," or "I'm not worthy." That belief then drives our behavior, because if you're not feeling worthy or good enough, you might reach for drugs or alcohol or whatever to mask that pain. Both beliefs and behaviors drive biological changes, for better or worse. It takes detective work and real courage to explore all of this as a mind-body-spirit adventure.*

In addition to the deep, emotional work that Palmer began that summer, she started taking a few vitamin supplements, which she and her mother had learned from Norman Cousins's book and from friends. These included omega-3s, vitamin C, and evening primrose oil (which her parents bought on trips to the U.K. since it was not available in the U.S. at that time). She tried to stay focused on the exciting opportunities the future held for her. As a naturally optimistic person, she trusted that good things would still happen to her, and she wanted the chance to see them happen.

*I didn't know exactly what I was going to do with my life, but I knew that something good would happen. It was instilled in me [by my parents] that life is good and that good things are going to happen. I was not 100 percent clear on what they were going to be, or how things were going to unfold, but there was something innate inside me that knew that good things would unfold in my life.*

Eventually Palmer was diagnosed with "relapsing-remitting MS," which means that her symptoms would come and go. It is the most common form of MS, with symptoms ranging from annoying to debilitating. A few days before Palmer's sophomore year was set to begin, the numbness retreated enough for her to be able to get on a plane and return to college.

Over the next two years, Palmer continued to meet with neurologists. She and her family firmly believed she could beat the disease, and they did not want to accept it as a foregone conclusion that she would continue to deteriorate until she was in a wheelchair. She went to libraries to read the few books she could find on the subject. She would question her doctors with the information she found, asking them, "What about evening primrose oil? Or maybe there's something to do with diet, like adding more salmon and omega-3 fatty acids?"

Unfortunately, her doctors told her over and over again that none of these remedies would help, and that there had not been enough double-blind placebo-controlled studies conducted to make any of her suggestions worth her time. They said the only thing she could do was take medication and avoid smoking or drinking too much. However, no doctor could ever explain the healing benefits of the medication. Instead, they used scare tactics, such as, "If you don't take the medication, you'll end up in a wheelchair, or potentially suffer a shortened life." Palmer's intuition warned her that medication would cause strong side effects. She was averse to needles, and the only medications for MS at the time were injectables. So, Palmer made the personal decision not to take the medication. Nevertheless, she refused to give up hope and began a series of intuitive experiments to determine if she could manage her MS symptoms on her own, without medication.

Throughout her healing journey, Palmer believes that empowering herself was absolutely key. Her doctors gave her little to no hope that there was anything she could do for her condition. It was Palmer's intuition and strong will to live that led her to take the reins and find her own solutions.

*We all need to be the CEOs of our own health and well-being. There's nobody else who has your best interest at heart. I questioned everything, and I encourage people to do the same. If you don't understand something, ask yourself,* Why? What is this medication actually going to do? How is that going to help me? What are the benefits? *Frequently, the medical community doesn't have enough time with its six-minute office visits to understand the latest medical literature and their patients. Now that we have the Internet with this magnificent information, there's a really good chance that you're going to be educating your doctor.*

Palmer already had a strong, intuitive sense that stress was contributing to her MS symptoms, and she traced it back to that pivotal childhood moment when she had decided to be her mother's protector. Over time, she noticed that her symptoms flared up every time she experienced a stressful event, so she actively worked on stress reduction.

*I thought that if I was hypervigilant, then I was going to need to learn how to relax. I noticed an immediate correlation between stress and the advent of symptoms. I mean, almost to the day or within a week, if I had conflict at home, difficult periods at school, or if I was feeling overwhelmed at work, I would notice—almost immediately—either new symptoms coming up or an exacerbation of flare-ups.*

Yoga proved to be a "godsend" for Palmer when she started practicing it in 1987. Palmer had grown up in the sunny climate of California, so year-round exercise was nothing new to her. However, she had grown up jogging, lifting weights, and doing aerobics, not doing calming exercises like yoga. Slowing down, via yoga and other modalities, was one of the best things she did to reduce her symptoms. In 1993, a boyfriend who was studying Soto Zen Buddhism introduced her to meditation. The effects were instantly palpable, both in her mind and in her body.

*When I would sit on my cushion and just follow my breath in a consistent practice, I noticed a lessening of MS symptoms. It was really striking to me that stress equals symptoms. It wasn't like I didn't have the MS anymore, it just made sense that relaxation equaled a diminishment of symptoms.*

Meditation practice helped Palmer develop a daily spiritual connection. Although she was raised in the Episcopalian faith and studied in a parochial school, she never considered herself to be very religious. She joined a local meditation group to support her new practice and found that meditating in a group was relaxing while bringing the best of the Eastern and Western worlds together.

*My spiritual life is having a meditation practice, getting out in nature, living with an attitude of gratitude, and being more mindful of what really matters. It is being aware that just going for a walk—not having to do a "type A" run through the forest, but just going for a stroll—is healing.*

Palmer's second intuitive experiment was with her diet. Her doctors told her repeatedly that changing her diet would not make a difference in her symptoms, but her intuition told her otherwise. She diligently continued with her research, and the few books on MS at the time recommended a low-fat, vegetarian diet for reducing MS symptoms. She had already grown up in a "low-fat" family, with tubs of margarine, nonfat milk, and nonfat ice milk lining her family's refrigerator and freezer, and she also followed these books' instructions by taking out meat, chicken, and fish and replacing them with more whole grains. Unfortunately, Palmer's body did not have a good reaction.

*Not only did I not notice a reduction in MS symptoms when I took out the meat, fish, and chicken, but I noticed an additional set of symptoms when I added more whole grains. I have dealt with constipation for as long as I can remember. I was told that constipation is just a symptom of MS, and laxatives and "living with it" were the only solutions. Nobody ever told me that what I was eating had anything to do with that. When I added whole grains into my meals, I would feel this gurgling, grumbling, unsettled stomach. I thought this was normal. I thought everybody had some tummy trouble after eating. I thought that was just what happened. It took me years to figure out that wasn't normal.*

Palmer's second experiment with intuition regarding her diet turned out to be a rockier path than her first experiment with stress reduction. Her MS and gastrointestinal symptoms continued to flare up, on and off, for the next two decades. During that time, she fell in love and got married, but chose not to have children as she advanced in a successful sales and marketing career with a series of telecom and technology companies. While her relaxation techniques, yoga, and meditation helped to relieve her stress to a large degree, they were not enough to completely elim-inate her MS symptoms.

Palmer had always considered conventional medicine to be her last resort. However, under pressure from various neurologists, she finally agreed to try it in the early 2000s—after nearly 20 years of dealing with MS symptoms.

*I was averse to taking medication. I avoided it for as long as possible. All of these neurologists would tell me again and again that the only thing I could do was take medication. It was a very tiresome refrain. Medicine was going to be my insur-ance policy for not going into a wheelchair, or even not dying early. Finally, one especially persistent neurologist at Stanford [University] insisted that I take one of the "ABC" injectable medications.*

"ABC" is a colloquial expression for the three popular MS drugs of that time: Avonex, Betaseron, and Copaxone. To this day, Palmer declines to share which of the three she took because she does not want to influence anyone else's decision. As part of her experiment with medicine, Palmer injected herself every day for four years with the MS drug as prescribed by her doctor. However, as with the diet experiment, her diligence did not pay off. Her symptoms did not improve, and she experienced additional side effects on top of her MS symptoms, even though she chose the drug that purportedly caused the fewest side effects.

*I will just say flat out that medicine didn't work for me. I did not notice any diminishment of symptoms and I acquired an additional three symptoms. I call them the three strikes. [First], I developed lipoatrophy, a condition where fat doesn't grow back where you inject yourself. The second strike was a wound on my hip where I injected myself that would not heal for six months. The third strike, and most concerning, was that I experienced symptoms of a heart attack 10 minutes after injecting myself one night. I took little comfort in the fact that the nurse had forewarned me that this was a known side effect of the medication. For me, it was a step too far.*

In 2008, after four years of injecting herself daily and seeing no benefits, only unwanted effects, Palmer decided to quit the medication. After quitting, her periods of remission continued to alternate with periods of intense, uncomfortable MS symptoms. By October 2010, Palmer was 45 years old, had been suffering from relapsing-remitting MS for 26 years, and her symptoms at the time included profound fatigue, uncomfortable tightness around her torso, and legs that felt like lead weights each morning.

Thankfully, Palmer's intuitive voice began nudging her about her digestive issues, which were still ongoing in the form of frequent constipation and rumbling after every meal. She decided to enlist a functional medicine nutritionist to join her team. The functional medicine approach appealed to Palmer because she wanted to work with a professional who could help uncover what was at the *root* of her illness instead of trying to mask it with symptom-reducing medications.

Using blood work to gauge Palmer's health, this nutritionist found that Palmer had a non-celiac gluten sensitivity (NCGS), which may affect about 30 percent of the population. This meant she did not have celiac disease, which may only affect a tiny fraction of people, but she was still sensitive to gluten. Palmer realized she had been eating gluten at almost every meal she could remember for her entire life. Along with fruits and vegetables, she would typically have a whole-grain cereal for breakfast, a sandwich on whole-wheat bread for lunch, and pasta or pizza for dinner, as well as an occasional beer on weekends—all of which have gluten. All of that gluten led to chronic inflammation, which was damaging her microbiome and intestinal lining. Her nutritionist informed her that she had intestinal hyperpermeability, commonly known as a leaky gut.

*My nutritionist educated me on the perils of eating gluten and what it might be doing to me to create a leaky gut. She had me remove all gluten and led me through a gut-healing protocol of herbs and other things to help heal and seal the lining of the gut. Within one week of removing the gluten, I stopped having all tummy trouble. After eating, I no longer had gurgling, rumbling, or anything like that. And within one month of removing the gluten, I noticed that my legs weren't heavy anymore, the tightness around my torso released—and I have never to this day experienced another MS symptom ever again. Period.*

Palmer is quick to point out that autoimmune conditions are multifactorial and that there are usually a combination of triggers involved. She now uses a healing framework with her clients that she calls F.I.G.H.T.S., which stands for "food, infections, gut health, hormone balance, toxins, and stress." Palmer says nearly everyone with autoimmune issues has gut issues, too, so the gut always needs to be addressed.

*For some, the unlucky combo might be chronic Lyme and hormonal imbalances; for others, nightshade vegetables and oral infections; still others, agricultural chemicals, candida overgrowth, and stress. For me it was a lifetime of chronic stress topped with the sensitivity to gluten. I'm clear that gluten was the linchpin trigger for me, but you don't just take out the bad stuff. You also need to heal the gut by supporting the microbiome and sealing a leaky gut. And you can do that in a variety of ways—with probiotics, fiber, bone broth, collagen, glutamine, zinc, and vitamin A, for example.*

Leaky gut, a condition once associated only with celiac disease, has attracted more attention in recent years, as it afflicts many people who have not been diagnosed with celiac disease but who suffer from other conditions, including irritable bowel syndrome (IBS), Crohn's disease, and rheumatoid arthritis.[24] When a gut becomes "leaky," the permeability of the intestinal wall increases due to inflammation. This in turn allows bacteria, viruses, and other toxic molecules to "leak" into the bloodstream, whereas normally these harmful things would not be absorbed into the body but rather passed through the intestines and expelled via a bowel movement.[25]

Imagine that the walls of your intestines are like mesh netting. When your intestinal walls are healthy, the holes in the mesh netting are small and tight, which means only those nutrients that are healthy and have been broken down fully may pass through into your bloodstream. When you have leaky gut, it is like having big, gaping holes in that mesh netting. Partially digested food, large gluten molecules, and bacteria that are supposed to live only in your intestines can suddenly seep into your bloodstream through the big holes in the netting, thereby causing inflammation, infections, and autoimmune conditions.

In 2010, Palmer began working with her functional medicine nutritionist to address her leaky gut, first by adjusting her diet to being gluten-free, and then by taking new supplements. She added to her regimen magnesium, vitamin D, and beneficial omega-6 oils like hempseed, borage seed, and flaxseed oils. It is interesting to note that, based on her research, Palmer "pulses" her supplements, or stops taking them temporarily, both by type and frequency, in order to ensure her body does not become dependent on any one.

After following her intuition for decades, Palmer finally discovered the two remaining lifestyle changes—a gluten-free diet and gut-healing supplements—that would control and ultimately eliminate her MS symptoms entirely, something her doctors said would never happen. Her earlier experiments with emotional expression, supplements, stress reduction, and meditation had helped to significantly reduce her symptoms over the years, but it was not until she changed her diet that she was able to keep her MS symptoms entirely at bay.

Over the decade since her final MS flare-up in 2010, Palmer has studied the causes of MS and other autoimmune diseases. Her research has led her to the field of epigenetics, which is an exciting field for cancer patients. Epigenetics is a relatively new field of science based on the concept that lifestyle changes lead to chemical changes in the bloodstream that, in turn, determine whether a gene is expressed or not expressed. While you may have inherited and therefore be "stuck" with a gene that makes you more susceptible to developing MS, cancer, heart disease, or Alzheimer's, it is ultimately your lifestyle choices that determine whether or not that gene gets expressed, or turned "on." Palmer explains:

> It turns out that genetics might be only 5 to 10 percent of the risk factor, while 90 to 95 percent is everything you are exposed to in your environment—what you eat, drink, and do. Something is causing the expression of these genes. I'll always have the genes for the MS. I'm saying they don't need to be expressed. For me, stress, gluten, and a perpetual leaky gut triggered my MS. I was continuously keeping my gut inflamed by eating gluten. In a vicious cycle, chronic stress was causing my gut to also be leaky.

In 2012, two years after healing, Palmer's research led her to tap into her body's intuition through muscle testing, a practice used in the BodyTalk modality which helps determine what the body needs. In her case, Palmer has learned how to test her body's reaction to food and supplements. In addition to muscle testing, BodyTalk helped Palmer to further understand her emotional trauma.

> BodyTalk was ideal because you can't fake it. It's like a lie detector test where your body tells the practitioner the truth, bypassing your conscious mind. The BodyTalk practitioner is the "midwife" for emotions and priorities for healing in your body. You lie on a table fully clothed and the practitioner has their hand on a certain body part while asking your body the questions silently and gauging the unconscious, deeper levels. BodyTalk opened me up to the whole idea that I had buried emotions that needed to surface.

Palmer has spent a lot of time working on forgiveness in general, because she felt like she was harboring resentments that had built up over the years and gotten lodged in her cells. To help forgive and release these stuck emotions, an additional technique Palmer uses is the Hawaiian Ho'oponopono prayer.

*The Ho'oponopono prayer is beautifully simple. It's four lines: "I'm sorry. Please forgive me. I love you. Thank you." If it feels good, you place one hand over the heart and the other hand over the belly. Then you envision people you need to forgive. Start with easy people, like somebody who cuts you off in traffic. You work your way up to the tougher ones. Finally, you say the prayer for yourself because often we need to forgive ourselves.*

During this time of critical emotional work, Palmer discovered her new life purpose: empowering people to reverse and prevent autoimmune conditions so that they could live their most vital lives. As a result, she decided to leave a successful career as a sales and marketing professional to help others find the path to healing and optimal well-being.

Today, Palmer is a certified functional medicine health coach, speaker, and author of *Beat Autoimmune*, in which she shares the full details of her decades-long healing journey. She lives in Northern California with her husband and cherishes their life together, hiking in the surrounding hills, still doing yoga, cooking delicious healthy meals, and laughing with friends. She also enjoys her new reason for living.

*I'm on a mission! I am really fired up about this empowering science of epigenetics, and this autoimmune equation, and the fact that we are way more in control of our health outcomes than we ever imagined possible. Helping people become empowered is what really gets me out of bed every morning!*

Palmer believes we are at a tipping point, in which educated, empowered patients will start to shift the medical paradigm. She is encouraged by the increasing number of health coaches and the number of people sharing their miraculous healing stories online, believing this will lead to more people taking charge of their own health. Like many radical remission survivors, Palmer wants to spread the message that healing is possible.

> *Hope is real. Healing is possible. I always want to transmit that certainty because I think there is a time, perhaps, where people don't yet know, where they haven't experienced that possibility for themselves. I know this [possibility of healing] to be true. We're not just an inconsequential n-of-1. Thousands of people have healed from conditions they had been told were "incurable" by doctors who have not yet learned or embraced the empowering science of epigenetics. Is it going to take hard work, and perseverance, and courage, and all of that? Yes. But I think the first step to really feel it is in your heart and adopt the growth mind-set to know you can, and then embrace the optimistic attitude that you will.*

Like many radical remission survivors, Palmer has learned, in hindsight, to see her illness as a gift. She views MS as the wake-up call she needed to follow her true path of helping others.

> *I know that it might sound trite, or it might sound virtually impossible to believe when you're in the throes of something, that this [disease] is a gift. You might say, "I'm bedridden. How can you possibly say this is a gift?" But just hold the possibility that this is happening for you rather than happening to you. It's an invitation to you to look at your life. Where are you living out of balance or incongruently? What requires more balance?*

Although Palmer survived MS and not cancer, she applied the 10 healing factors of radical remission and, with persistent intuitive experimentation, healed herself completely of multiple sclerosis. Over her 35-year journey, Palmer saw half a dozen neurologists at six leading institutions. Each new expert confirmed her diagnosis of MS by her symptoms, MRIs, and clinical office visits. Not one of them offered any hope that her condition would improve. Their goal was to slow the progression of her inevitable decline, which they believed would lead to life in a wheelchair followed by early death.

Recently, Palmer had a blood test and another MRI to confirm her remission: All the antibodies to her neurological tissues were in the normal range, and her MRI showed no new lesions and a disappearance or fading of old ones. Her neurologist declared, "This couldn't be a better story."

Palmer defied her dire prognosis and today she inspires hope in thousands of other patients with autoimmune disorders. Her inspirational story and continued research provide further evidence that the body can heal from conditions that the conventional medical world still considers "incurable." To learn more about Palmer, visit PalmerKippola.com.

# Action Steps

We all possess an intuitive sense that connects our brains and our bodies. Some people have learned to pay closer attention to it than others. Accessing your intuition is like exercising any other mental muscle—if you don't use it, you lose it.

I outlined several techniques in *Radical Remission* for accessing your intuition, including quieting your mind and asking yourself, *What do my body, mind, and soul need in order to get well again?* Other suggestions included guided imagery, meditation, journaling, and dream work. Here are some additional action steps to help you strengthen your own intuition "muscle."

## Try Energy Healing

- **Traditional Chinese medicine**, which includes acupuncture and other energy-based treatments, is believed to improve the flow of your chi while releasing any stagnant energy that may be contributing to your illness. You can find a licensed acupuncturist in private practices, group clinics, hospitals, or day spas. Some insurance plans will cover these treatments.

- **Reiki** is a form of energy healing that does not involve any physical contact. The practitioner taps into your energy and shifts blockages by moving their hands a few inches above your body, although this type of energy work can also be performed remotely. Look for a certified Reiki practitioner in a private practice, wellness clinic, or hospital.

- **Yoga** was developed centuries ago as a way to prepare the mind for meditation. All physical yoga practices, known as asanas, can help relax your body and mind so that you move into a quieter place where it is possible to hear your intuition. Kundalini yoga is a specific type of yoga that is focused on awareness, enhancing intuition, and strengthening your energy field. You can find yoga classes in most cities at yoga studios, community centers, and gyms, or you can take classes online or via apps.

- **Find an energy healing practitioner** to help guide your way. Technology has greatly assisted our ability to find and work with energy healers and teachers. Many energy healers continue to teach in-person workshops, but now there are online courses, videos, coaching, and training with leading experts like Donna Eden or Machaelle Small Wright, or in modalities such as BodyTalk, healing touch, and Matrix Energetics.

## Listen to Your Body

- As you move forward with decisions, start to test your body's reaction to each decision, whether big or small. Notice if your stomach is clenched or relaxed when you think about each possible outcome. Does one outcome make your heart race, while the other option does not? Do you get nauseated when you think about a decision, or do you feel at ease? Your intuition—as it communicates to you through physical sensations—can help guide your decision-making. You just need to learn its signals.

## Remove Yourself from Distraction

- When you need to make a decision and want to listen to your intuition, it is important to remove yourself from distractions (e.g., TV, radio, computer). To tap into your body's natural intuition, take a shower, go for a walk without earbuds, or go for a drive without the radio. In this empty, quiet space, your intuitive voice will not have to fight as much to be heard.

Researchers who study the intuitive areas of the brain know that there is a part of you that often knows the right answer before the rest of your brain knows what is happening. This is your intuition—you were born with it and there are simple ways to make it stronger and more present in your everyday life. Radical remission survivors show us that when our everyday lives become threatened by a scary health diagnosis, our intuition often becomes loud and clear and speaks to us through strong gut feelings, sudden insights, or a calm, internal voice. And although society tends to brush off such intuitive guidance as illogical or impulsive, studies have shown that this guidance comes from a part of our brains that is concerned with only one thing: survival.

CHAPTER 6

---

# RELEASING SUPPRESSED EMOTIONS

## Alison's Story

*We cannot create a new future by*
*holding on to the emotions of the past.*

— Dr. Joe Dispenza

When you touch a hot stove accidentally, your body remembers the pain the next time you see a stove. You stay away from the stove instinctively for fear of burning yourself. Emotional pain works the same way. Your mind and body remember the emotional pain you felt in a particular moment in your past, and that memory is filed away—sometimes buried—for your own protection. It is a useful self-defense mechanism because it helps us to function. However, scientists have shown that suppressing emotions can suppress the immune system, which contributes to disease and hampers the body's ability to heal.[1]

As I discussed in *Radical Remission*, suppressed emotions are any emotions you hang on to, whether negative or positive, conscious or unconscious. They include stress, fear, grief, worry, and nostalgia, and radical remission survivors believe that releasing such emotions has been vitally important for their healing journeys.

In this chapter, we will review the key points on releasing suppressed emotions, looking at the cultural developments that have occurred in the past few years related to this topic. Where there is increased societal interest, scientific interest usually follows, so we will discuss the new research that has been conducted regarding the connection between emotions and the immune system. Next, we will dive into the healing story of Alison, a radical remission survivor of brain cancer who beautifully illustrates the power of releasing suppressed emotions. We often hear in our interviews that releasing suppressed emotions is one of the most difficult parts of a healing journey, so we will also provide you with a few simple action steps to give you a starting point for your own emotional healing journey.

More than a decade ago, when I first set out to look for common factors among radical remission survivors, I expected to hear about physical things like diet, supplements, and exercise. No one was more surprised than I was when every interview circled back to mental, emotional, and spiritual healing factors. I certainly did not anticipate the importance of past emotions and their connection to current physical health. But repeatedly, radical remission survivors have described their need to release their emotional baggage in order to fully heal.

Radical remission survivors and their healers have a theory that "blockages" can eventually lead to illness if not addressed. According to this theory, these blockages can be physical, emotional, or spiritual. Within this framework, health is achieved when all three levels of the body-mind-spirit system flow freely, both in terms of energy (chi) and blood flow. Radical remission survivors view cancerous tumors as physical blockages that need to be cleared. To do this, the root cause of the blockage needs to be addressed, otherwise the tumor may come back. This is why radical remission survivors focus on clearing out anything that is "stuck" in their lives, be it physical, emotional, or spiritual.

Research has demonstrated time and again that stress weakens the immune system—the same system that is responsible for detecting and removing cancer cells from the body. Stress negatively affects every cell in your body, not just your immune cells. Fortunately, hundreds of studies have shown that releasing feelings of stress, anger, or fear can *strengthen* your immune system. Finding methods to manage stress while in the midst of a health crisis therefore becomes an essential step for radical remission survivors.

Like stress, fear is another emotion that weakens or "freezes" the immune system. Given the severity of a cancer diagnosis, it is not surprising that fear is one of the most commonly suppressed emotions among radical remission survivors. The fear of death, in particular, challenges cancer patients from the moment they are diagnosed. While facing fear is not always an easy thing to do, healers and radical remission survivors agree that it helps bring the body back into balance, whereas holding on to fear causes the body to "tighten" and creates an energetic blockage. Alison's story, which we will share in depth later on, provides a great example of a radical remission survivor who has learned how to accept and manage her fear.

Feeling emotions fully such as stress and fear and then releasing them fully allows the body to relax in such a way that it enhances the immune system's ability to heal. Many radical remission survivors liken it to standing under a waterfall. Emotions pour onto you in response to a situation, but then they flow out and away from you. If you always stand under an "emotional waterfall," it means you will feel life and all its emotions to their fullest but never accumulate any emotional baggage. This will enable you to experience whatever emotions you may be feeling in the present moment, unencumbered by the past.

## Recent Developments

In the past few years, we have seen the value of releasing suppressed emotions brought to the forefront of our collective consciousness. It has become more and more acceptable to discuss your emotions with others and to find new ways to deal with them. A few things that have recently risen to prominence in popular culture are a deeper understanding of fear and trauma, the importance of self-love, and the emergence of both tapping and eye movement desensitization and reprocessing (EMDR) as tools to help with unresolved trauma.

## A Deeper Understanding of Fear and Trauma

Every time you have a fearful thought, your self-healing mechanism turns off. Stressful emotions such as fear trigger a stress response within your body that puts you into fight-or-flight mode, which suppresses your immune system. My friend and colleague Lissa Rankin, M.D., *New York Times* best-selling author of *Mind Over Medicine* and *The Fear Cure*, does not shy away from talking about fear's role in illness.

> *If we wish to live long, optimally healthy lives, addressing our fear is arguably more important than what we eat, whether we exercise, how many vitamins we take, or how many bad habits we have. I understand that it's radical to suggest that unchecked fear may lie at the root of many diseases. I'm not suggesting that these diseases don't also have biochemical roots, but I am suggesting that fear predisposes you to harmful biochemical influences, which inactivate the body's natural self-healing mechanisms. Even more important, I'm suggesting that you can do something about this. Coming into the right relationship with your fear requires befriending it, getting curious about it, listening to your scared parts without letting them hijack your whole system, and helping to calm the parts that are frightened so the hormones of stress dissipate and the biochemical soup of intimacy, which are healing hormones, sets the hormonal stage for the possibility of radical remission.*

Rankin, like many other healers and radical remission survivors, suggests that if you are willing to view life's challenges as a learning opportunity, then you can start to release your fears and move toward more curiosity and self-understanding. Two specific fears that radical remission survivors have described having to face in their healing journeys are the ongoing "scanxiety" they feel before every scan or doctor appointment and the omnipresent fear of death.

Both fears are real and justified. However, you do not have to be paralyzed by them. Instead, you can work on accepting those fears and find ways to make them loosen their grip. One of Dr. Rankin's "prescriptions" for fear is meditation.

*If you're able to distance yourself from the voice of fear [e.g., through meditation], you'll find a place that's very still and peaceful. Accessing this place of absolute stillness requires being in the present moment, and in this place of stillness, fear doesn't exist. When you're in this state of consciousness, even your own death doesn't scare you.*

Fear may suppress our immune systems, but we can diffuse it with practices like meditation. We do not need to be victims to our fears but can accept and manage them as a natural part of any healing process. Mindfulness-based stress reduction (MBSR) is an effective strategy for releasing suppressed emotions, and I am happy to report that the research continues to advance in terms of understanding the myriad ways MBSR can improve your health.

For example, a recent study of breast cancer patients found that taking a six-week MBSR course led to a significant increase in the length and activity of telomeres, which protect the ends of your DNA in the same way that the little plastic cap at the end of your shoelaces keeps them from fraying. As you age, your telomeres naturally shorten each time the DNA in a cell is copied to make a new cell. The shorter your telomeres, the "older" your cells are, and consequently, the older you feel and the greater your risk of disease. Breast cancer patients in this study not only received the well-known psychological benefits of MBSR (e.g., reduced depression, anxiety, and fear of cancer recurrence), but also improved their cellular health via increased telomere length and activity.[2]

In addition to understanding the impact of fear on the immune system, scientists are also beginning to understand the long-term consequences of adverse childhood experiences, including their impact on physical health in adulthood.[3] Stressful experiences in childhood can heighten your default response to stress, which, as we have discussed, suppresses immune function, thereby putting you at higher risk for chronic illnesses later in life.[4]

And thanks to the recent #MeToo movement, we are in a pivotal moment of recognizing the severity of suppressed emotions that stem from past trauma and assault. Given the facts that 50 percent of sexual assault survivors will experience post-traumatic stress disorder (PTSD) in their lifetime[5] and that one in five women will be raped during their lifetime,[6] it is only logical that sexual abuse will be at the root of suppressed emotions for many cancer patients. The #MeToo movement's lasting impact for cancer patients who have experienced such trauma is that society has finally acknowledged the importance of speaking up and releasing any long-held emotions that surround such trauma, thereby allowing these patients to get the help they need to process their emotions. EMDR and EFT, described in detail below, are two emerging therapies that have been shown to be very helpful in releasing past trauma.

## Self-Love

These days, whether you open a magazine, listen to a podcast, or scroll through social media, chances are you will run across someone talking about the importance of self-love. The concept of loving yourself has been around for decades, started in large part by Louise Hay, considered by many to be the founder of the self-help movement. Louise healed herself naturally from cervical cancer in 1978 using a self-designed program of affirmations, visualizations, nutritional cleansing, and psychotherapy, after which she dedicated her life to helping others improve their own lives by learning to love and appreciate themselves. When more people love themselves, they have more love to give, and therefore the world is a better place. In Louise's words, "Loving ourselves works miracles in our lives."

The self-love movement has risen in popularity in recent years thanks to social media. In our 24/7, social media–obsessed world, we now have an open window into the (highly idealized) lives of friends, acquaintances, and celebrities. People rarely post on social media about their bad days or the more mundane parts of their lives. Instead, most people tend to share their most "Insta-worthy" moments, such as glamourous vacations, happy children, professional milestones, fascinating people they have met, or volunteer work. Unfortunately, this endless stream of perfection can lead to false comparisons, envy, and feelings of being "less than." Study after study has shown that use of social media contributes to symptoms of anxiety and depression.[7]

In this context, the self-love movement is experiencing a resurgence, helping to counterbalance our natural tendency to compare ourselves to others. Look for social media posts with the hashtags #selflove and #selfcare alongside images of people taking time to do something special for themselves that relieves their stress and restores happiness. Radical remission survivors have reported going on "social detoxes" by taking a few days (or weeks) off of social media and going on "self-love retreats"—a few days all to themselves designed to restore peace and self-esteem. By taking these actions, they have been able to increase their feelings of self-love while releasing feelings of self-loathing and/or stress. Most important, radical remission survivors believe that connecting to such feelings of self-love and worthiness helps their bodies heal.

One such radical remission survivor is Anita Moorjani, a cancer survivor, international speaker, and *New York Times* best-selling author of *Dying to Be Me* and *What If This Is Heaven?* In April 2002, Anita was married to her husband and living a cosmopolitan life in Hong Kong when she was diagnosed with stage 2 lymphoma (cancer of the lymphatic system). She made the personal choice to refuse chemotherapy, because she had watched both a dear friend and a family member die from cancer despite chemotherapy in the years just prior to her diagnosis. Instead, she chose to go on a four-year healing journey that included hypnotherapy, meditation, prayer, diet change, traditional Chinese medicine, ayurvedic medicine, yoga, and naturopathic medicine. Unfortunately, this healing journey did not keep the cancer at bay, and it continued to ravage Anita's body.

Almost four years after her diagnosis, Anita's cancer had progressed so significantly that she had toxic lesions all over her body, was too weak to walk or move on her own, and was confined to her bed or wheelchair. She was in significant pain and on a constant supply of oxygen. On February 2, 2006, Anita slipped into a coma while at the hospital, and her major organs began to fail. During the coma, Anita had a strange sensory experience in which she felt that she was able to perceive everything that was happening around her, even things far away. For example, she could "hear" conversations about her happening in faraway hallways, was able to "see" her brother traveling to make it to the hospital in time, and could "feel" the intense pain her parents and husband were feeling.

Anita experienced what researchers call a near-death experience (NDE). In an NDE, a person who is unconscious experiences a profound spiritual journey, and many people who have experienced NDEs report similar elements, such as a "white light" or deep emotional insight. In Anita's case, she realized during her NDE that being fearful her entire life and suppressing her true nature and emotions had contributed to her illness and was preventing her from healing fully.

Her fear had its roots in a lifetime of trying to live up to everyone else's expectations in the restrictive Indian culture of her childhood. This culture expected women, Anita included, to be subservient and docile—which conflicted with Anita's modern mind-set and opinionated nature. In addition, growing up as a Sindhi Indian who practiced Hinduism while living in Hong Kong and attending British schools meant that Anita spent her whole life trying (unsuccessfully) to fit into multiple cultures. Amid this pressure, Anita says she lost sight of her true self. By suppressing her emotions, she believes that cancer became a physical manifestation of her disconnection.

*I was a people-pleaser and feared disapproval, regardless of the source. I bent over backward to avoid people thinking ill of me, and over the years, I lost myself in the process. I wasn't expressing my true self, because my worries were preventing me from doing so. [During my NDE], I understood that the cancer wasn't a punishment. It was just my own energy, manifesting as cancer because my fears weren't allowing me to express myself as the magnificent force I was meant to be.*

Her NDE brought Anita a deep-seated understanding that she deserved unconditional love—that we *all* deserve this love and are part of the same universal consciousness. During her NDE, Anita realized she had nothing more to fear.

*In that expansive state [during the NDE], I realized how harshly I'd treated myself and judged myself throughout my life. This understanding made me realize that I no longer had anything to fear. I saw what I—what all of us—have access to. I made one powerful choice: to come back. That decision, made from that awakened state, was the single most powerful driving force in my return.*

When Anita decided to "come back," she defied medical expectations with a rapid and complete recovery. Within six months, she went from being in a coma to being a lively, healthy woman completely free of disease. Anita's case has been documented and confirmed by multiple oncologists, none of whom can explain her recovery, but Anita believes she healed because she released her fears and embraced unconditional love—both for herself and for others.

Anita has been cancer-free since 2006. Today, she travels the world sharing her message of universal love and self-acceptance. While the near-death experience aspect of her radical remission is unusual, her message of letting go of fear and negative self-talk and replacing it with self-love is common among radical remission survivors.

## EMDR

The population that gets the most attention for PTSD is military veterans—and with good reason. The U.S. Department of Veterans Affairs estimates that between 11 and 20 percent of military veterans are currently dealing with PTSD, while 30 percent of Vietnam veterans, in particular, are expected to suffer from PTSD in their lifetime.[8] As if this were not bad enough, other researchers have shown that people suffering from PTSD have a significantly higher chance of developing cancer,[9] a finding that makes treating PTSD all the more urgent.

The Department of Veterans Affairs has adopted a technique called EMDR (eye movement desensitization and reprocessing) as its go-to psychotherapeutic method for helping veterans with PTSD. The VA's embrace of this technique has greatly increased its popularity over the past few years, although it has been practiced by psychologists for many decades.

Briefly, EMDR is a psychotherapeutic technique that uses alternating bilateral brain stimulation (e.g., via eye movements or sounds) to promote the reprocessing of dysfunctionally stored information (e.g., traumatic memories) related to a traumatic event.[10] During an EMDR session with a trained psychotherapist, you recount the trauma experienced in detail while moving your eyes back and forth in a clockwork-like fashion, holding hand buzzers, and/or listening to alternating sounds in your right then left ear (think of the 1980s video game Pong). Recounting these traumatic events while the brain's attention is being drawn to the right-left stimulation is believed to reprogram the brain and reshape the traumatic memory.

Although researchers are still working to understand exactly *how* EMDR works, they have confirmed that it *does* work and is an effective treatment for PTSD.

Major progress has been made in EMDR research over the past few years because scientists can now use neuroimaging techniques, such as electroencephalography (EEG) or functional magnetic resonance imaging (fMRI), to show exactly how this therapy changes our brains. Such neuroimaging studies have shown that EMDR, as well as other therapies like trauma-focused cognitive behavioral therapy (TF-CBT), significantly decreases activity in the brain's amygdala, prefrontal cortex, and hippocampus. Reduced activity in these areas helps to reduce cortisol levels.[11]

In another study, a team of researchers reviewed 15 studies on PTSD and found that EMDR was one of the quickest and most effective treatments for PTSD[12] compared to other interventions such as antidepressant drugs, biofeedback-assisted relaxation training, or prolonged exposure with cognitive restructuring. In a different study of breast cancer patients suffering from PTSD, a team of Italian researchers looked at EEG scans before and after EMDR treatment and found that EMDR was highly effective in relieving post-traumatic stress disorder for breast cancer patients, as compared to a control group.[13]

In another study that aimed to find ways to reduce stress for stomach cancer patients, participants were randomly divided into two groups. The first group of cancer patients received the standard cancer treatment, while the second group received the standard cancer treatment plus two one-on-one EMDR sessions with a trained nurse. The results showed a significant stress reduction in the EMDR group but none in the group that received only standard treatment.[14] Collectively, these studies show that EMDR is a safe and effective way for cancer patients to release suppressed emotions such as stress or trauma.

## Tapping

Another technique showing promising results in helping to alleviate conditions such as PTSD, anxiety, and depression, is tapping, also known as EFT (emotional freedom technique). Tapping is a healing technique based on the principles of both traditional Chinese medicine and modern psychology. Tapping is similar to acupuncture in that it taps into meridians (the energy pathways of the body in traditional Chinese medicine) in order to improve energy flow. However, instead of using needles as in acupuncture, with tapping you use your fingertips to gently and repetitively tap on specific acupressure points (meridian endpoints) of the body. Tapping is a way to stimulate acupuncture points without needles. While tapping these points, you bring in psychology by focusing on reframing certain emotions or physical symptoms that are associated with that particular acupressure point.[15] The good news is that while acupuncture requires seeing an acupuncturist, tapping is something you can do safely at home at a time that works for you.

The main goal of tapping is to release a negative emotion or physical symptom you may be experiencing in the present moment, whether it be fear, physical pain, forgetfulness, or anything else that is bothering you. According to EFT practitioners, tapping on an appropriate acupuncture point while mentally repeating an affirmative phrase (e.g., "I am at ease") helps to release suppressed emotions because it engages both the brain's limbic system and the body's energetic system at the same time.[16]

As with EMDR, researchers are seeing equally positive results from tapping/EFT. Dozens of studies have demonstrated the efficacy of tapping for emotional release,[17,18,19] but one group of researchers that included renowned EFT experts Peta Stapleton, Ph.D., and Dawson Church, Ph.D., set out to prove that tapping can lead to improvements in the physical body.[20]

In the study, the subjects took part in a four-day EFT training workshop led by certified instructors and learned tapping through clinical demonstrations, practice sessions, and instructor feedback. In addition to taking comprehensive surveys designed to gauge any psychological benefits of the workshop, the researchers wanted to measure the effects of EFT on the central nervous system by measuring heart rate variability, on the circulatory system by measuring resting heart rate and blood pressure, on the endocrine system by measuring cortisol levels, and on the immune system by analyzing saliva samples.

After the 12-hour tapping workshop, participants reported significant declines in anxiety, depression, PTSD, and pain levels.

In addition, self-reported happiness levels increased significantly among the participants. However, most revealing were the participants' physical changes. Following the EFT workshop, the participants experienced significant reductions in cortisol levels, blood pressure, and resting heart rate—all signs that they were successfully out of fight-or-flight and into rest-and-repair mode.[21]

Two additional studies have found that tapping can actually change gene expression in health-promoting ways. As previously discussed, just because you have a certain gene does not mean that gene will be expressed, or turned "on." Instead, the field of epigenetics has shown that lifestyle factors, including diet, emotional patterns, or exercise habits, can turn healthy genes on (or unhealthy genes off) in a matter of weeks or even days.

One study looked at war veterans suffering from PTSD. After participating in hour-long EFT sessions once a week for 10 weeks, there was a significant change in the expression of six genes related to reducing inflammation and strengthening the immune system among the veterans who received the EFT, compared to a waitlist control group of veterans with PTSD. Perhaps more meaningful to the participants, the veterans who received EFT showed a more than 50 percent reduction in their PTSD symptoms.[22]

A second, small pilot study compared the effects of a single hour-long EFT session with socializing for an hour. Researchers found that the expression of 72 genes related to enhancing immunity and reducing inflammation changed significantly after just one hour-long tapping session. Researchers analyzed both blood and saliva samples from the participants and found that many different genes were affected, including those that control the synthesis of red and white blood cells, metabolic regulation, and the suppression of cancer tumors. This small yet promising study shows the potential power of using tapping for making significant and health-promoting changes to your genetic expression.[23]

Lastly, while few studies have been conducted specifically on EFT and cancer, one study found that EFT helped reduce the side effects of two hormonal therapies for breast cancer. This is important because adverse side effects are the reason most women stop taking these drugs, a choice that may lead to cancer recurrence. In this study, participants took an EFT course in which they received tapping instruction for three hours per week for three weeks.[24] The participants completed a number of questionnaires before the course began, as well as 6 and 12 weeks after the course ended. Thanks to the EFT course, the study participants showed significant reductions in anxiety, depression, fatigue, and hot flashes.

Nick Ortner, author of *The Tapping Solution* book series, has dedicated his life to making tapping accessible to everyone. In studies, tapping has been shown to regulate the amygdala (the stress center of your brain) and lower levels of cortisol (the "stress hormone")—both of which will strengthen the immune system and increase its ability to remove cancer cells.[25] Tapping has been shown to "turn off" the amygdala, thereby cutting off the stress response and allowing your brain synapses to be rewired for a more appropriate emotional response to any given situation.[26] About EFT, Nick says:

> Today, the fight-or-flight response is rarely activated by a physical threat. Most of our fight-or-flight responses today are triggered by a negative memory or [negative] thought that has its roots in past trauma or conditioned learning from childhood. When you think of something that causes you anxiety or other uncomfortable feelings, the thought sets off the amygdala "fire alarm." Tapping as you trigger your fight-or-flight response sends the message that the amygdala can deactivate, even though the threatening thought is still present. With repetition, the hippocampus gets the message—this thing that was previously filed as "dangerous" is not, in reality, a threat.

Researchers are just beginning to understand and measure the benefits of tapping/EFT, but these early studies show that it is a quick and effective way to release suppressed emotions, change your gene expression to be more health-promoting, and strengthen your immune system. Because of its broad scope, ease of use, and fast results, tapping has become a therapy of choice among radical remission survivors who want to release suppressed emotions.

## Releasing in Groups

Not all techniques for releasing suppressed emotions will work for all people. Each person finds their own way to release suppressed emotions—perhaps by attending a meditation, MBSR, or tapping class; punching a pillow; or banging a drum. For some, releasing emotions is easier in a group setting. A growing number of organizations have developed community music interventions designed to improve mental health. One group of researchers set out to determine if such a musical therapy group had any measurable psychological or physiological benefits.

In this study, the participants attended a 10-week group drumming course that met once a week. The researchers wanted to see if the course could improve symptoms of depression, anxiety, and social resilience compared to a control group who took part in other weekly social activities but were not actively involved in music interventions.[27] Impressively, significant improvements across all three emotional measures were found in the drumming group—but not the control group—in as little as six weeks. What's more, the beneficial effects lasted for three months *after* the group drumming course ended.

To take the study a step further, researchers analyzed saliva samples from the participants to see if the group drumming course led to any physical changes. The researchers measured the participants' levels of cortisol and cytokine (immune cell proteins that reduce inflammation) and found that after the 10-week group drumming course, participants showed a significant reduction in stress and inflammation levels—both of which are good news for anyone who wants a stronger immune system. In addition to its psychological and physiological benefits, this study incorporated the healing factor of social support, because the drumming was done in a group setting. It would be interesting to see, perhaps in a

RADICAL HOPE

future study, if participants would experience such positive results if they learn the drumming in a one-on-one lesson, as opposed to in a group setting.

One radical remission survivor who has tried to release her suppressed emotions in many ways—including drumming—is Caryn Murray, an appendiceal cancer survivor from Chicago who is a trained shaman and has been studying the mind-body-spirit connection for more than 20 years. In the year leading up to her diagnosis, Caryn went through a painful divorce, filed for bankruptcy, and had to move in to take care of her elderly mother who was suffering from severe Parkinson's disease and dementia. Caryn's two adult children, ages 20 and 22 at the time, were away at college.

After this extremely difficult year-and-a-half period, Caryn was diagnosed in 2013 with stage 4 appendiceal cancer, the same cancer that Bob (from our chapter on empowerment) faced. Caryn's treatment began with emergency surgery to remove the 15 pounds of tumors pressing on her abdominal organs. After-ward, Caryn asked if she could try healing her cancer naturally from that point forward, but her doctors told her the cancer was too advanced and that they needed to take immediate action.

Caryn agreed to four rounds of chemotherapy over three months followed by a 12-hour HIPEC surgery. In addition, she embraced all 10 radical remission healing factors, although she found releasing suppressed emotions to be her critical factor.

> Releasing suppressed emotions is a juicy and liberating topic. As a trained shaman, I went on my own journey by lis-tening to a drumming tape. During one particular session, I discovered a "soul contract" I had in place that was leaking my life-force energy. During that journey, I was able to rewrite that existing contract and replace it with a new soul contract [that helped me heal].

During the years of healing that followed her conventional treatment, Caryn worked with many energy healers.

*I worked with an EnergyTouch practitioner to identify the core emotion attached to my cancer diagnosis—shame! This awareness allowed me to look at myself and examine how I was caring for myself. I wasn't at the top of the list—I was depleted. I was a giver, a caregiver, a mom, a sacred space holder . . . for others. I had to learn to love and nurture myself the way I cared for others. I had to give myself radical self-care and self-love, breaking old patterns, and love myself as I love my children.*

Caryn looked into her childhood to see what emotional patterns she may have established early on that she needed to release as part of her healing.

*In our household growing up, the one who was sick got all the attention. During my self-healing, I was able to recognize that I used my illness to gain the attention and nurturing I desperately yearned for. I repeated the affirmation, "I no longer have the need to use my condition to receive love and attention." It is crucial to get to the core issue or trauma that stops the flow of energy or prana in one's physical body, which can allow "dis-ease" to enter our experience.*

It has been more than six years since Caryn was diagnosed with stage 4 appendiceal cancer, which has a less than 25 percent five-year survival rate. By combining groundbreaking conventional medical treatments like the HIPEC surgery along with the 10 radical remission healing factors, including releasing the emotion of shame from her past, she has been able to overcome tremendous odds and lead a healthy, normal life. She now gives back to cancer patients as a certified Radical Remission workshop instructor and health coach.

Another radical remission survivor who felt that releasing her suppressed emotions was key to her recovery is Alison, an energetic woman from rural Colorado. In addition to the other nine healing factors, Alison credits her recovery from a rare and terminal brain cancer to the emotional work she did to help deal with her childhood trauma.

## Alison's Story

In 2013, 48-year-old Alison Gannett was living her "perfect" life. At the time, she was a world champion extreme freeskier and pro mountain biker, had a "real" job as a climate change scientist, and ran a side business leading outdoor adventures for women. To top it off, she lived on an idyllic 80-acre farm with her husband, where they grew their own organic food.

But then Alison started having physical and mental symptoms she could not explain. When she almost burned the house down cooking bacon, her husband rushed her to the emergency room. They and the doctors were shocked to learn that a tumor the size of a baseball was taking up more than half her brain. Just like that, Alison became a cancer patient, diagnosed with hemangiopericytoma, a rare type of brain cancer.

Alison's doctors told her she would need surgery, chemotherapy, and radiation, and then everything would be "great." However, Alison's intuition told her they were not sharing the full story, so she pushed to understand what "great" meant for her type of cancer. Through Internet searches, she discovered that with the standard protocol of surgery, chemotherapy, and radiation, she would not likely live much longer than without any treatment, and she would have to deal with serious side effects such as the risk of getting a secondary cancer. Neither option was enough for Alison. She desperately wanted to live a happy life with her husband and die of old age.

After the diagnosis, Alison's first reaction was shock, followed quickly by denial. Her reasons for living were too strong for her to accept the grim prognosis. She thought, *I'm not going to be a victim of this. I want to live and I need to find out how I can live.*

Since the tumor was pressing on blood flow to the brain and could kill her at any moment, Alison agreed to have immediate surgery. Unfortunately, the surgeons could not remove all the small tumors that had sprung up near the baseball-size tumor. More worrisome, the surgery had injured her brain such that her doctors did not want her to start chemotherapy or radiation or have a second surgery for a few months, so that her brain could heal from the trauma. Alison considers this additional period of time a blessing, because it gave her half a year to "really hit Google hard."

In her research, Alison learned that the average survival time for her exact type of cancer was 6.8 months—and that was *with* conventional medical treatment. Each time she saw that depressing statistic, she thought about how she wanted to spend the last six or seven months of her life. Eventually, she decided that she wasn't going to spend her last days undergoing futile treatments. Instead, she would create better statistics by healing herself. Against her doctors' wishes, Alison refused the recommended chemotherapy and radiation, as well as a follow-up surgery to remove the smaller tumors they had missed.

Instead, Alison dug more deeply in her research to find a different path back to health. She found radical remission survivor Dr. Nasha Winters, a licensed naturopathic doctor (N.D.) and fellow of the American Board of Naturopathic Oncology (FABNO), to help guide her in her healing journey. Dr. Winters is a 25-year radical remission survivor of stage 4 ovarian cancer and a proponent of the metabolic theory of cancer. Like many radical remission survivors, after healing herself, Dr. Winters dedicated her life to helping other cancer patients find their own way to heal, either in conjunction with conventional medicine or as an alternative. Dr. Winters worked with Alison to determine the likely causes of her cancer and then recommended a multifaceted healing strategy, including reversing the root causes of her cancering process and suggesting nontoxic treatments. Alison recalls:

*When I was diagnosed, I had a short period of morbidity and [thinking] crazy death thoughts. It was totally overwhelming and scary. But once I learned from Dr. Winters that cancer is just about the root causes, and there were other people out there who had completely reversed the root causes of their cancer, I had the seeds of hope that I could reverse my cancer and that my body might be able to heal itself.*

Working with Dr. Winters, Alison came to understand that a variety of conditions may have led to her cancer. For example, she learned she had an imbalanced gut microbiome, most likely due to years spent taking antibiotics after multiple knee surgeries, not uncommon for a professional athlete. She also had a compromised immune system, most likely due to a childhood punctuated by frequent ear, chest, and sinus infections, and heavy metal poisoning from her drinking water. After getting genetic testing, Alison discovered that she had genetic variations that made her not able to process dairy, grains, toxins, or saturated fats very well, which likely led to a lifetime of low-grade gut inflammation and intestinal hyperpermeability. In addition, she had been exposed to various viruses in her life (e.g., Epstein-Barr, cytomegalovirus) and was experiencing prediabetic blood sugar levels after years of being vegan/vegetarian. Years of overexercising had led to massive inflammation and adrenal fatigue, which were compounded by exposure to endocrine disruptors, such as from plastic water bottles and plastic hydration devices (for skiers), all of which taxed her thyroid and led to hormonal imbalances.

Alison believes that another important root cause of her cancer was being a "type A overachiever" her whole life, which led to undue amounts of stress. This stress showed up in her labs as elevated cortisol, which can drive up insulin, thereby driving up glucose levels. This means that stress, not just a sugar-filled diet, can increase the supply of cancer's preferred fuel, glucose. For Alison, this stress started early as a child of an alcoholic and neglectful father, which caused her to strive for perfection as she grew to adulthood.

*I was a fat, dorky, math geek. I was teased as a child and I think I eventually overcompensated for that by becoming a world champion extreme skier, jumping off cliffs for a living. I wanted to say, "See me? I'm now amazing."*

In addition to these mental and emotional stressors, Alison learned through her blood testing that she was deficient in certain vitamins and minerals. Through genetic testing, she learned that she was born with a genetic variation that made it hard for her to absorb vitamin D$_3$, which research has shown to be vitally important for one's immune health and hormone regulation.

Since so many factors had potentially led to her cancer, Alison believed she had to address all of them in order to heal, and that there was no *single* change that could reverse her cancer. Instead, she understood she had to address what Dr. Winters calls the "Terrain Ten," which are similar to the 10 healing factors of radical remission. (Note: You can learn more about Dr. Winters's Terrain Ten in her book, *The Metabolic Approach to Cancer.*) Alison worked diligently with Dr. Winters on all aspects of her life, including customized nutrition, sleep, supplements, exercise, intestinal permeability, detoxification, treating viruses, meditation, genetics/epigenetics, and her emotional and spiritual life. However, Alison came to believe that childhood traumas and her pattern of lifelong stress were the largest root causes of her cancer, and therefore the most essential factors for her healing.

*It's kind of like peeling layers of the onion. You can think of [the radical remission healing factors] as layers that you're peeling away, and you can't deal with everything at once. I might have reformed my diet, but if I hadn't changed my stress-a-holic ways, I would still be giving the cancer cells potential fuel, because cancer cells ferment glucose or fructose and other carbohydrates. By being a stress-a-holic, I was giving them what they wanted—and I really had to get away from that. So what I did is EFT and meditation. I've also done extensive counseling, psychotherapy, and have a full-time meditation coach—trying to deal with my past, stop worrying about the future, and focusing on clearing my head, enjoying the present moment.*

In her process of healing, Alison came to believe that childhood trauma was a big part of her disease process. In her willingness to open up about her painful past, Alison discovered she had many repressed emotions of grief, shame, and trauma.

*It's hard dealing with emotional trauma. It was probably the hardest part of that cancering process for me. I hadn't dealt with any of those [emotions and trauma] and I think that's hugely important. A lot of people don't dig into the emotional possibilities that could be involved with their cancers, and for me, that was a huge one. My way of dealing with emotions was to build a fortress around myself and become impermeable to the rest of the world, but it wasn't actually dealing with the trauma of my childhood. I just stored all that pain in different parts of my body.*

Alison came to understand and appreciate that her repressed childhood emotions had shaped her professional career choices (extreme athlete, entrepreneur, nonprofit founder, driven scientist) as well as her unhealthy survival mechanisms.

*I was a child of an alcoholic, and I didn't [emotionally] process what it was like to grow up in that situation. As a youngster, I just ate and became overweight. That was my way of dealing with the trauma. Then, in my 20s, I discovered exercise and I was like, "Oh, this is a way to not be fat." It was also a great way to literally run away from my problems. When you're running and you get in that state of bliss, you never have to deal with anything. So that's what I was doing to deal with my trauma. I was addicted to exercise to literally run away from my problems.*

Dealing with suppressed emotions from her abusive childhood and learning how to better manage her stress were key to Alison's recovery. Slowly she learned how to process her emotions in a healthier way, create new emotional habits to sustain her health, and become more empathetic.

*I had to learn to deal with the grief and the pain. Processing the feelings, as opposed to avoiding them, was really important. When I'm having a bad day—for instance, because of the deaths of my pets this year—I let myself feel into the grief, whereas before I would have just packed it away. I learned to feel into the emotion and really experience the abandonment and loss. I was never able to be a child—always playing the role of mother while my mother played the role of father and mother. And there was significant abuse in the family, as well as addictive behaviors, bipolar [disorder], and depression. No emotions were shared, and everyone pretended there were no elephants in the living room. I remember spending a large chunk of time afterschool in the bathroom crying by myself. [Those experiences] have become my best teachers, because going through those things enables me to be a stronger person. But they also enable me to feel into the suffering of other people, and help guide them through a process [of healing] that I went through.*

While working through her suppressed emotions, Alison addressed the other nine radical remission healing factors. She embraced her reasons for living, including her husband, family, friends, idyllic farm, and her newfound interest in customized cancer nutrition. These friends and family, including her husband, mother, and three siblings, provided strong social support during her recovery, flying in, if needed, to help care for her. As a professional athlete, overachiever, and someone who had always dealt with stress by overexercising, Alison discovered to her surprise that she actually needed to exercise *less* in order to heal. She learned this lesson the hard way.

*I tried to start running as soon as I was able. I was an idiot! I hadn't learned. Because I was so scared of the diagnosis, I wanted to run away from my problems again. But immediately the inflammation and cancer markers across all my [blood] labs went through the roof.*

Instead of her usual long-distance running, mountain biking, backcountry skiing, and other extreme sports, Alison had to learn to ease back into exercise with gentler types of movement, such as walking in nature, surfing in the ocean, and paddleboarding on rivers, all of which helped her get more of her much-needed vitamin $D_3$ from sunshine. The genetic variation that inhibited Alison's vitamin D absorption meant that she needed more time in the sun and more vitamin $D_3$ supplementation than most people.

Nature became Alison's "church," as she used gentle outdoor exercise to keep her mind clear. She grew spiritually during her healing journey by developing a meditation practice. Inspired by her new meditation teacher, Alison explored different religions and types of spirituality and started to conceptualize divinity as love, treating everything and everyone with as much love as she could. She describes this newfound peace and sense of loving-kindness:

> *Through cancer, I changed my relationships with my friends and family for the better. I'm just a different person. I was really tough [before], and not vulnerable at all. I'm completely vulnerable now in a good way. I'm softer. I'm less the "captain of my ship" and more "part of the ocean."*

Under Dr. Winters's careful direction, supplements played an important role in Alison's recovery. To this day, Alison takes numerous supplements to reduce inflammation (e.g., Boswellia), build up her immune system (e.g., vitamin $D_3$), balance her hormones (e.g., melatonin), and work on her microbiome (e.g., Bifidobacterium). During her time of recovery, she took additional supplements to help detoxify her body of infections, viruses, and heavy metals.

Diet was another major change for Alison. She thought she had created the optimal life by growing her own food. But in reality, her vegetarian diet—which included numerous grains and carbohydrates—may have been contributing to her cancer, at least according to the metabolic theory of cancer. This is how she describes it:

*I was a "carb-a-holic." I was growing grains on my farm—I was growing all my carbs. I thought,* Since I'm growing my own food, and I'm a professional skier, I just have this perfect life. *But once I reviewed my blood work with Dr. Winters, I realized I was not only not the "picture of health," but I was a health disaster on every single front.*

Alison's detailed blood work revealed that her protein, albumin, and ferritin levels were dangerously low, which indicated she needed to add meat or other protein sources back into her diet. She learned that her specific type of brain cancer may be sugar- and fructose-dependent, and that cancers in general prefer to metabolize fructose, glucose, and other carbohydrates. She chose to eliminate fruits and carbs from her diet and go on a therapeutic ketogenic diet a month after her diagnosis. Under Dr. Winters's supervision, Alison began closely monitoring her ketones, glucose, and glucose ketone index (GKI). To do this, she would first eat a meal, and then four to six hours later would test her blood ketones and blood sugar with an at-home finger-prick test to determine how her body was metabolizing her food.

Alison did further genetic testing to determine how her body processes food, through which she learned that her body does not process dairy well. The smallest amounts of dairy would send her blood sugar through the roof and her ketones plummeting, which is viewed (in the metabolic theory of cancer) as "feeding" her cancer. Other genetic variations did not allow her to metabolize caffeine, catechins (think green tea), sulphur/brassica vegetables (think kale), or saturated fats (think coconut oil) very well.

As her knowledge grew regarding potential causes of cancer and as she learned how her body reacts to certain foods, exercise, and other treatments, Alison continued to make lifestyle changes, monitor her progress, and make appropriate adjustments with her healing team to become her own knowledgeable health CEO whose constant goal was full remission. "Test, assess, and address. Don't guess," is Dr. Winters's motto, which Alison has fully embraced by testing around 100 of her blood chemistry markers every month for the last six years, and which she will continue to do in the future.

Alison took her time building her healing team. She works with about 14 different doctors and healers, including a neurological oncologist, three neurosurgeons, a neurologist, two naturopaths, three general practitioners, a psychotherapist, a massage therapist, an EFT coach, a somatic experience coach, a meditation teacher, and an acupuncturist. One of the things she was most shocked to learn was that medical doctors in the U.S. are not permitted to discuss alternative cancer treatments that are not part of the "standard of care" without risking losing their medical license. Therefore, while she believes her conventional doctors are just as important as the rest of her team members, she has learned not to rely solely on their specific expertise.

> *A lot of people don't know that with the American Medical Association, [medical] doctors are only allowed to talk about surgery, chemo, radiation, clinical trials, or [FDA-approved] immunotherapy. If they even mentioned the ketogenic diet, or some kind of customized diet, or emotional therapy, or supplements, they can lose their license. So we have to be understanding that they can't discuss those things. Does that mean I'm going to drop them as part of my team? No. They run my MRIs, are great surgeons, and they're helpful in that regard.*

When asked if intuition played a part in her healing, Alison acknowledged that she was not in touch with her intuition at first, because she was so obsessed with achievement before she got diagnosed. Alison believes that modern society rewards those who are overachievers, so that is what she did—at all costs. She feels that this pursuit of achievement suppressed her intuition about her health. For instance, she ignored many warning signs that her immune system was "off." She thought it was normal to have chronic bronchitis, yeast infections, and thyroid imbalances. In addition, she assumed her chronic arthritis was from jumping off cliffs or just getting older. She never knew that arthritis was actually chronic inflammation of the joints.

Alison discovered that when she changed her mind, body, and spirit with the 10 radical remission healing factors, her chronic conditions went away. This list was long and included arthritis, bladder infections, yeast infections, polycystic ovarian disease, fibrocystic breasts, Hashimoto's thyroiditis, hormone imbalances, Epstein-Barr virus, cytomegalovirus, intestinal permeability, fatty liver, prediabetes, chronic bronchitis, and ear and tooth infections. Because of the significant improvements she experienced both physically and emotionally, Alison now sees cancer as a gift that helped her heal every aspect of her life. She is still using a low-dose naltrexone supplement to balance her immune system and an at-home infrared sauna to detoxify her massive heavy metal poisoning.

As Alison outlived her dire prognosis over the next few years, she continued to experiment and make changes to create the healthiest life possible. She became more attuned to elevations in her stress and cortisol levels and would promptly address any mental or emotional stressors to bring them back down. As a result of this learning process, she made the difficult decision to sell her business teaching women extreme freeskiing and mountain biking, because running it proved to be too stressful for her mind and body. As Dr. Winters told her, "Just because you love your job doesn't mean it isn't killing you."

In 2014, one year after her diagnosis, Alison became a student of her naturopath, Dr. Winters, taking a yearlong program through the International Cancer Advocacy Network (ICAN) in order to dive more deeply into the individualized root causes of people's cancer. In 2015, she founded Customized Oncology Nutrition, which specializes in creating personalized wellness plans based upon each client's DNA, blood chemistry, and health history. In her new work, she helps people prevent or conquer cancer with nutrition for the body, mind, and spirit.

Today, Alison's cancer is stable, although she still has the small tumors in her brain. As she puts it:

*You can have tumors, but they can either be "cancering"
or they can just be a collection of dormant cells in your body. I
have a couple of tumors in my head that they missed [during
the surgery], and at first I was super angry about that, but I now
use them as a reminder any time I even think about cheating
[on my new lifestyle].*

To keep her tumors dormant, Alison continues to monitor her-self regularly. She runs around 100 comprehensive blood tests at her local lab (via prescription from her general practitioner) every month to determine whether there are any increases in her inflammation markers or any changes in other markers that would indicate that her cancer could potentially be fueled. Alison has found that her inflammation levels increase any time she overexercises, experiences a stressful situation, catches a virus or bacterial infection, or eats a food to which she is sensitive (e.g., dairy) or which throws off her blood sugar.

To satisfy the scientist within her, Alison has funneled her energy into maintaining a detailed spreadsheet that is "probably two yards long," which tracks her blood test results so that she can see trends as they occur. She creates a similar spreadsheet for each of her clients, including a column that explains what each lab could indicate. She says these labs empower her so she's not just sitting around waiting for the next scan. Each month she can make adjustments because, as she puts it, "There are no such things as 'good' labs or 'bad' labs, just information."

Alison adjusts her supplements to deal with any stressors that pop up and practices meditation every day to reduce her stress levels. She has consciously stopped overexercising. She spends a lot of time outdoors, her main activity being an hour-long dog walk each day. When she has some extra time, she enjoys activities like ocean surfing, river rafting, and stand-up paddleboarding, all of which keep her heart rate low and bring her endless joy. She makes time to connect with friends and family.

Alison loved her life before cancer but realizes now that certain aspects of her life were not as healthy as they could have been—otherwise, she would not have gotten cancer. In response, she drastically changed every aspect of her life.

*I loved my life before cancer. I was blessed with jobs that I loved, being outside, and traveling around the world, but it didn't mean that it was a healthy life. I thought I had the perfect life, but that normal [life] gave me cancer. Everything about my life that I thought was normal had to be reinvented into what I now call the "new normal." And actually, it is a much better version of myself. I feel healthier six years later than I did in my 20s. I am a lot more balanced and no longer prone to extremes.*

Alison has come to see cancer as a wake-up call that has helped her live a better life and give back to others through her coaching.

*My check engine light was on, and I had to dig in and find out what was going on. I did and have continued to do so to make every day better than the last. Cancer is the single greatest gift that's ever been given to me. I wouldn't be the person I am today [without cancer]. I'm six years into it. I think it's a journey. It's not like you ever get there, but I feel like I'm making tons and tons of progress.*

Alison continues to eat a strict ketogenic diet to maintain her health, but she does not consider it restrictive.

*You can have your cake and eat it, too! I've invented so many great recipes so that I can enjoy my keto bread, dairy-free keto ice cream, and keto brownies. I would never go back to what I was eating before. The way I eat now is better. My skin feels better, my body feels younger, and I don't have any signs of the cancering process or of any inflammation in my body. My immune system has fixed itself. My liver is renormalized and my blood sugar is balanced. It's super exciting!*

As part of her ketogenic diet, Alison eats in time-restricted eating windows (known as intermittent fasting), where she eats only within a certain time frame each day to help control her blood sugar/insulin spikes and to enable her ApoE4 gene to create a long life instead of a shorter one with potential Alzheimer's. In addition, she does a full water fast three days per month because of her specific genetic makeup and because people with the ApoE4 gene benefit greatly from periods of fasting, which Alison can see in her lab results. Alison has found that a fast helps to reboot her immune system, stimulate autophagy (cell "recycling"), and rebuild mitochondria.

Above all, Alison believes that the key to any radical remission is to reverse the root causes of the cancer. She feels that a strong root cause of her own cancer was the suppressed emotions she was holding on to from her childhood, which is why she worked so diligently to process and release her childhood trauma.

> *We can put a Band-Aid on all our traumas and root causes, but there's no amount of treatment—whether you do a futuristic standard of care, integrative, combination of both, or nothing—that will work if you don't reverse the root causes of cancer. The cancer is always going to have an opportunity to come back, so you can rip the Band-Aid off, or you can peel it off slowly. That's what I had to do, and I was willing to go there, but it's not for everybody. However, I love what I've found underneath the Band-Aid.*

More than six years after she had only 6.8 months to live (according to statistics), Alison's medical doctors are blown away by the fact that she is still alive—although Alison is not. She used her overachieving personality to dig deep into the root causes of her cancer, including doing deep, intense emotional work to release her buried emotions from childhood. Alison is an inspiration for all people who are willing to do the hard work of releasing suppressed emotions, which can contribute to tremendous healing results. To learn more about Alison, visit AlisonGannett.com.

# Action Steps

While releasing suppressed emotions in the body-mind-spirit system is no easy task, radical remission survivors have told us repeatedly that it is well worth the effort. In *Radical Remission*, I suggested the following action steps, which still remain relevant: (1) Keep a "thought journal" to discover your underlying thoughts and beliefs; (2) Make a list of all the emotions you experience in a day to uncover themes; (3) Practice daily forgiveness; (4) Enroll in a stress management course; (5) Make an appointment with a qualified psychotherapist, energy healer, or energy kinesiologist; and (6) Try eye movement desensitization and reprocessing (EMDR) or hypnosis to deal with any trauma held in your body.

In addition, here are a few more ways to help you kick-start emotional release and boost your immune system.

- **Take a self-love retreat.**

    When you are in the middle of a health crisis, it can be difficult to find the time and energy to tackle your emotional baggage. If you need a helping hand, many institutions are dedicated to helping you enhance your body-mind-spirit connection with daylong, weekend, or weeklong workshops on topics such as "A New Pathway to Recovery," "Well Woman: A Restorative Retreat for Women Touched by Breast Cancer," and "Free Your Energy, Transform Your Life." If the thought of a retreat sounds cost-prohibitive, be aware that many centers have scholarships available. In addition, local libraries, wellness centers, hospitals, and nonprofits may offer local workshops.

- **Try tapping.**

    Because of the increased popularity of EFT and tapping, many resources are now available. If you would like to teach yourself how to tap, *The Tapping*

*Solution* book series and EFTuniverse.com offer easy-to-follow guides. You'll also find several guided tapping videos for free on YouTube. If you prefer in-person instruction, many libraries, wellness centers, hospitals, and therapists now offer courses to help guide you.

- **Write a letter to those who hurt you.**

  A powerful method of emotional release is to write a letter to the persons who have hurt you, regardless of whether they are dead or alive. Pour your pain, frustration, resentment, and anger onto the paper. The physical act of writing down your emotions and addressing them directly will begin to release the emotions from your body. You do not need to send the letter; in fact, many radical remission survivors have found that writing the letter is all they needed to do. Once written, you can ceremonially burn the letter, tuck it in a drawer for occasional rereading and releasing, or just throw it away.

- **Let it out in a group.**

  Taking a class or joining a group whose mission is to release your emotions can be greatly beneficial to your healing. Examples include drum circles, dance groups like Gabrielle Roth's "5Rhythms" classes, yoga classes, chanting classes, and art therapy groups. Check your local resources at libraries, yoga studios, newspapers, or local online groups to help you find the right group for you.

- **Make social media work for you.**

  As we try to manage our emotions better and release things like stress, anxiety, or depression, it is important to reflect on how our screen time and social media use affects our emotional states. Here are some simple tips to get you started:

1. Take two days completely off from social media and notice how you feel during and after those two days. Consider taking every other day off from social media.

2. Learn how to unfollow, block, or "mute" people whose posts lead you to feel negative emotions.

3. Make an effort to follow people on social media who lift your spirits and are authentic about their entire lives, both good and bad (as opposed to sharing only their best moments).

4. Try using apps to track and limit your social media time, such as Screen Time for iOS or Digital Wellbeing for Android.

Note: If you choose to approach this healing factor intensively, be aware that a big emotional release may bring about physical side effects. For example, a sudden release of emotional "toxins" can also cause temporary, physical symptoms like strong fatigue, sleep disruption, night sweats, digestive upset, or headaches. However, do not let this alarm you. Knowing what to expect and understanding that these are normal side effects will help you to accept them and let them run their course without worrying about them and adding to your stress.

To help get you through any physical symptoms, holistic healers typically recommend drinking plenty of water, spending time in nature each day, and eating unprocessed, unrefined, organic foods. Finally, Epsom salt and/or baking soda baths can gently help to detoxify your physical body.

Dealing with emotions that you are avoiding, either consciously or unconsciously, may not sound like fun, but think of it like jumping off a high-dive. At first, it is intimidating and scary to climb up the ladder, walk to the edge of the diving board, and look down at the pool far below. Your heart may be pounding with fear. However, once you face your fears and take that plunge, the water is refreshing and you realize that it was not so hard after all. It is the same with releasing suppressed emotions—it may seem intimidating at first, but it will be well worth your efforts in terms of lightening your emotional load and strengthening your immune system.

---

## CHAPTER 7

# CHANGING YOUR DIET

---

## Jeremiah's Story

*Eat food. Not too much. Mostly plants.*

— MICHAEL POLLAN

Nothing in the integrative cancer world today sparks a fiercer debate than what type of diet is best for cancer patients. On one side are the plant-based advocates, who contend that vegetables, fruits, and whole grains provide all the nutrients one needs to heal. On the other side are advocates of the trendy ketogenic diet, which is a high-fat, limited-carbohydrate diet originally developed to help with epilepsy, but which has gained traction among integrative health practitioners who are using it to help people with cancer and Alzheimer's.

This debate can make it difficult to figure out which diet is best for you. Research has shown that plant-based, ketogenic, and other diets such as the Mediterranean diet provide significant health benefits. However, there is also evidence that shows some shortcomings for each diet. What this implies is that there may be no single diet that is best for every human—no one-size-fits-all solution. We realize that this is not exactly what you want to hear, especially if you have recently been diagnosed with a disease such as cancer.

Keep in mind that radical remissions occur with people who follow all three of the diets mentioned above. Survivors tend to rely on three criteria when determining which diet is right for them. They look at (1) the results of testing (e.g., blood tests, food sensitivity tests, etc.), (2) symptom reduction while trying out a new diet, and (3) the benefits of the diet (e.g., increased energy, a healthier weight, etc.). Finally, it is important to note what these three diets have in common: eating whole, organic vegetables while reducing your intake of sugar, refined grains, and processed foods. Research shows that making these types of dietary changes can reduce your inflammation and strengthen your immune system, thereby helping your body to remove cancer cells more effectively.

In this chapter, we hope to provide some guidance and clarity as you chart your own dietary path. We will share some of the latest developments and research in this quickly evolving field of study. After that, we will share the full healing story of baby Jeremiah, whose mother made radical changes to his diet—in addition to incorporating the other nine healing factors—to help him achieve a radical remission from a rare form of lymphoma. We will end the chapter with a few simple action steps that we hope will inspire you to begin making improvements to your own diet.

# Recent Developments

## Cancer Rates and Trends

For the past two decades, the World Cancer Research Fund International (WCRF) and the American Institute for Cancer Research (AICR) have issued cancer prevention guidelines for diet, weight management, and physical activity.[1] Their recommendations appear to be paying off, because the latest *Annual Report to the Nation on the Status of Cancer* showed that overall deaths from all cancers combined continue to decline slightly each year (which they have since 1999), with some notable exceptions.[2] But let's talk about the good news first.

The report, written by several leading government agencies, found that new cancer cases and deaths from lung, bladder, and larynx cancers have continued to decrease in tandem with the long-term decline in tobacco smoking.[3] Also notable was the rapid decline in the death rate for melanoma, likely due to the impact of new therapies such as immune checkpoint inhibitors for late-stage melanoma patients.[4]

Unfortunately, the report contained some disheartening news. For example, cancer used to be a disease associated with older people, but in the past few decades, we have seen a rise in cancer among people ages 20–49.[5] The most common cancer diagnosis for women in this age group was breast cancer, followed by thyroid and melanoma.[6] Meanwhile, for men ages 20–49 the most common cancer diagnoses were colorectal, testicular, and melanoma.[7]

Given the importance of diet to overall health, one would hope that diet and nutrition would be found in the tool kit of every practicing doctor. After all, diet leads all the other risk factors for disability and premature death, easily beating smoking, high blood pressure, obesity, and physical inactivity.[8] Unfortunately, the average number of hours devoted to nutrition education in medical school has declined over the last 20 years, even as the incidences of diet- and lifestyle-related chronic diseases have continued to rise.[9,10,11] A new study conducted by the Indiana University School of Medicine found that medical students and physicians agree that the nutrition education currently provided in medical school is sorely inadequate,[12] showing that it is not that doctors *disbelieve* in the healing power of food. Rather, they simply don't know much about it.

This is unfortunate because the research has demonstrated again and again that *we are what we eat*. From a scientific standpoint, the cells of our food are broken down and converted into fuel that our bodies' cells need in order to function properly. If we put in "bad fuel," our bodies cannot function optimally. If we put in "good fuel," we can fundamentally change the state of our health.

Radical remission survivors radically changed their diets and believe these diets were absolutely essential to healing their cancer or other life-threatening diseases. While the specifics of their healing diets vary (e.g., vegan, ketogenic, paleo, etc.), the vast majority of radical remission survivors have made the following key dietary changes. I discussed these in detail in *Radical Remission*:

- Greatly reducing (or sometimes eliminating) their consumption of sugar, meat, dairy, and refined foods
- Greatly increasing their vegetable intake (and sometimes fruit)
- Choosing organic foods
- Drinking filtered water

As a reminder, making dietary changes can be emotionally stressful, whether due to the loss of comfort foods and traditional family recipes, the time required to learn a whole new way of eating, or body image and weight-loss issues. You may be the kind of person who can jump right in and make major changes overnight, but if you are not, know that many radical remission survivors made small changes over time. Either way, it is worth the time and effort to improve your diet given its benefits.

## An Unhealthy Diet Can Cause Cancer

A team of researchers at Tufts University recently isolated diet alone as a cause of cancer. The researchers found that a suboptimal diet accounted for 5 percent of invasive cancers in adults older than 20, while 4–6 percent of cancer diagnoses were attributed to alcohol intake, 7–8 percent to excessive body weight, and 2–3 percent to physical inactivity.[13] In this study, a "suboptimal diet" meant eating too few vegetables, fruits, and whole grains and too much highly processed meat, red meat, and sugar-sweetened beverages. Of these factors, high intake of processed meat and low intake of whole grains (i.e., not enough fiber) were the two factors associated with the largest number of new cancer diagnoses. Because the colon is so sensitive to changes in diet, it is not surprising that colon cancer comprised the highest proportion of diet-related cancer cases (38 percent) in this study, followed by cancer of the mouth, pharynx, and larynx (all parts of the digestive tract).[14]

But there is hope that changing your diet can reduce your risk of getting cancer. For instance, in a study of over 48,000 post-menopausal women ages 50–79, researchers found that among women who were originally overweight or obese, reducing their total fat intake and increasing their intake of vegetables, fruits, and grains led them to reduce their risk of being diagnosed with pancreatic cancer by 29 percent.[15]

While being overweight has been shown to increase your risk of getting cancer, the opposite issues of malnutrition, weight loss, and being underweight are dangerous side effects of chemotherapy and radiation.[16] It is imperative that cancer patients fill their bodies with nutrient-rich foods, but there is not yet a research consensus on which diet is best.

## A Healthy Diet Can Prevent Cancer

So what exactly is a healthy diet? After reviewing hundreds of dietary studies, journalist Michael Pollan summarized his research with his famous quote, "Eat food. Not too much. Mostly plants." In the studies he reviewed, the subjects derived the most benefit when they ate unprocessed foods in their wholest forms, when the majority of their diets were vegetables, and when they maintained a low daily calorie intake. Coming to a similar conclusion, the WCRF, American Institute for Cancer Research, and American Cancer Society recently reviewed the leading diet research and recommended that people looking to avoid cancer should eat a largely plant-based diet, with limited amounts of red and processed meat, as well as limited alcohol.[17]

In a similar review, research teams in Europe and the U.S. analyzed more than 90 studies with more than 85,000 subjects and concluded that adhering to a healthy diet has the potential to significantly reduce one's cancer risk, especially for colon, breast, and lung cancers. The researchers determined that a healthy diet includes mainly vegetables and fruit, with small amounts of Western foods (fatty, salty, sugary, refined, and animal products). The opposite was also found to be true: Unhealthy dietary patterns (those consisting of mostly Western foods) were associated with an increased risk of cancer.[18]

Some of the latest research shows that a healthy diet reduces the risk of getting cancer in the first place, specifically colon cancer.[19] A group of researchers reviewed the studies on various diets, including the Healthy Eating Index-2010, the Mediterranean diet, the Alternative Healthy Eating Index-2010, and the Dietary Approaches to Stop Hypertension (the DASH diet). Their review analyzed close to 200,000 subjects ages 45–75. Across the board, high-quality diets were associated with a significantly lower risk of colorectal cancer across all racial/ethnic groups.[20] For this study, "high-quality" meant a diet high in fruits and vegetables, whole grains, legumes, nuts, and healthy oils, while low in red meat, sugary beverages, alcohol, and sodium.

The Mediterranean diet centers on vegetables, fruits, nuts, seeds, legumes, potatoes, whole grains, bread, herbs, spices, fish, seafood, and olive oil. It contains limited amounts of poultry, eggs, cheese, and yogurt, and very small amounts of red meat, sugar-sweetened beverages, added sugars, processed meat, refined grains, refined oils, and other highly processed foods. It is based on the traditional foods typically eaten in countries like Italy, Spain, and Greece. Epidemiology researchers have noticed that people from these regions are exceptionally healthy compared to people in other developed countries and have a lower incidence of many diseases, including cancer, diabetes, and heart disease.

A team of researchers set out to evaluate the preventive effect of the Mediterranean diet on breast cancer. They recruited more than 4,000 women ages 60–80 who were at high risk for cardiovascular disease and had no prior history of breast cancer. The women were randomized into three different diet groups and followed for five years to see who (if anyone) developed breast cancer.[21] The study participants were randomly assigned to either (1) a group that was told to eat a Mediterranean diet supplemented with additional extra-virgin olive oil (EVOO), (2) a group that was told to eat a Mediterranean diet supplemented with additional mixed nuts, or (3) a control group that was told to reduce their dietary fat intake. (Note: The researchers asked the two treatment groups to supplement with EVOO and nuts, respectively, because they hypothesized that these foods might provide additional protection against cancer.)

The researchers found that the group that ate a Mediterranean diet supplemented with EVOO had an incredible 62 percent relatively lower risk of getting malignant breast cancer compared to the control group.[22] This is one of the first randomized controlled trials to show that a long-term dietary change—such as eating a whole-foods, plant-centric diet—actually helps prevent cancer.

## A Healthy Diet Can Help You Survive Cancer

Of particular interest to cancer patients, recent research shows that diet can improve cancer survival rates. An Australian study examined the association between the diet of women with ovarian cancer and their overall survival rate by examining diet questionnaires that had been completed by these women at the time of their diagnosis, and then tracking their five-year survival rate.[23] The women who ate the most fiber increased their chances of surviving ovarian cancer by 31 percent, compared to those who ate the least amount of fiber. There were significant survival advantages for women who ate more green leafy vegetables, fruit, fish, poly- and monounsaturated fat, and cruciferous vegetables, and who drank green tea. Participants who ate a diet with a higher glycemic index (higher in sugar) had a lower survival rate.[24]

Another study analyzed Hispanic breast cancer survivors and found that a healthy diet reduced the risk of cancer recurrence. In this study, a group of breast cancer survivors attended a nine-session program that met for a total of 24 hours over the course of 12 weeks. The program included nutritional education, hands-on cooking classes, and food-shopping field trips. The control group received only written dietary recommendations.

After analyzing blood samples at the start of the study, as well as at 6 and 12 months later, the researchers concluded that the short-term intervention led to long-term dietary changes, including increased fruit and vegetable intake. In addition, these dietary changes led to significant changes in biomarkers that are associated with reducing the risk of a cancer recurrence.[25]

## Plant-Based Diets

While you were growing up, you probably heard the phrase "eat your veggies" all too often. Yet in our modern age of fast, convenient, and processed food, we do not actually eat enough vegetables. Radical remission survivors repeatedly emphasize the vital importance of increasing their intake of healthy, organic vegetables and fruits. One such survivor is Kris Carr.

Before Kris Carr was a documentary star and *New York Times* best-selling author, she was a 31-year-old actress and photographer living in New York City. Her life was filled with late-night parties, never-ending work stress, and the carefree immortality of youth. This all changed on Valentine's Day 2003, when Kris was unexpectedly diagnosed with stage 4 epithelioid hemangioendothelioma (EHE), a rare sarcoma that affects less than .01 percent of cancer patients. To make matters worse, there were no well-researched, conventional medicine treatments available for her type of cancer. Her doctors believed her cancer to be incurable and told her that all she could do was watch and wait until her cancer became aggressive, at which point one doctor told her she may need a triple organ transplant of her liver and both lungs.

Kris quickly discovered that healing her cancer was going to be a full-time job, so she ventured out on "the greatest journey of her life" to find wellness and filmed herself along the way, ultimately creating her award-winning documentary, *Crazy Sexy Cancer*. Kris came to view the grocery store as her personal pharmacy and went back to school to study nutrition. She worked on resolving her chronic insomnia, stopped making excuses for not exercising, and completely upended her fast-paced life, especially her diet.

*Because my diet had been based on what to eat to stay slim for the camera as an actress, I had no idea how to be healthy. So I swapped martinis for organic green drinks and a compassionate vegan diet. My diet is now based on an anti-inflammatory, plant-based approach that focuses on whole foods, low-glycemic fruits, copious amounts of veggies, and proper hydration—including delicious green drinks and superpowered smoothies.*

Kris believes that eating raw and living foods helped heal her body and keep her cancer stable. Today, more than 16 years after receiving a terminal diagnosis, Kris's cancer remains small and stable. She has dedicated her life to encouraging people to take control of their health with a plant-based diet and healthy lifestyle and has written five books on this topic, including the *New York Times* best-sellers *Crazy Sexy Kitchen* and *Crazy Sexy Diet*.

The scientific research on plant-based diets backs up Kris's lifestyle choices. Looking at a collective body of research on the impact of diet on illness over a 15-year time span, a team of researchers from across the United States determined that a diet rich in vegetables, fruit, plant-based proteins (e.g., beans), and whole grains significantly decreased the risk of illness, cardiovascular disease, and cancer by 12–28 percent.[26] In a similar meta-analysis, a team of researchers in Canada studying the relationship between colon cancer and diet found that eating either a meat-centric or sugar-centric diet significantly increased one's risk of getting colon cancer, while eating a plant-based diet significantly decreased that risk.[27]

Canada as a whole has taken a keen interest in keeping its citizens healthy by promoting a healthy diet. In 2019, Health Canada updated *Canada's Food Guide* so that the "what you should eat plate" is now composed of 50 percent vegetables and fruits, with water as the drink of choice instead of milk.[28] Specifically, the report recommends eating "plenty of vegetables and fruits, whole grains, and protein foods, and to choose protein foods that come from plants more often."[29] What makes Canada's report different from most other countries' reports is that Health Canada purposefully excluded industry-commissioned studies when coming up with the new guidelines, due to the potential conflicts of interest.[30] Go Canada!

One plant-based diet advocate who seconds Canada's findings is Liana Werner-Gray, a holistic health and nutrition coach and author of the best-selling books *The Earth Diet* and *Cancer-Free with Food*. Liana healed herself naturally of early-stage throat cancer through diet and lifestyle changes. She was inspired by the Aboriginal elders near her childhood home in Australia who ate only whole, organic foods from the earth, lived long lives, and rarely got sick. Liana believes everyone can benefit from eating highly nutritious foods, especially if you are in a health crisis.

*Health is a choice we make from moment to moment. Raw, whole, plant-based foods—those that are consumed in their natural, unrefined state—provide us with the enzymes and life-force energy we need to survive and thrive. Foods that come to us relatively intact have more nutrients. Eating whole foods from the earth that are chemical-free strengthens the immune system and increases energy.*

Eating a plant-based diet can seem like an obvious choice when you consider that nature has provided everything we need to survive as a species. Increasing your intake of fruits and vegetables is one of the easiest dietary changes you can make because of their wide availability at grocery stores and in restaurants. You can even grow your own. Of course, eating more fruits and vegetables will require a mind shift if you grew up in a meat-and-potatoes home. Start by gradually increasing the fraction of your plate devoted to vegetables and fruits until they make up half of every meal. This small change will make a big difference by giving your body an optimal amount of healing nutrients, while naturally reducing the portion of your diet devoted to meat and potatoes.

## The Ketogenic Diet (featuring Bone Broth)

The ketogenic diet has surged in popularity over the past few years. The keto diet strictly limits carbohydrates (typically only 50 grams per day, or the equivalent of two apples), thereby greatly reducing your glucose levels. The diet also increases the amount of fat you consume. Making these changes forces your cells to get their energy from fat instead of from glucose. When your cells derive their energy from fat, the process is called ketosis, in which ketones (acids) are released into your bloodstream.

The ketogenic diet remains controversial because there are no long-term studies on its healthfulness. Over the short term, though, it has helped some patients achieve remission and has been shown to ease chemotherapy- and radiation-related side effects. Cancers that seem to respond well to the keto diet include glioblastoma,[31] neuroblastoma, colon, pancreatic, lung, and prostate cancers.[32] In addition, the diet has helped patients with neurologic diseases like epilepsy and Alzheimer's.[33] One recent review in Austria concluded that the keto diet was a beneficial addition to conventional cancer therapy that could be used safely alongside conventional radiation treatment and chemotherapy.[34]

When two pediatric brain cancer patients were switched to a ketogenic diet, researchers found a 21.8 percent average decrease in glucose uptake at the tumor site in both subjects.[35] Since cancer cells metabolize, or "feed on," glucose, a decrease in glucose uptake indicates a decrease in cancer cell activity. In a similar case report, a 65-year-old woman with glioblastoma multiforme—an extremely lethal type of brain cancer—was suffering from progressive memory loss, chronic headaches, and nausea.[36] She was given a combination treatment of water-only therapeutic fasting; a calorie-restricted, four-to-one ketogenic diet (four parts fat to one part carbohydrate and/or protein, with a maximum of 600 kilocalories per day), and supplementation with personalized vitamins and minerals. After only two months on this treatment, no discernable brain tumor tissue was detected using PET and magnetic resonance imaging (MRI). Her body showed reduced levels of blood glucose and elevated levels of urinary ketones. Unfortunately, when the patient stopped this strict diet therapy, she experienced a tumor recurrence 10 weeks later.

Bone broth, one of the superstars of the ketogenic diet, reflects a centuries-old tradition valued for its health benefits. The French call it *consommé*, Latinos and Italians call it *brodo*. Your mother may have made you chicken soup—with bone broth—when you were sick. Before the invention of canned/boxed broths and stocks, you would likely find a pot of bone broth brewing in every grandmother's kitchen. You will still find it in most restaurant kitchens today because a good bone broth/stock is every chef's secret weapon to add delicious depth and fatty flavor to soups, stews, gravies, and sauces. Today, savory bone broths have regained popularity for their nutrient and mineral density.

Proponents of bone broth for health believe the broth's amino acids, gelatin, and collagen help boost immunity, fight inflammation, and repair the digestive tract.[37] Traditional Chinese medicine practitioners recommend bone broth to support digestive health, strengthen the blood, and fortify the kidneys.

However, many vegetarian and vegan advocates disagree with aspects of the ketogenic diet, particularly its reliance on fat, since most ketogenic followers get their fat from meat sources. It is possible, although more difficult, to eat a ketogenic diet from entirely plant-based sources, such as avocados, nuts, and coconuts. A best-selling book on this topic is *Ketotarian* by Will Cole.

Many radical remission survivors have had success with the ketogenic diet, including Alison from Chapter 6, but it is not the right diet for everyone. It is important that you first consult with your doctor, naturopath, or nutritionist to determine if it is an appropriate diet for you and to learn how to monitor your ketones for safety, as having too many ketones in your bloodstream can be dangerous.

## Cancer as a Metabolic Disease

If modern medicine has learned anything about cancer in the last 50 years, it is that cancer is not a simple disease. In fact, it is not a single disease, but hundreds of different diseases, each with mitochondrial dysfunction at its center. In *Radical Remission*, I wrote about the German biologist Otto Heinrich Warburg, who won the Nobel Prize in medicine for his discovery that cancer cells are healthy cells that have been damaged in such a way that they now feed on glucose instead of on oxygen. Because of this discovery, Warburg theorized that cancer is a disease of improper cell metabolism, and his theory is what has inspired the idea—currently popular among scientists—that cancer is a metabolic disease. In brief, Warburg's metabolic theory of cancer states that damage to a cell's mitochondria is what causes a cell to become cancerous.

Mitochondria are the "energy factories" of our cells, and they are in charge of using oxygen to produce energy, telling the cell when to reproduce, and telling it when to die. A cell that has become cancerous does the exact *opposite* of a healthy cell—it reproduces uncontrollably, does not die when it is supposed to, and gets its energy from glucose instead of oxygen.

A leading expert on the metabolic theory of cancer is Dr. Nasha Winters, the naturopathic oncologist we read about in Alison's story and co-author of *The Metabolic Approach to Cancer*. I first learned of Dr. Winters via her own radical remission story. Dr. Winters was diagnosed with stage 4 ovarian cancer in an emergency room when she was only 19 years old, and her doctors gave her only a few months to live. Crippled with severe pain, ascites, nausea, the inability to eat, and being severely cachectic due to her cancer, Nasha was uninsured and out of options. She scoured her local library for holistic healing options and ultimately charted her own healing path, which evolved into a 28-year journey that continues to this day.

Nasha started naturopathic medical school five years after receiving her terminal diagnosis. Because she was still dealing with her own health issues, she was able to apply everything she learned to herself first before later recommending it to her patients. Now a highly respected expert, Dr. Winters trains doctors on the metabolic approach to cancer treatment. She says:

> *Study after study shows that only 5–10 percent of cancer is caused by damaged DNA. These inherited mutations cause cancer only if said mutations also alter mitochondrial function. The remaining 90–95 percent of cancer cases are caused by poor diet and unhealthy lifestyles that also damage mitochondrial function. A stunningly effective cancer treatment is available right at the grocery store: food! I have been using low-glycemic [i.e., blood-sugar lowering], calorie-restricted, fasting, and keto-genic dietary approaches with my patients for several decades, with incredible results.*

Today, Dr. Winters still has tumors present in her body, but she has managed to keep them small and stable by treating her cancer as if it were a metabolic disease.

The idea that we have the power to repair damaged mitochondria and thereby reverse cancer through diet and lifestyle changes is highly empowering, and researchers are studying it intensely. The diet that is most often recommended by those who subscribe to the metabolic theory of cancer is the ketogenic diet.

## Intermittent Fasting

When was the last time you went hungry for more than an hour, whether you were sick or not? In the developed world, hunger is an unfamiliar feeling. Yet fasting—the voluntary practice of not consuming food for a period of time—is one of the most ancient healing traditions. Virtually every culture and religion on earth has practiced fasting in some shape or form. For example, around 400 B.C., Hippocrates recorded prolonged periods of fasting as a medical therapy,[38] supposedly saying, "To eat when you are sick is to feed your sickness." When animals get sick, including dogs and cats, most curl up somewhere safe to sleep, refusing food (but not water) until they feel better. Humans are the only species that forces food consumption when sick, and it has only been in the last 50 years that we have been able to eat quick, processed meals at any time of the day or night.

Proponents of intermittent fasting believe that our bodies have not evolved quickly enough to handle this steady stream of high-calorie food. Some researchers have been studying the effects of intermittent fasting, which mimics the way humans ate more than 300 years ago, when food was not so readily available.

Intermittent fasting gives your digestive system a break by restricting your food intake for a limited time period so that it can process the food you have eaten, absorb its nutrients, and allow your body to focus on other functions, including healing, rest, and repair. Food digestion in your small intestine requires approximately 40 percent of your body's energy,[39] leaving limited energy to focus on other things.

Intermittent fasting (IF) is a critical component of the ketogenic diet because it can induce ketosis. The break from eating leads to a break from glucose, which causes your body to burn fat for its energy, thereby creating ketones. Researchers of the ketogenic diet believe that ketones may be an evolutionary survival mechanism that protects against genetic damage[40] and may reduce glucose, insulin, and IGF-1 (insulin-like growth factor 1) levels,[41] all of which improve your health and immune system.

The most straightforward method of intermittent fasting is time-restricted intermittent fasting, in which you limit your eating windows to 12 hours a day (or 10, or 8). In this scenario, you might eat your dinner at 6 P.M. and not eat again until 6 the next morning. During the 12 hours when your body is not eating, it has the time it needs to digest your dinner before you go to sleep and can focus on rest and repair for the remainder of the 12 hours. People who practice IF with shorter eating windows might start their day with a late breakfast or end it with an early dinner.

Another method of fasting is the 5:2 intermittent fast, in which you restrict yourself to 400–600 calories a day for two days per week, and then eat normally the other five days. Yet another method is to do a full water fast one day a week. If you decide you want to try intermittent fasting beyond the basic, 12-hour time-restricted method, you should consult with your doctor or health professional first to determine which IF methods are safe for your body.

Researchers have only recently begun to study the impact of intermittent fasting on cancer. The initial studies show that intermittent fasting greatly helps during chemotherapy. One such study found that intermittent fasting enhances the ability of nerve cells to repair DNA, protects DNA from damage caused by chemotherapy, and switches on a number of DNA repair genes.[42] Another study revealed that fasting cycles slowed the growth of cancerous tumors and made a range of cancer cell types more vulnerable to chemotherapy.[43] In yet another study, fasting was shown to enhance the patient's responsiveness to chemotherapy, as well as reduce its side effects.[44]

One promising study on fasting followed nearly 2,500 women with early-stage breast cancer (but who did not have diabetes) and analyzed their dinner and breakfast times over the course of four years.[45] The researchers found that a fasting window shorter than 13 hours per night was associated with a 36 percent higher chance of breast cancer recurrence, compared with fasting 13 or more hours per night. In addition, markers for insulin, chronic inflammation, and sleep duration were positively impacted by longer nightly fasts.

Researchers who wanted to understand the effects of a fasting-mimicking diet, that is, a diet very low in calories,[46] created a study with 100 healthy people and randomly divided them into two groups. One group followed an unrestricted diet (the control group), and a second group followed an unrestricted diet except for five consecutive days per month when they ate a low-calorie, fasting-mimicking diet. After three months, those who had been on the fasting-mimicking diet experienced a significant reduction in body weight, total body fat, blood pressure, and IGF-1 (which has been implicated in aging and diseases) compared to the control group participants, with no adverse effects reported.[47]

The fasting studies conducted thus far have indicated that a nightly fast of more than 13 hours is safe and highly beneficial for most people and that additional fasting protocols—such as the 5:2 intermittent fast or a restricted-calorie diet for five consecutive days per month—bring with them health benefits that can help strengthen your immune system and may slow the growth of cancer.

## Gut Health and Your Microbiome

There has been a lot of press in recent years about the gut and the role of the microbiome, and with good reason. Discovering the gut's connection to health has been one of the most important advances in health research during the past few decades. What we find most exciting is that you can take concrete action steps to improve the state of your microbiome and the way your body digests food.

Consider the fact that 70 percent of your immune system resides in your gastrointestinal system.[48] The human digestive tract hosts trillions of bacteria, some helpful and some harmful.[49] The good bacteria help your immune system prevent infection, produce vitamins, and metabolize hormones.[50] The bad bacteria cause infection, reduce nutrient absorption, and lead to poor digestion and elimination.

Your intestines are absolutely key to the health of your body. If you were to cut open and lay flat all your intestines on the ground, they would cover an incredible 400 square meters, which is about the size of a tennis court![51] That's a lot of surface area to protect. Therefore, it is not surprising that the intestinal tract requires about 40 percent of your body's energy to do its dual job of digesting and absorbing nutrients while simultaneously preventing the absorption of harmful substances, bacteria, and viruses.[52]

In a sense, the intestinal wall is the "bouncer" of your body, and the important security role it plays determines your intestinal permeability. The small intestine provides an interface between your body and the outside world. On the other hand, this barrier must be open enough to absorb essential nutrients and fluids from your food and liquid intake.[53] When this function breaks down, it can lead to severe immune system deficiency and an increased risk of disease, including cancer.[54,55]

Many things can damage your intestinal wall, including aspirin, ibuprofen, or naproxen; alcohol, milk, or a diet high in carbohydrates and/or fats; and chronic stress, nutrient deficiencies, or treatments like chemotherapy and radiation.[56] Each person's body is different, though, and not everything on that list will damage your microbiome. When your intestinal wall is too permeable and allows things to be absorbed into your body that should not be absorbed, you suffer from a condition known as leaky gut. (We talked about leaky gut in Palmer's story in Chapter 5.)

Just as having healthy intestinal permeability is a crucial component of a strong immune system, so is having a healthy microbiome, the trillions of bacteria and microbes that live permanently inside your intestines.[57] An unhealthy microbiome has been shown to significantly and directly impact your mental and physical health and can increase your chances of developing a wide range of conditions, including cancer, cardiometabolic diseases, allergies, and obesity.[58]

Several studies have illustrated the direct connection between your brain, gut, and microbiome.[59] Did you know that your gut microbes can communicate directly with your central nervous, endocrine, and immune systems?[60] In one study, researchers gathered data from the gut microbiomes of 2,000 people over the course of six years[61] and reviewed the subjects' lifestyle factors, along with taking stool, serum, and urine samples. By analyzing the changes in the subjects' gut microbiota over time, the data suggest that poor lifestyle choices can lead to an unhealthy microbiome, which in turn promotes the progression of cardiometabolic diseases, including obesity.[62]

Esophageal cancer, one of the most deadly forms of cancer,[63] may be caused by several factors, including the use of antibiotics, poor dietary choices, and cigarette smoking[64]—all of which are known to disrupt the gut microbiome. A group of researchers who reviewed numerous studies on the role the microbiome plays in esophageal cancer found that the gut microbiome of people with a healthy esophagus was significantly different from the gut microbiome of people with esophageal cancer, with the cancer microbiomes containing far more bad bacteria than non-cancer microbiomes.[65]

Other factors can negatively impact your microbiome. Due to our culture's obsession with cleanliness, cosmetics and hand sanitizers that include the antibacterial chemical triclosan are very popular, but this chemical has been shown to stimulate the growth of estrogen-dependent cancer cells (like those found in many breast cancer patients).[66] In addition, taking broad-spectrum antibiotics kills not only the bad bacteria that make us sick but also the beneficial bacteria that keep our microbiomes in balance. As a result, taking antibiotics unnecessarily or too frequently can allow opportunistic, bad bacteria and fungi (such as candida) to flourish in our intestines, which can cause health complications long after we finish our final dose of antibiotics.

While we don't yet fully understand the microbiome, scientists are working to fill in the gaps in our knowledge. Research is underway regarding the connection between the microbiome and cancer risk, treatment, and side effects.[67,68,69]

The good news is that there are many actionable dietary and lifestyle changes you can make to keep your microbiome healthy. For instance, eating a vegetable-rich diet that is high in natural fiber has been shown to support microbial diversity in your gut, while a diet made up of mostly refined carbohydrates and starches has not.[70] This is because fiber is technically a prebiotic, which is not digestible by the human body and is never actually absorbed into your bloodstream.

However, the trillions of healthy microorganisms that make up your microbiome *can* digest that fiber, so they feed on it in order to grow and diversify. In this way, eating food that is high in fiber is a way to feed the microbiome. There are many delicious, naturally fermented foods that are probiotic in nature and can therefore help feed your microbiome, including sauerkraut (fermented cabbage), kimchi (fermented cabbage and radish), and kombucha (fermented tea).

If you're ready to throw in the towel on changing your diet because it's just too confusing, keep in mind that hundreds of studies have shown that we can change our health with basic food choices. Dean Ornish, M.D., a recognized leader in medicine for more than 40 years and author of six *New York Times* best-selling books, including *Undo It! How Simple Lifestyle Changes Can Reverse Most Chronic Diseases*, summarizes radically changing your diet for health in this way:

> *We often have a hard time believing that the simple choices that we make in our lives each day—what we eat, how we respond to stress, how much exercise we get, and how much love and intimacy we have—can make a powerful difference in our health and well-being, but they do. For more than 33 years, my colleagues and I have found that a whole-food, plant-based diet, moderate exercise, stress management techniques such as yoga and meditation, and learning to give and receive love more fully could often reverse the progression of coronary heart disease, early-stage prostate cancer, type 2 diabetes, high blood pressure, obesity, depression, and other chronic diseases.*

After reviewing the medical literature on diet as it relates to cancer and health, we can offer some general advice:

- Regardless of whether you and your health team decide that a plant-based, ketogenic, or Mediterranean diet is best for you, remember that these diets encourage eating whole, unprocessed foods that are high in fiber and rich in vegetables (though on the ketogenic diet, only specific vegetables are allowed).

- Talk to your health team about experimenting with periods of fasting, whether intermittently (between dinner and breakfast), or for a few days per month.

Changing your diet may seem daunting at first, but we hope that our breakdown of the latest diet trends and research studies have helped clarify some of the confusion around this topic and inspired you to take action. Changing your diet is hands-on and highly actionable—it is something you can *do*—which is why it has been the first step for so many radical remission survivors.

One such survivor is Jeremiah whose parents, Tanya and Gene, utilized the 10 radical remission healing factors to help heal their baby boy's rare lymphoma, although changing his diet was one of the most major changes they made.

# Jeremiah's Story

A cancer diagnosis is terrifying for anyone, but when it is your child, it is even more gut-wrenching. And when the diagnosis is for your newborn baby, it is excruciating. This is what happened to Tanya Gomez and her partner, Gene, when their son Jeremiah was born in 2010.

Initially, Jeremiah was healthy and happy, and their hearts were bursting as he began to smile, coo, and laugh with them in their Southern California home. Tanya had always followed a healthy diet and lifestyle herself, so she was determined to give Jeremiah the healthiest food she could once he was old enough to eat solid food. As Jeremiah grew bigger and bigger each day, Tanya reveled in his milestones. But one month after his standard immunizations, when Jeremiah was five months old, Tanya and Gene noticed a lump on his chest about the size of a dime. The lump was harder and bulkier than the rest of his baby-soft skin, so although Jeremiah seemed otherwise happy and healthy, they took him to see a doctor right away. Their doctor was concerned enough that he biopsied the lump.

As soon as the doctor entered the room with the biopsy results, Tanya knew it was something serious, but she never in her wildest nightmares imagined it would be cancer. Unfortunately, it was. Jeremiah was diagnosed with subcutaneous panniculitis-like T-cell lymphoma (SPTCL), a rare form of skin lymphoma. Tanya remembers:

> My tears came down and I only had one question: "Is it curable?" In that moment he said, "There are options for chemo. You're going to need to talk to the oncologist. We're going to do further studies." And I said, "Okay." But as soon as I left and we were driving away, I told Gene, "We're not doing chemo."

Tanya did not dismiss the potential effectiveness of chemo, but was concerned about its efficacy and the side effects it would have on her little baby. Jeremiah's doctors told Tanya and Gene this rare cancer was one that was ordinarily diagnosed in 15- to 35-year-olds. That meant that there were no well-researched chemotherapy regimens for children as young as Jeremiah, so the doctors did not have a clear idea about how effective the treatment would be or how harmful the side effects would be. The chemotherapy regimen typically used for this kind of lymphoma is so strong that the doctors said it would kill a baby; therefore, they were going to use a child leukemia regimen instead.

Tanya knew from reading the fine print of the side effects of the chemotherapy the doctors were suggesting that Jeremiah could end up with permanent and severe vision and immunodeficiency problems. They also told her Jeremiah would need around 40 spinal tap procedures to deliver all the chemo treatments, which could lead to brain damage. Because the doctors were uncertain if this chemotherapy would cure Jeremiah's cancer—they even asked Tanya to sign a waiver of responsibility in case Jeremiah died during treatment—Tanya's intuition told her to begin researching alternative options.

Right away, many of her friends called her "crazy" for trying to find other ways to help her son. Gene wanted to follow the doctor's recommendations and just go with the chemotherapy. Nevertheless, Tanya listened to her intuition as a mother and researched as much as she could about Jeremiah's cancer. Tanya's father was the only person to initially support her holistic approach.

By the time Jeremiah's doctors finally tested his bone marrow to help them understand the extent of Jeremiah's lymphoma, an entire month had passed since his original diagnosis. At this point, multiple skin lesions had appeared on his body and Tanya was becoming frantic. The results of the test showed that his bone marrow was comprised of 7 percent cancer cells, as opposed to the 3 percent considered normal. Tanya felt let down by the delays and lack of research behind the suggested chemotherapy treatment.

*I said [to the oncologist], "He's not an animal. And I feel that you are treating us like a number. I love my son and it's my job to make sure he gets the proper treatment, and I just don't feel like he's getting it here. I need you guys to splice the biopsy samples because I'm going to be sending them to other hospitals. I want to know what they have to say about it. And I'm going to choose whoever's going to give us the proper service, because I feel you guys are dropping the ball." So immediately— the next day!—they gave me an appointment. I don't know how [the hospital] fit that in 'cause they always would say it takes about two weeks because they're so full.*

Tanya fully explained chemotherapy's long-term side effects, which Jeremiah would have to live with for the rest of his life, to Gene and their families so they could understand where she was coming from. Gene was understandably wary of using alternative methods against the recommendations of their conventional medical doctors, so she overprepared for every medical appointment, including requesting advance copies of any test results, which was her right as the mother of the patient. Through her research, she also found a case report on PubMed.gov of a two-year-old child in Croatia with Jeremiah's same diagnosis who was now in remission.

This was a case that the doctors had either not found or chosen not to share with them. Tanya never viewed her son's doctors as superior or smarter than she was; instead, she just saw them as specialists who had a knowledge base that she did not have.

In addition to intravenous chemotherapy, the doctors were suggesting approximately 40 spinal taps on Jeremiah in an attempt to directly treat his brain with chemotherapy by infusing it into his spinal fluid. This concerned Tanya for two reasons: First, Jeremiah did not show signs of cancer in his brain; and second, multiple spinal taps could leave him with brain damage, impairing him for the rest of his life. Every doctor they went to suggested this, and Tanya wanted Gene to know exactly what this would do to Jeremiah.

> *What I started to ask was, "What's going to happen? What are the side effects [of the spinal fluid chemotherapy]?" And they said, "If he reaches for a cup, he'll think it's to the left, but the cup will be on the right side—so his vision will be distorted. He might have some kind of brain damage as a result. With his kidneys, he'll probably urinate blood. And he'll get sick a lot." And I said, "Well, if he'll get sick a lot, can't I just quarantine him and keep him in the house?" And they said, "No, that's not going to help because it's all going to come from his own body." And I'm like, "What do you mean, 'from his own body'?" And they said, "Because we're going to kill off his immune system"—which was already compromised! And as soon as we drove out of there, Gene told me, "I'm sure I don't want to do chemo anymore."*

At this point, it had been three months since Jeremiah's diagnosis, and Tanya had been using that time to search for clinics outside of the United States. She searched for these clinics discreetly, as she had talked to other parents who wanted to give their children an alternative to chemotherapy and heard awful stories. One mother, whom Tanya calls "Sarah," reached out to Tanya to warn her of what might happen if they decided to have Jeremiah treated outside the United States with alternative treatment. Sarah recounted how a child was taken by the authorities and that chemo was forced on the child.

Tanya was shocked to hear these stories, and they made her more wary of the U.S. health care system. She talked to a social worker in her family and learned that as long as both parents consented, they could theoretically treat their child wherever they wanted. Tanya intuitively knew that treating Jeremiah abroad was the right thing to do and she was willing to give up her U.S. citizenship and her entire life to do so, but she needed to make sure that Gene was fully on board before leaving the country to treat Jeremiah.

Another obstacle was Jeremiah's age. He was only eight months old when Gene agreed to treatments other than chemotherapy, and most of the clinics abroad were wary of treating an infant, because Jeremiah's immune and digestive systems were not yet developed enough to withstand the clinics' standard treatments. Just as large doses of chemo would be more harmful than helpful to Jeremiah, the clinics that focused on alternative treatments were equally wary that their typical doses would be harmful. Tanya searched for clinics primarily in Mexico and South America and finally found one in Chile that agreed to treat baby Jeremiah. As soon as she described Jeremiah's case, they told her they were hopeful they could help him heal.

Thankfully, Jeremiah's whole family rallied behind his parents' unorthodox decision. Tanya recalls:

*Once Gene agreed to go to Chile, it took us two days to organize a fund-raiser. His whole family and my whole family came together for this cancer thing. It was amazing! My brother had a huge backyard. So we organized what's called a kermés. A kermés is when everybody brings something either to sell or to purchase. Some sold drinks, tamales, posole, etc. We invited everyone we knew. My brother sold carne asada tacos. A family member of Gene's owned a bakery, and they brought cakes to raffle off. My cousins knew how to make muffins with really cool designs, which they sold. People did raffles for me. It was* *amazing to see all the help during these moments. That day of the kermés we raised about $12,000.*

Thanks to the generosity of friends, family, and strangers, Tanya was able to book tickets for herself, Gene, and Jeremiah two days later. The plan was for Gene to accompany them for one week while she stayed for 45 days in Chile with Jeremiah. So, on a sunny day in December 2010, they got on a plane with eight-month-old Jeremiah to begin his 45-day treatment regimen. Although Jeremiah had three large, cancerous skin lesions, Tanya felt hopeful and was determined not to let her family down.

This particular clinic followed the teachings of Don Manuel Lezaeta Acharán, a pioneer of natural medicine in Chile who passed away in 1959. Tanya's father had a book she had read that outlined his teachings, so Tanya had an idea of what to expect. Essentially, the clinic would focus on giving Jeremiah's body the tools to fight off disease naturally, instead of using treatments to fight the disease directly. This appealed to Tanya because she was already familiar with the importance of a healthy diet and life-style, the cornerstones of the clinic's treatments.

Upon arrival, the doctors recommended a strict diet change, which Jeremiah began immediately. The first change they made was to put him on a vegan diet, asking him to consume specific foods in a specific order throughout the day. The clinic was very focused on optimizing digestion and on the negative effects an overworked stomach can have on the body. In order to optimize nutrient absorption, the clinicians aimed to keep his stomach's internal temperature low, since a higher temperature would indicate (according to their theory) that the stomach was overworking.

Tanya had stopped nursing when Jeremiah was four months old. The doctors at the clinic told her that breast milk would have been the best milk for Jeremiah at this time, but that there were other options. On his new diet, baby Jeremiah drank home-made, blanched almond milk blended in a baby bottle with oatmeal, apples, and raisins every morning, and throughout the day as needed.

Jeremiah began eating solid foods while at the clinic. He had oatmeal and apple about an hour later for breakfast, a basic meal of potatoes, spinach, and other vegetables mashed together in broth for lunch, and a similarly vegan meal for dinner. The center prepared three fresh green juices a day for Jeremiah in between meals. Getting an infant to drink three green juices a day made with kale, green apples, spinach, and carrots was a huge challenge, and Tanya had to use every strategy she could think of to incentivize him to drink the juice.

A worker at the clinic would come in every mealtime to help Tanya prepare the food for Jeremiah and would help clean and maintain the cooking supplies. Tanya was more involved than most caregivers at the clinic because she wanted to learn how to make the food for Jeremiah at home after his time at the clinic was over.

In accordance with the clinic's theories on optimizing stomach and intestinal temperatures, Jeremiah received a variety of daily thermal treatments. First, the nurses would wake him early each morning to assist Tanya with the first thermal treatment. Tanya would run a cold, wet cloth over Jeremiah's body in a specific way that was meant to shock his body while releasing toxins and activating his lymphatic system. Immediately after, Tanya would wrap him in blankets and put him back to sleep. Warming the body again was essential, according to the clinic doctors. Later, when Jeremiah awoke naturally, he would eat his breakfast.

Around noon, the patients at the clinic were usually due for a steam bath. Jeremiah was too small to have a steam bath, so instead he was wrapped in a warm, damp towel and then in layers of blankets, at which point he would fall asleep. This made him sweat profusely, simulating a steam bath. After an hour, the wrap was removed and Jeremiah would usually sleep a bit more. When he awoke, he would receive a clay pack treatment that involved covering his skin with a thin layer of clay brought in from nearby mountains.

To put the clay on Jeremiah, Tanya would take a clean square cloth the size of his belly, spread the wet clay on the cloth, and place it on Jeremiah's belly. She would then wrap his belly with a fleece cloth and, on top of that, a receiving blanket. This would keep his core body temperature cool, and the blankets were to avoid any airflow getting into the belly area. He stayed like this for two hours, during which Tanya would give him a bottle of almond milk (blended with oatmeal, apples, and raisins) to hold him over until lunch. If it was warm enough, he would often crawl around outside to absorb vitamin D from the sun and walk barefoot (with Tanya's help) to absorb the energy of the earth. In between treatments, Jeremiah would have time to practice his walking around the clinic with Tanya or play outside, and he would eat his last meal around 6 P.M. before going to sleep.

Jeremiah's cancer helped supercharge Tanya's and her family's spirituality and their Catholic faith. Right after Jeremiah's diagnosis, Tanya and Gene would host rosaries and invite their families over to join them in prayer. Tanya prayed every morning and every night for Jeremiah's health, and she says she talked with God regularly. As a result, Jeremiah grew up praying every night as well.

Tanya questioned God a lot in the beginning, but she never lost faith. She would often break down crying and ask God, "Why Jeremiah? Why choose *him* to have cancer?" Tanya came to believe that Jeremiah's cancer had a divine purpose.

> *I knew then that God chose me for a specific reason. He knew what I was going to do for Jeremiah and He knew the outcome. He had chosen me for this purpose. He knew that if Jeremiah had this, that it would be one less child that suffered through chemo because of what I was going to do for him. It's so important that people know there's another option.*

Tanya remembers vividly a time during Jeremiah's treatment in Chile when she feared that he would not survive the cancer and that the treatment would not work. One of the nurses Tanya had come to know well stopped her and said,

> *Tanya, everything that happens in this hospital is because of that guy [pointing upward]. We just help Him. So, you keep*

*your faith and you keep asking Him what you need, because if
you don't ask, you won't receive.*

Tanya took the nurse's advice and continued to ask God for
help. Shortly after that, on day 35 of their 45-day treatment, one of
the doctors came to check on Jeremiah. Tanya expressed concern
that one of his lesions was changing—it appeared to be breaking
up into three sections, with soft skin in between. The doctor told
her that was a sign of the cancer retreating. Tanya felt instantly as
if God had answered her prayers, and she couldn't hold back her
tears of joy and relief.

She and baby Jeremiah continued with the intensive schedule of two to three thermal treatments, three juices, and three
vegan meals a day. Jeremiah was a star patient, crawling around
and cheering up everyone with his baby smile.

*[Jeremiah's] cells regenerate at a much faster rate than
adults' [cells]. So whatever Jeremiah was doing, it was working
10 times faster than it would on an adult's body. That's the
difference with Jeremiah. The doctor said that Jeremiah was the
best patient he'd ever had in terms of how his cells turned over.
It was amazing to see! Everybody was so amazed. By the 45th
day [at the clinic], all three of his lesions had disappeared. Most
people don't have those [kind of] results before they leave the
clinic. Jeremiah had those results at the clinic.*

Tanya and Jeremiah returned to the U.S. after the 45-day treatment
was finished, but she waited a year after their return from the clinic
to have Jeremiah's U.S. doctors conduct another bone marrow
test, from which they would gauge what was happening with
his cancer. She was hesitant, since it is a very painful procedure
for anyone, much less a toddler. When Jeremiah was eventually
tested, his oncologist was shocked to discover that Jeremiah had
fewer cancer cells (less than 3 percent) than a healthy patient.

*The doctors said, "Everyone's bone marrow has about 3 percent abnormal cells. Your son tested less than 3 percent! Your son went from being one of the sickest children we've ever seen to one of the healthiest. We did all the tests and we can't find any cancer in his blood or bone marrow, and the lesions are all gone. At this point, we do not recommend doing any chemo. You may come back for annual testing."*

After hearing that there were no more cancer cells in Jeremiah's bone marrow, Tanya thanked God for letting her son live and for giving him a chance at a normal life. Tanya credits her spiritual faith and her father for keeping her focused and confident throughout the process. She faced doubts from everywhere—from doctors, friends, family, and even herself—but her faith in God kept her determined to carry on and seek the best life possible for her son.

Once Jeremiah's treatment at the Chilean clinic ended, the clinic doctors recommended that he maintain his vegan diet for three years, after which point he could ease up on the restrictions little by little. However, Tanya wanted to be extra cautious, so she kept Jeremiah on the vegan diet for five more years, until he was six years old. By that time, he was happy to continue eating just as he had his entire life.

Jeremiah's U.S. doctors recommended yearly check-ins. However, Tanya intuitively felt that if she followed the same strict diet and monitored his health via his skin, nails, and countenance, she would not need to subject Jeremiah to testing so often. Therefore, she waited until 2018 to subject him to another blood test and examination. Once again, the test results confirmed that Jeremiah was still cancer-free eight years after his diagnosis and subsequent natural treatment. The doctor said, "Whatever you're doing, keep it up!"

Today, Jeremiah is a happy, easygoing, and cancer-free nine-year-old boy and fourth grader who loves baseball, basketball, drawing, and being silly. To this day, he has never tried beef or pork. Tanya added limited quantities of organic, farm-raised chicken, wild-caught fish, and organic cheese to his diet when he was around six, but he still mostly keeps to a vegan diet. He drinks fresh green juices frequently, but what is most important to Tanya is that Jeremiah is learning how to eat healthfully. Jeremiah loves vegetables and proclaims that his mom "makes some mean veggie tacos." They have fruit trees outside their house, from which they pick fresh fruit almost daily, and Tanya still makes homemade almond milk.

*I try to make things for him that are [sweet]. I'll make crepes, my own version of them, and I'll make a nice blueberry jam. If it's healthy, yummy, and sweet, it takes effort, because it doesn't have the syrups or the bad, refined sugars in it. So I try to give him as much of a normal life as possible, but just my version of it. He has tasted sweets and does like them, but I tell him we can't have them here [in the house] and we can't take them home with us, but that he can have unlimited fruit. He loves fruit, especially honeydew melon and tangerines.*

Exercise was not officially prescribed by the clinic when Jeremiah was being treated because he was still a baby at the time. However, Tanya has always strongly encouraged Jeremiah to maintain movement and exercise as a core part of his life. She believes that staying active will help keep her son's cancer from coming back.

*He's a different kid when he's playing—very competitive, very mobile, very agile. He gets into it! Even playing one-on-one basketball with him, he gets aggressive when he drives [the ball]. It's the opposite of him talking [in normal life]. I'm very athletic myself, and Jeremiah gets a lot of extra help with athletics from both his dad and me. I love CrossFit and he's gotten into it, so he does his own little workout by my side. It is really neat to see him work out—he gets so into it!*

Jeremiah's friends and family have played a key role in his continued good health. It is not easy for a young child to live with significant dietary restrictions. Thankfully, Jeremiah's friends and family have supported him by not eating sweets in front of him. His journey has inspired his entire family—both his mother's and father's sides—to change their lifestyles. He has influenced both sides of the family to go organic and start juicing. This willingness to adapt to and accommodate Jeremiah's diet has not only helped him fit in better but has also given Tanya more peace of mind. She knows she can count on her family and friends to support Jeremiah, no matter what.

> *It all comes down to self-motivation and the support group you have around you. It comes down to you, because nobody can see if you're cheating [on the diet] or not. When [Jeremiah] was a baby, or when he was growing up and we were at family functions, his dad, family, and the cousins would never eat candy in front of him. If someone ate cake, they wouldn't eat it in front of him. For little cousins' birthdays, they would bake something different for Jeremiah. They are so supportive of his health and his diet. Stress is a big problem when fighting cancer. I believe the fact that Jeremiah had no clue of any of this was a huge help to his own body.*

Tanya and Gene ultimately split as a couple, but have remained friends and are in alignment when it comes to maintaining Jeremiah's healthy diet and lifestyle. Thanks to dietary changes, thermal treatments, and the love and support of his mother, father, and extended family, Jeremiah was able to recover from severe cancer when he was only 10 months old. Now nearly 10 years old, he remains cancer-free.

Jeremiah does not remember anything about his treatment because he was so young at the time, and as a result he may not fully appreciate his radical remission. However, every time Tanya watches him throw a baseball, run around outside with his friends, or pick up a fork for a bite to eat, she is grateful for the normal, healthy life her little boy gets to live.

# Action Steps

In *Radical Remission*, I noted that some people are able to go "cold turkey" and completely change their diets overnight. However, most people cannot change that quickly and therefore need to tackle it in stages. One way to do this is by eliminating one thing at a time (e.g., one less dessert, portion of meat, or serving of refined grains per day) or adding in at least one more vegetable or fruit to every meal. You can start small by making sure you buy organic fruits and vegetables—at least when it comes to the Dirty Dozen (the 12 fruits and veggies with the highest exposure to pesticides from conventional farming)—easing back your alcohol consumption, or adding a select few organic, grass-fed, hormone-free meat or dairy products to your weekly shopping.

In addition to the major diet changes described in this chapter, which you should discuss with your doctor, here are some additional ideas to get you started on improving your diet:

- **Make every meal 50 percent.**

   This is by far the easiest diet adjustment to make and will provide significant benefits. Make sure that half your plate at every meal is made up of vegetables and/or fruits. Some easy ways to do this are: (1) For breakfast, make a fruit and veggie smoothie in your blender; (2) for lunch, put your meal on a bed of lettuce and see how colorful you can make the salad; (3) and for dinner, shrink the size of your protein to that of a deck of cards and increase your vegetable sides so that they cover half the plate.

- **Try intermittent fasting.**

    You can start off by not snacking between dinner and breakfast. This method alone could launch you into time-restricted, 12-hour fasting if you finish dinner by 7 P.M. and eat breakfast at or after 7 A.M. the next day. As your body adjusts, you may be able to further shorten your "eating window" each day. Alternatively, you could try a water fast for one day a week, if approved by your doctor. Lastly, consider trying a 5:2 weekly schedule in which you eat normally for five days of the week and then eat only 400–600 calories for the remaining two days. You can easily track your calorie intake via various tracking apps on your smartphone. One popular free app is MyFitnessPal.

- **Find a good nutritionist.**

    Radically changing your diet can feel overwhelming, which is why a qualified nutritionist—especially one who specializes in working with cancer patients—can help you navigate your dietary options, get you tested for food sensitivities, and recommend a diet that is right for your body at this time. In today's age of video conferencing, you can search the Internet for a nutritionist you like and not be limited to ones only in your local area.

- **Support your microbiome.**

    To encourage more healthy bacteria to grow in your gut, try eating more high-fiber vegetables and adding probiotic-rich fermented foods into your diet. You can easily make your own sauerkraut by chopping up an organic cabbage, adding filtered water and some salt, packing it tightly into a glass jar, screwing the lid on tight, and letting it sit for a week at room temperature, out of the sun. Be sure to refrigerate it after opening. Another way to support your microbiome is to reduce your use of antibacterial soaps, gels, and wipes, which include microbiome-degrading chemicals. Instead, just use regular soap and water.

- **Consult the Environmental Working Group (EWG).**

    The EWG is a nonprofit group dedicated to improving our environmental health. Its website provides decades of research on the Dirty Dozen (those foods you should seek out from organic growers), the Clean Fifteen (conventionally farmed foods that are safe to purchase), and the least toxic household cleaners and cosmetic products. The EWG houses its immense database of products and information at EWG.org, as well as on two apps that you can download: EWG's Healthy Living (for insight into the most eco-friendly products to buy) and EWG's Food Scores (to make healthier food choices by looking at food ingredients and labels).

Radically changing their diet is typically one of the first actions radical remission survivors take to improve their health. Your diet is completely under your own control and is therefore one of the easiest things to change. While conventional medicine doctors may not receive much training in nutritional health, there is a large body of scientific evidence to back up the benefits of shifting away from the standard American diet in order to reduce inflammation and strengthen your immune system.

## CHAPTER 8

# HERBS AND SUPPLEMENTS

## Tom's Story

*Remedies from chemicals will never stand in favorable comparison with the products of nature.*

— Thomas Edison

Many radical remission survivors report that supplements are a key part of their recovery, but it is important to understand that this factor must be uniquely customized for each person. No two radical remission survivors take the same supplements, even if they have the same cancer. For this reason, we strongly recommend that you consult with a nutritionist, naturopath, herbalist, or functional medicine or integrative doctor before taking any action. This is the one radical remission healing factor you should not explore on your own.

Radical remission survivors have noted that in addition to the need for personalization, the quality of supplements varies widely, which is why it is important to have a health professional on your team who can guide you toward trustworthy and effective brands.

You will find a lot of people making sweeping claims about the "hottest" new herbs and supplements for curing cancer or other ailments. For instance, you have probably heard that we are all deficient in vitamin D, or that we should all take curcumin as an anti-inflammatory. This may indeed be true for you, but given your specific health status, blood work, and nutritional intake, taking herbs and supplements without knowing what your body *actually* needs could do more harm than good.

Be aware that this personalized advice may not come from your M.D. We previously discussed the fact that doctors do not get adequate training in nutrition. Similarly, few M.D.s receive training in nonpharmaceutical herbs and supplements. In fact, radical remission survivors have reported that their M.D.s have often tried to discourage them from taking any kind of nonprescription supplements. Although it is crucial that you consult with your M.D. to ensure that supplements will not interfere with any of your prescriptions, it is equally important to find someone who has been trained in herbs and supplements who can make recommendations for your specific body. In an ideal world, your herbalist and oncologist would be on the same healing team and communicate with each other directly. The real world, of course, is not so simple.

Despite your doctor's fear of the unknown, the good news is that most herbal supplements taken during cancer treatment are safe and very unlikely to have negative herb-drug interactions with your conventional medical therapies. A recent study found that about one-third to one-half of all cancer patients use some form of herbs or vitamin supplements during their conventional treatment[1] and that the potential for negative herb-drug interactions was either unlikely or not expected in 95 percent of the subjects' herb-drug combinations and of low clinical relevance in the other 5 percent.[2]

In this chapter, we will share some encouraging trends and the latest research findings related to herbs and supplements, followed by Tom's inspiring story of radical remission from stage 4 colon cancer, in which supplements—alongside his specialized chemotherapy—played a starring role. Lastly, we will suggest some simple action steps to inspire you to bring this powerful healing factor into your own life.

In *Radical Remission*, I noted that the main difference between chemotherapy and vitamin or herbal supplements is that most chemotherapy is designed to kill cancer cells directly, while most supplements are designed to strengthen the immune system so that it can remove cancer cells on its own, as it was designed to do.

In general, radical remission survivors take supplements for one of three reasons. First, they may want to boost their immune system and overall health (i.e., add something to the body that it is lacking, such as vitamin D or melatonin). Second, they may wish to detoxify their body of something that should not be there, such as parasites, heavy metals, harmful bacteria, or toxins. Last, they may take supplements to help them digest their food better, such as prebiotics, probiotics, or digestive enzymes.

Radical remission survivors emphasize that neither supplements nor diet alone can serve as a single solution for healing. Americans have grown accustomed to the idea that pretty much any medical problem can be solved by a pill. This is not how supplements work. While the right supplements can provide critical support during your healing process, they are more of a Band-Aid than a magic bullet. Supplements will not do you much good unless you are also willing to make radical changes to your diet, mind-set, and lifestyle. That being said, after fully implementing the other nine healing factors, many radical remission survivors did find that taking targeted supplements was the missing link in their healing journeys. The supplements provided their bodies with the nutrients and minerals they needed to fully heal.

One possible reason is that due to large-scale farming and breeding practices and pesticide use, today's fruits and vegetables lack many of the trace minerals our bodies need and contain lower amounts of vitamins and nutrients than they did 50–100 years ago.[3] For example, scientists at Washington State University found that there has been an 11 percent decline in iron, 16 percent decline in copper, and 25 percent decline in selenium content among wheat varieties grown from 1842 to 2003.[4] Similar studies conducted in countries around the globe have found comparable declines in the micronutrient content of crops.[5] Global climate change isn't helping the problem, since scientists have found that rising carbon dioxide levels in the air have led to decreased levels of zinc, iron, and protein in food crops.[6] Finally, the presence of pesticides and chemicals in our food supply and drinking water irritates and disrupts our gut microbiomes, which means we need to take special gut-healing supplements to get our microbiomes back on track.

Integrative oncology physician Keith Block, M.D., whose comprehensive, individualized treatments we will learn about later on in Tom's healing story, believes strongly in the importance of an anticancer diet complemented by targeted nutraceuticals (i.e., supplements). His supplement recommendations are based on the results of a patient's microenvironment, terrain, and molecular laboratory testing, the specific type of cancer they're facing, and their conventional treatment regimens, which he routinely gives using time-sensitive protocols. These supplement recommendations are then modified as the patient progresses through treatment.

Dr. Block favors supplements based on food concentrates and whole herb extracts. For example, his supplemental interventions include a highly concentrated formula of green tea[7] with reishi and chaga mushrooms and an organic green drink supplement, both made in the U.S. and laboratory tested for purity. He uses a multivitamin-mineral supplement that—unlike what is readily available on store shelves and online—he has tailored specifically to cancer patients. This customization includes omitting iron and copper, both of which can fuel oxidative stress and angiogenesis, and adding cancer-fighting food and botanical extracts.

## Recent Developments

More and more cancer patients are seeking out information about herbs and supplements, asking their doctors about which ones to take, and seeking an integrative provider if needed. One recent study found that among breast and gynecological cancer patients, one-third of the women had worked with their medical teams to add either herbal supplements, homeopathy, or vitamins to their healing regimens.[8]

Hundreds of supplements are being studied at the moment, and scores of them have already been proven to be helpful to the immune system. For example, researchers found that patients with multiple myeloma who were undergoing chemotherapy and stem cell transplantation were able to significantly strengthen their immune systems by taking the mushroom supplement AndoSan.[9] Another study of prostate cancer patients who had high prostate-specific antigen (PSA) levels (which is indicative of a prostate cancer recurrence) found that white button mushroom powder lowered PSA levels and increased other blood markers related to strengthening the immune system.[10]

And it's not just mushrooms. One probiotic kefir product was found to induce the death of cancer cells (apoptosis).[11] Vitamin D supplementation has been shown to inhibit the growth of certain breast cancers (e.g., estrogen-receptor-positive breast cancer),[12] while ginseng has been shown to significantly boost immune function in non–small cell lung cancer patients.[13] Lastly, researchers have found that supplementing with lycopene (found in tomatoes) helped to lower PSA in prostate cancer patients in just three weeks.[14] These studies on various supplements demonstrate that, just as with prescription drugs, herbs and supplements can provide significant health benefits when taken in the right dosage and under the right circumstances.

## Increased Toxins

One of the reasons radical remission survivors choose to take supplements is to detoxify their bodies of carcinogens. Cancer rates have soared since the Industrial Revolution began in the late 18th century,[15] and hundreds of studies have linked many man-made toxins to cancer.[16] For example, since World War II ended, the global production of pesticides has increased by an estimated 26-fold, from 0.1 million tons to 2.7 million tons,[17] and alongside that the number of pesticide-linked cancer cases has increased.[18] This is not surprising, considering that only 5 percent of the 80,000 commercially manufactured chemicals created since World War II have been tested for safety.[19] However, whenever chemicals *have been* tested in safety trials by organizations like the IARC (International Agency for Research on Cancer), almost 50 percent of those tested since 1971 have been found to contribute to cancer.[20] And a recent study concluded that more than 100,000 lifetime cancer cases could be due to carcinogenic chemicals in tap water that is considered "safe to drink" by public water authorities.[21]

Thankfully, things are starting to change, albeit slowly. Several recent lawsuits have started to hold manufacturers of toxic chemicals accountable for their contribution to the global cancer epidemic. For instance, the company Monsanto, which makes the common pesticide Roundup, has recently lost three lawsuits in which juries determined that there was sufficient evidence to show Roundup was a direct cause of the plaintiffs' non-Hodgkin's lymphoma. The IARC recently classified Roundup—which contains the chemical glyphosate, the most widely used herbicide in the world—as a "probable carcinogen."[22]

In addition, Johnson & Johnson, the maker of Johnson's baby powder and many other talc products, currently faces more than 14,000 lawsuits claiming that its talc products contained asbestos fibers, which led to ovarian cancer or mesothelioma, both very aggressive cancers. Several juries have already found Johnson & Johnson liable for such cancer cases, forcing the company to pay millions of dollars to the plaintiffs or the deceased plaintiffs' families.

When certain radical remission survivors have discovered (through extensive blood, urine, and hair testing) that they have been exposed to possible cancer-causing agents, they have worked with qualified health professionals to determine the appropriate detoxifying supplements to take. For some people, that may mean intravenous chelation therapy to remove lead, mercury, or arsenic from their bodies, while others may take supplements such as nystatin (to remove the fungus *Candida*), black walnut or berberine (to remove parasites), or garlic or echinacea (to remove harmful bacteria).[23] And, of course, the ultimate goal is to eliminate toxins from our environment, air, and drinking water, so that no one needs to take detoxifying supplements in the first place. This is an idealistic goal, to be sure, but one that voters and consumers should keep in mind whenever they are voting or buying consumer goods.

## Homeopathy

In Latin, the word *homeopathy* means "same suffering." Homeopathic doctors use extremely small amounts of plants and minerals, typically diluted thousands of times in water, to stimulate an internal healing process. More specifically, homeopathic doctors administer extremely diluted versions of a substance that—if you were to take it while healthy and in an undiluted form—would produce the same symptoms you are currently experiencing. That is where "same suffering" comes in. The theory is that because it is in such a diluted state, the substance will not produce symptoms in your body, but rather will teach your body about that substance, therefore reducing your symptoms. In this way, homeopathy is purported to work similarly to vaccines.

Clinical studies of homeopathic remedies used in combination with conventional medical treatment have shown that homeopathic remedies can improve patients' quality of life, reduce symptom burden, and improve survival time in cancer patients.[24] For example, homeopathy has been shown to reduce the severity of the difficult side effects of chemotherapy, radiation, and surgery, including nausea, fatigue, and foggy-headedness.[25] Meanwhile, researchers at the Medical University of Vienna found that patients suffering from advanced stages of cancer who used homeopathy enjoyed significantly longer survival time as compared to a control group.[26]

In one very impressive study conducted in India, 15 patients with a variety of advanced brain cancers were treated with a homeopathic dilution of Ruta 6 (isolated from the plant *Ruta graveolens*) as well as calcium phosphate.[27] They drank two drops of

Ruta 6 in a teaspoon of water and a small dose of calcium phosphate twice a day. All the patients gradually improved, as tracked by regular CT (computed tomography) scans and clinical exams. Amazingly, eight of the nine patients with glioma showed a complete regression of their tumors, while the ninth showed a partial regression. One of three patients with meningioma showed a complete regression, while the other two have enjoyed a prolonged period of tumor stability. One patient with neurinoma enjoyed a prolonged period of tumor stability, while one patient with craniopharyngioma and another with a malignant pituitary tumor both showed complete regression. The time it took from the first homeopathic treatment to complete regression and/or a stable state ranged from three months to seven years.

Meanwhile, across the globe, researchers at the MD Anderson Cancer Center who were working in collaboration with the Indian researchers decided to investigate the effects of Ruta 6 and calcium phosphate on brain cancer cells in vitro (i.e., in petri dishes).[28] They discovered that the homeopathic treatment caused the brain cancer cells in the petri dishes to die by eroding their telomeres while allowing healthy white blood cells to survive. This promising pilot study indicates that homeopathy may be a potential cancer treatment with minimal side effects that warrants further study, especially for brain cancer patients.

## Cannabis

The medical use of cannabis (marijuana) is one of the hottest topics in the cancer world right now. Proponents of medicinal marijuana claim it is a wonder drug that can be used for hundreds of conditions, including irritable bowel syndrome (IBS), multiple sclerosis (MS), sleep disorders, HIV/AIDS, rheumatoid arthritis, fibromyalgia, epilepsy, and cancer.[29] They contend that it is safe, easy for patients to use, and relatively inexpensive compared to pharmaceutical drugs.[30,31] In fact, no recorded cases of overdose deaths from cannabis have ever been found, even after extensive literature reviews.[32]

Opponents of medicinal cannabis argue that there are not yet enough randomized trials to confirm its benefits, harms, or potency. They point out that cannabis impairs coordination and judgment, and that there is potential for dependence, addiction, and abuse.[33] Despite these objections, the fact that marijuana has proven invaluable in easing numerous symptoms—nausea, pain, motor dysfunctions, gastrointestinal problems, etc.—helps explain why so many states in the U.S. have already legalized it for medicinal use.[34] In fact, a recent Gallup poll reported that two in three Americans believe that cannabis should be legalized.[35]

Cannabis use dates back to ancient religious ceremonies, but it has also been widely used in textiles, nutrition, and medicine.[36] The earliest evidence of medicinal cannabis use dates back to around 400 A.D.[37] The cannabis plant contains more than 500 different biologically active compounds,[38] including tetrahydrocannabinol (THC), which is psychoactive and gets you "high," and cannabidiol (CBD), which does not produce the "high" that THC does.

Cannabis affects your body by stimulating your endocannabinoid system, a complex cell-signaling system in your central nervous system, internal organs, connective tissues, glands, and immune cells—in other words, nearly everywhere.[39] A variety of processes occur when you ingest cannabis and your cannabinoid receptors are stimulated, including regulation of sleep, increased appetite, and reductions in stress, pain, nausea, and inflammation.[40] In general, your endocannabinoid system helps your body eat, sleep, relax, forget, and protect.[41] Given this range of health benefits, it's no surprise that the endocannabinoid system has been in the anticancer spotlight for the last decade.[42,43]

While cannabis is perhaps best known for reducing the side effects of chemotherapy, it is helpful to know that cannabis itself produces very few side effects, and even those are mild. In a recent study, the World Health Organization reported that CBD is generally well-tolerated, with a good safety profile, and no addictive effects.[44] In a different study looking at the effects of medical cannabis over a 40-year period,[45] the researchers found that less than 15 percent of all study participants had any side effects at all, and the few side effects reported were dizziness, vomiting, and urinary tract infections.[46] Most fascinating, there were *no significant differences* in the side effects reported between the people who received medical cannabis and those who received either a placebo or no cannabis.[47]

## Cannabis and Cancer

The use of cannabis in the palliative care of cancer patients is well-established, with hundreds of clinical studies showing a significant improvement in treatment-related symptoms such as nausea, being underweight, and pain.[48,49,50] When it comes to nausea, cannabis is especially helpful. In a review of 23 randomized controlled trials, patients who received cannabis experienced significantly less nausea and vomiting than subjects who received a placebo.[51]

In addition to reducing the side effects of chemotherapy, cannabis has been shown to improve the effectiveness of chemotherapy.[52] In one study, researchers found that THC and CBD significantly increased the effectiveness of many common chemotherapies, including cytarabine, doxorubicin, cisplatin, and others.[53] Similarly, a recent phase 2 randomized, placebo-controlled trial looked at the effects of cannabis on cancer patients with recurrent glioblastoma multiforme (GBM), a particularly aggressive brain tumor with a very poor prognosis.[54] These cancer patients took either chemotherapy plus THC and CBD, or chemotherapy plus placebo. After one year, 83 percent of the patients in the THC/CBD group were still alive, while only 53 percent of the patients in the placebo group were still alive.[55]

Recent studies have shown that cannabis can do more for sick patients than just alleviate side effects or boost the power of chemotherapy. One study of HIV patients found that cannabis activates immune function and reduces systemic inflammation.[56] Anything that can reduce inflammation and boost immune function can help your body heal. If cannabis reduced inflammation and boosted immune function in patients with HIV, it may have similar health-promoting benefits for cancer patients.[57]

The most promising cannabis studies, in our opinion, are those that look at cannabis's direct, anticancer properties. Several studies have shown that cannabis has a strong effect on tumor reduction and cancer cell death (apoptosis), and can act as a direct, antitumor agent.[58] In mouse studies, CBD has been shown to inhibit the progression of many types of cancer, including glioblastoma, breast, lung, prostate, and colon cancer.[59] Other studies with mice have found that CBD inhibits breast tumor growth and reduces tumor size, which leads to significantly longer survival time.[60] One mouse study showed that CBD inhibited the growth of triple-negative breast tumors,[61] while yet another found that THC slowed the growth of breast tumors by inducing apoptosis.[62] Humans are different from mice, of course, so we will need to wait for human trials to be conducted before declaring cannabis an official anticancer supplement. In the meantime, CBD appears to fall into the category of "can't hurt, will help with treatment-related side effects, and might help inhibit tumor growth and/or kill cancer cells."

## Mistletoe

Another promising supplement that is gaining in popularity is the liquid extract from mistletoe berries, leaves, and stems. We covered mistletoe briefly in Chapter 3 in Bob's story of healing from appendiceal cancer, and it has been used for decades in Europe and Asia, both as a first-line cancer treatment and as an adjuvant therapy to help alleviate the side effects of chemotherapy and radiation. In fact, mistletoe extract is one of the therapies that European doctors prescribe most to cancer patients.[63] Usually given by self-injection under the skin every two days, the benefits of mistletoe therapy include reducing tumor activity and increasing survival time, all with fewer side effects than with conventional treatment alone,[64] as well as improving one's quality of life by increasing energy and reducing nausea.[65]

In a phase 2 safety trial of mistletoe therapy in Germany, a group of bladder cancer patients received weekly injections of mistletoe for six weeks, *instead of* chemotherapy or surgery. (Note: There was no control group in this study.) Amazingly, more than half the patients receiving the mistletoe were in full remission after only 12 weeks.[66] In addition to these highly encouraging results, the side effects of the mistletoe were very mild, including a rash at the site of injection and a few low-grade fevers.

Another study looked at melanoma in mice to evaluate the effects of Korean mistletoe as a cancer treatment. Researchers found that the mice who were given the mistletoe had a significant reduction in tumor size and a significantly higher survival rate compared to the control group of untreated mice. In addition, the mistletoe extract induced both early- and late-stage apoptosis (i.e., natural cell death), which is crucial in cancer healing because one of the ways cancer cells malfunction is that they "forget to die" when they are supposed to and then accumulate into bulky, cancerous tumors.[67]

Currently, mistletoe therapy is not FDA-approved in the U.S. for oncologists to use as part of the official standard of care for cancer. However, in an exciting development, Johns Hopkins University School of Medicine is currently running the first phase 1 clinical trial in the United States to analyze the effects of mistletoe on cancer patients. A phase 1 trial means that researchers are testing a therapy to evaluate its safety, determine an appropriate dose, and identify any side effects.

This clinical trial represents a key milestone in the U.S. medical community's acceptance of mistletoe. Not only is it the first step toward getting FDA approval as a first-line cancer treatment, but it also helps the therapy to be reimbursed by health insurance companies. As of this writing, the trial is still accepting new participants. You may find out more about mistletoe and your eligibility for this trial at BelieveBig.org, a nonprofit organization that supports the use of mistletoe therapy and nutritional-based healing in the United States.

BelieveBig.org was started by the vivacious radical remission survivor Ivelisse Page. In 2008, Ivelisse was a happy wife and mother of four with a deep faith when she was diagnosed with stage 4 colon cancer. She was 37 at the time, the exact same age her father had been when he was diagnosed with advanced colon cancer. Because Ivelisse was deeply affected by her father's two-year decline and ultimate death from cancer when she was only 13, she and her sisters had vowed to be hypervigilant about preventing the disease. For years, Ivelisse had received routine colonoscopies, eaten organically, and exercised regularly.

Ivelisse was understandably shocked when she was diagnosed with a rare, asymptomatic, yet highly aggressive form of metastatic colon cancer, despite doing everything she could to prevent it. She agreed to have immediate surgery to remove 15 inches of her colon and 28 lymph nodes, the biopsies of which confirmed her cancer diagnosis. Five weeks later, she had a second surgery to remove 20 percent of her liver, because scans showed that the cancer had already metastasized there.

At this point, her surgeon recommended immediate and aggressive chemotherapy. However, Ivelisse pushed back because she felt that chemotherapy was "burning down the forest for one rotten tree." In addition, her intuition told her that chemotherapy would kill her because she was so chemically sensitive.

During this time, Ivelisse's husband had been on a search for complementary therapies. Ultimately, their searching (plus a little serendipity) led Ivelisse to find Peter Hinderberger, a homeopathic medical doctor working near Ivelisse in Baltimore, Maryland. He had received his medical degree in Europe and was therefore trained in mistletoe therapy. After careful evaluation, and always keeping her four children in mind, Ivelisse felt she had everything to gain and nothing to lose by trying mistletoe.

*In nature, mistletoe grows on a host tree but doesn't kill the host tree as most parasitic plants do. It also blooms in the winter when most things are dead. It's interesting that what it symbolizes and how the plant responds in nature is similar to what mistletoe does for cancer.*

For Ivelisse's cancer, her every-other-day mistletoe injections, along with the other nine radical remission healing factors, helped to keep her cancer at bay without the use of chemotherapy. In terms of her diet, she limited her consumption of meat and processed foods, eliminated all dairy, and kept eating the large amount of organic fruits and vegetables she already ate. Exercise came back into the picture as soon as she was strong enough after surgery, and staying alive for her family provided her with ample reasons for living. She experienced a huge emotional release during a time of prayer her friends held for her, focused on staying positive about the future throughout her treatment, and empowered herself by building a team of both naturopathic and conventional doctors. Finally, Ivelisse continued to follow her intuition and deepened her already strong spirituality by surrendering her healing outcome to God.

Ivelisse's surgeon was strongly opposed to forgoing chemotherapy, and her oncologist was "cautiously optimistic" until three years later, when her scans continued to show that she was still in full remission post-surgery—something they had not imagined possible given the aggressive nature of her cancer. They told her not to change a thing and to continue whatever she was doing, including the mistletoe injections. To this day, more than 11 years later, Ivelisse's cancer has never returned.

For those wishing to follow in her footsteps, Ivelisse warns:

*Mistletoe is not just a supplement; it is definitely a science. You need to go to someone who is trained. Because it's a natural substance, everyone's body is going to respond differently. There are different types and strengths of mistletoe. There's mistletoe grown on ash trees, pine trees, apple trees—they're all different based on the type of cancer you have. In addition, as your body*

*is healing, you may need different grades or formulations. So
you really need to be seen by someone who is trained.*

Ivelisse is still on mistletoe therapy, which often surprises people. However, to Ivelisse, stopping the mistletoe is not an option
because of its effectiveness and relatively low cost ($140 per
month). Today, more than 11 years after being given an 8 percent
chance of surviving her stage 4 colon cancer, Ivelisse is as energetic as ever and a vibrant wife and mother of four who spends her
days running BelieveBig.org, the nonprofit she co-founded with
her husband.

Now that we have covered the latest in trends and research
regarding herbs and supplements, we would like to share with
you the in-depth healing story of Tom, a courageous father and
husband who used many herbs and supplements, as well as a novel
chemotherapy treatment and the other nine radical remission
healing factors, to overcome stage 4 colon cancer.

# Tom's Story

In 2012, Tom Melzer was a happily settled 62-year-old living and
working in a Midwestern town with his wife of 43 years. Their
two adult children, both in their 20s, had started their own
lives. He and his wife happily watched from afar as their grown
children began to build their careers and find loving, supportive
relationships.

For 40-plus years Tom had held relatively stressful jobs in
production management for railroad, railcar leasing, and locomo-
tive equipment manufacturing. Despite the inevitable stress that
comes with this profession, Tom had always enjoyed his work. In
his free time, he enjoyed catching up with his children, spending

quality time with his wife and friends, reading, or engaging in three of his favorite hobbies: winemaking, golfing, and gardening.

If you had asked him at that time, Tom would have told you that he considered his lifestyle to be relatively healthy. Regular exercise and a good night's sleep provided him with a solid foundation. While his jobs were stressful at times, they kept him satisfied, and he had a great support system in his family, friends, and faith. He had even regularly consulted a nutritionist to identify the right vitamin supplements for his body and age. However, in hindsight, he realized:

> *My meals were usually meat-based. I thought I was eating correctly since the 1970s. After all, we had our own 60-by-60-foot garden. We knew to eat fruit before meals, as their digestion generally takes place in the small intestine. We made meals to be balanced to include salad greens and vegetables, and were also aware of the benefits of favorable food combining (for example, proteins and vegetables, or carbohydrates and vegetables), and what to avoid in other combinations (proteins and carbs). But, in addition to various meats, we were also not excluding much sugar, as we enjoyed desserts. Now I am well aware of the links between meat diets and colon cancer.*

In addition to eating meat and desserts, Tom enjoyed the occasional glass of homemade wine.

> *I have been a lifelong winemaker. . . . I buy California grapes every year that are shipped into the area. I've got the process down and I'm making good wines now. But I don't drink much. I may have a glass of wine in the evening but that's about it.*

Little did Tom know that his peaceful, winemaking life would change overnight. On a weekday in January 2012, Tom headed to the office in the morning as usual. His stomach began to hurt and, unfortunately, the pain did not go away all day. It was bad enough that he made a point to work late and get fully caught up, so he could get checked by his family doctor the next morning.

Despite being in considerable pain, Tom did not expect the doctor to find anything serious. At his previous annual physical only five months earlier, his blood tests had come back normal, with the exception of a slightly elevated PSA (prostate-specific antigen), which his doctor said they would watch. At that time, 62-year-old Tom had never had a colonoscopy.

Two hours and multiple tests and scans later, Tom's doctor walked into the room accompanied by a surgeon and slowly closed the door. Tom knew that whatever the doctor was about to say, it wasn't good.

The doctor broke the news that Tom had a sizable tumor in his large intestine. Tom tried his best to focus as the doctor continued his explanation. The tumor had most likely been growing undetected for years. Because it was situated at the top of Tom's large intestine, feces had still been able to pass by underneath it, giving the cancer more time to grow and spread to a significant portion of his abdomen before causing any symptoms.

Tom was still trying to absorb all of this when his doctor told him the worst news yet: Based on the scans they had just taken, Tom's large intestine was in danger of bursting at any moment. The doctor wanted Tom to have emergency surgery that very night. Tom agreed, and in a matter of minutes the surgeon was scrubbing in, a nurse was calling his wife, and medical assistants were prepping Tom for surgery. He remembers:

*I realized that this was very serious and that the cancer was very far along. And yet, I was thankful that I did not have a burst large intestine, which was the fear of the surgeon and why he wanted to act on me immediately—due to how the large intestine was stretched and filled [with the tumor]. He was quite concerned that, if [the intestine] burst, it would be a much more difficult and much more serious surgery. So I was thankful for the detection before a possibly worse situation.*

When they opened him up, Tom's surgeons were dismayed to find that the cancer had already spread to several other organs in his abdomen. They ended up removing two-thirds of his large intestine, one-quarter of his pancreas, a significant portion of his stomach, and all of his spleen and gallbladder. Even so, they still were not able to remove all the microscopic cancer cells. Tom's surgeon tested almost two dozen lymph nodes in Tom's pelvis and abdomen and most of them contained cancer cells, which meant that Tom would definitely need chemotherapy and perhaps radiation to remove the remaining cancer.

A few hours later, Tom awoke from surgery to find his wife and doctor by his side. Tom and his wife listened to the news that he had stage 4 colon cancer and that several of his organs were now smaller or gone altogether. In just one day, Tom had gone from feeling healthy and happy to recovering from surgery and facing stage 4 cancer. His wife tearfully called their two children to let them know the news as Tom tried to process it all.

After the surgery, Tom worried that he would be more susceptible to infections and diseases since so many of his organs had been removed, particularly his spleen (which helps to filter the blood and fight off infections). His doctors addressed his concern by giving him preventive vaccinations, but Tom had an intuitive feeling that he would need to take additional supplements and radically change his diet for the rest of his life to make up for the fact that he now had fewer organs than usual.

> *I was on antibiotics and whatever other medications they gave me for the 7 to 10 days following the surgery. But I came through it okay. At the hospital, the doctors also gave me four shots. They gave me a flu shot—I never get a flu shot, but they insisted on a flu shot. And they insisted on three other immunity shots. I asked [the doctor], "Do these things need to be boosted at some time in the future?" He said no, but I was very concerned.*

Back at home after the surgery, Tom's battle with cancer had only just begun. His doctors said he would need chemotherapy to remove the remaining cancer cells in his body, so Tom knew he would have a hard road ahead of him. Some of his friends had reached a state of being "cancer-free" after going through chemotherapy, only to have it recur a few years later. This led Tom to believe that chemotherapy would not be enough to keep his stage 4 cancer at bay in the long run.

Watching his friends battle cancer had taught Tom about the stress that chemotherapy puts on the body. As soon as he felt well enough, he called a naturopath friend—Dr. Robin Sielaff in Portland, Oregon—to ask about alternative cancer treatments (such as intravenous vitamin C, which one of Tom's friends had used to treat his cancer). Dr. Sielaff warned that Tom's cancer was too far advanced to use only natural healing methods, so she urged him to find an integrative oncologist, that is, a board-certified physician who uses natural healing treatments and chemotherapy at the same time.

> *I looked at somebody in New York City, I looked at MD Anderson, I looked at the Cleveland Clinic, I looked at Cancer Treatment Centers of America. But I concluded that the Block Center [for Integrative Cancer Treatment] would probably be my best option. I came to that conclusion by reading Dr. Block's book, Life Over Cancer. I first jumped to the section [in the book] on how to deal with cancer naturally once you have it. . . . That helped me make a decision to use Dr. Block. When I visited the Block Center, I again asked about a more natural way of doing the treatment by using, say, intravenous vitamin C. I could see their hesitation and they said, "You're pretty far advanced." So they recommended their integrative chemotherapy program.*

Tom was drawn to the Block Center because of its natural approach to healing combined with its utilization of the latest conventional medical treatments. The doctors at the Block Center thoroughly tested Tom's blood, genetics, urine, saliva, and hormone levels, and analyzed his mental health and stress levels. They then recommended that he receive integrative chemotherapy treatments twice a month for six months.

Tom began his treatment days with an early-morning intravenous vitamin infusion that contained numerous vitamins and immune boosters to help mitigate the toxicity of chemotherapy and to prevent side effects that might result from the chemotherapy. He would then have a few hours before starting his chemotherapy to take advantage of the other healing treatments offered at the Block Center.

Tom always had a strong belief in God, but during his treatment, his faith took on a whole new meaning. As Tom participated in the guided meditation sessions at the Block Center, he focused on God and on coming to terms with his health and mortality. For Tom, believing in God reassured him that whatever the outcome of his treatment may be, he would be at peace, allowing him to focus on relaxing deeply and increasing positive emotions such as peace and love.

*If I had to summarize my spirituality, it's that I'm looking to God as my Source. I'm praying for a long life, and I am confident that I'm being heard and that those prayers are being answered. I am asking for continual healing and continual support. Probably the greatest thing in my prayers has been thankfulness. I would be thankful even if God determined that He didn't want me to live that long—I would still be thankful for all that He has done for me. So yes, it's really God [is my] Number One. And the Block Center directives [are my] number two.*

The Block Center offered private psychotherapy sessions that focused on releasing suppressed emotions and group discussions that included laugh therapy sessions focused on increasing positive emotions. The group psychotherapy sessions allowed Tom and the other cancer patients at the Center to express how they were feeling and to support each other around their shared experiences.

In addition to these mental-emotional-spiritual offerings, the Block Center has a large, modern kitchen that serves healthy food to its patients and offers cooking classes and demonstrations so patients can learn exactly how to cook the food that will be in their recommended diet plan. These cooking classes and lunches helped to ease Tom into the radical diet changes he would need to make.

About two to three hours after his morning vitamin IV infusion, and after his mental health and cooking sessions, Tom would start his chemotherapy infusions, during which calming music would be played and a physical therapy massage would be administered. After a few hours of receiving chemotherapy at the Center, his doctors would send him home with a portable chemotherapy device (worn in a fanny pack and infused via an under-the-skin port on his upper chest) that allowed him to receive the chemotherapy in timed infusions for the next 48 hours.

The Block Center doctors schedule the flow rate of this portable chemotherapy so that the dose is the strongest at the time of day (or night) that will affect the cancer cells most effectively. Interestingly, every cell in your body—whether healthy or cancerous—has its own circadian rhythm that dictates when the cell is "awake" (active and dividing) versus "asleep" (resting and not dividing). These active times vary based on cancer type and do not always coincide with our bodies' diurnal clocks.

Giving a person chemotherapy at the time of day (or night) when their cancer cells are most "awake" allows that person to reduce the standard chemotherapy dose while still yielding the same (or better) results, all with significantly fewer side effects.[68] This technique is called chronomodulated chemotherapy; the Block Center imported this method from Europe in the 1980s, becoming one of the first clinics in the U.S. to offer it.

As soon as Tom arrived at the Block Center, the doctors conducted numerous tests to determine which oral and intravenous supplements would best mitigate the side effects of his particular chemotherapy and aid his overall healing. They took into account his unique cancer type, physiology, genetic makeup, and microbiome status to help him find the right combination of supplements for his body at that particular time. Tom explains:

*I had been supplementing [with vitamins] to a much lesser extent prior to my cancer. Post-cancer, I changed my diet and started to take more specific supplements—the Block Center really helped with that. They did metabolic testing and extensive blood panels and that sort of thing. As a result, they instructed me in a protocol that included not only anticancer foods and supplements, but also [foods and supplements] specific to my metabolic terrain. For example, I now begin my day with a smoothie. I usually make the smoothie with strawberries and blueberries and often pineapples as well for the base, and then I load it up with four different types of [supplemental] oils and four powders.*

The four oils he currently adds to his morning smoothie are (1) a high-lignan flaxseed oil, (2) hemp oil, which contains omega-3 and omega-6 fatty acids in a healthy ratio, (3) MCT (medium-chain triglyceride) oil, which is derived from organic coconut oil and helps balance blood glucose levels, and (4) a few drops of tangerine oil. He adds tart cherry concentrate to help reduce his internal inflammation. Finally, he adds four supplemental powders: (1) organic whey protein powder, (2) L-glutamine powder, (3) taurine powder, which supports the nervous system, and (4) a blended powder of organic, freeze-dried vegetables, including broccoli, cabbage, kale, parsley, tomatoes, chlorella, spinach, carrots, wheatgrass, beets, and sweet potatoes.

*I feel that [the morning smoothie] is really a helpful thing for me. I know I'm getting a healthy dose [of vitamins] right off the bat to begin the day. I never did smoothies before and these smoothies are great. I really do enjoy them!*

Tom drinks filtered, alkaline water to reduce inflammation in his body. Internal inflammation creates an environment that encourages the growth of cancer cells,[69] so anything a person can do to reduce internal inflammation is considered cancer-preventive.

In terms of dietary changes, Dr. Block recommended that Tom cut out sugar, white-flour bread, pasta, meat, dairy, and alcohol from his diet as soon as possible. For Tom, these changes were very difficult to make given that he had eaten the standard American diet his whole life. His new diet limited him to mostly fresh veg-etables and fruits, since most of the products at the grocery store contain added sugar of some kind, and those that do not often contain something else that Tom is no longer supposed to eat. He was up for the challenge, though, and made a mental shift to focus on the positive aspects of the diet change.

> I've replaced [meat] with fish. Prior to a main meal, I will often consume some fruit. I eat colorful salads, with lots of varied peppers, celery, carrots, tomatoes, and often broccoli and cauliflower on them, along with the typical lettuce and spinach. Sometimes I will even top it off with vinegar and oil and put on some roasted pecans. Now that's a really good and healthy salad! My fruit intake has also gone up significantly.

The body-mind-spirit treatments offered at the Block Center, along with the chronomodulated chemotherapy, allowed Tom to take control of his health while not at the Center by focusing on other aspects of his recovery such as diet, supplements, positive emotions, and spirituality. By the time his six months of low-dose, chronomodulated chemotherapy had ended, he was cancer-free according to his scans, and he was well in the habit of living his new, cancer-preventive lifestyle.

> I had another office visit with Dr. Block after I was done with the 12 sessions [of chemotherapy] over 24 weeks, and he gave me five or six directives. He said, "Everything looks good! Your vitals are good, your metabolic balance looks good. Now I want you to concentrate on these five or six things." Number one was diet. Number two was supplementation. Number three was exercise. Number four was quality sleep. And number five was sweating and detoxification. I have followed that program quite diligently and I think incorporating the entire protocol has been a major factor in my health.

While celebrating the fact that he was now in remission from stage 4 colon cancer, both Tom and his doctors knew he needed to be vigilant about keeping his body-mind-spirit as healthy as possible. The cancer could come back at any time. Therefore, Tom made the decision to retire from his high-stress job in order to reduce stress and focus entirely on his health and on moving forward in his new life. He followed Dr. Block's directives faithfully and stuck closely to his new diet and supplement regimen.

Dr. Block emphasized the importance of getting quality sleep and regular exercise. Now retired from his job, Tom had less stress and more time, which allowed him to focus on getting more sleep and exercise. He found that focusing on his spiritual connection and positive emotions helped him to be at peace with any outcome of his treatment, which helped him to relax deeply and therefore get high-quality sleep.

Tom made movement a part of his daily routine, whereas before his diagnosis he had not exercised daily. Now that he was retired, he did a lot of yard work each day, one of his favorite hobbies, including clearing brush and deadwood, mowing his lawn with a push mower, composting, and gardening. He occasionally went on walks, bicycled with his wife, or participated in walking golf with friends.

> *I found that I had a whole lot of energy for the first six sessions [of chemotherapy]. I felt really good, but starting around sessions eight and nine the chemo was building up in my system and the addition of these chemo infusions was really starting to be debilitating. I understood that that was part of the necessity of going through the whole battle, but that was probably the lowest point I've had in the ability to exercise. Post-chemo, I got back on a regular program. There are just a whole host of benefits to exercise. If I were not exercising, I do not think I would be feeling as well as I do—it's as simple as that.*

Tom's wife and two adult children and their families were his reasons for living and gave him the motivation he needed to stick with his new lifestyle. Thankfully, his wife has been very supportive of the changes in his lifestyle, diet, and supplement regimen, and has been by his side from the moment he was wheeled into emergency surgery. She accompanied him to the Block Center for his first few chronomodulated chemotherapy infusions until he became more accustomed to it. According to Tom, she was and is an indispensable part of his healing team.

Tom's two adult children were also key supports. When the chemotherapy started taking a real toll on Tom, his son began driving down on weekends to help out, which was a tremendous help. During Tom's six months of treatment, his daughter was working and living far away overseas, but her frequent phone calls and his desire to see his children's lives unfold helped him stay committed to his healing process.

> *We visit [our daughter] occasionally, and she will do some traveling on vacations, so at times we will join her and her husband in various spots. Thanks to her, we have really increased our international exposure to various places around the world! My daughter and son were big reasons for living—you know, to be a part of their lives as they're growing their careers. Our daughter just recently had a child, so that was our first grandchild! We're getting daily updates of pictures and texts coming from her. . . . It's so wonderful. Now she is expecting again. . . . I am so thankful to God for being alive."*

It has been eight years since Tom's initial diagnosis and emergency surgery. Despite being diagnosed with stage 4 colon cancer, which has only a 14 percent five-year survival rate, today Tom is feeling stronger and happier than ever. He does not attribute his healing to any one factor, but rather to *all* the changes he made and treatments he tried after being diagnosed. From changing his diet and supplements to completing a full course of chronomodulated chemotherapy to trying new meditation and relaxation techniques, Tom made radical changes in every area of his life. As he sees it, he put in the work and did whatever he could to stay alive, and thankfully the work paid off. For him, that payment came in the form of the sweetest reward of all—getting to gaze into the eyes of his first baby grandchild.

One of the most important healing factors for Tom was finding the right combination of supplements—supplements that gave his immune system the boost it needed to stop the progression of his stage 4 colon cancer. While supplements alone did not lead to his remission, supplements combined with chronomodulated chemotherapy and the other nine radical remission healing factors turned out to be the right recipe for Tom's complete healing.

## Action Steps

Radical remission survivors take three main categories of supplements to aid their recovery:

1. **Digestive supplements**—To help digest your food, including digestive enzymes and prebiotics/probiotics to assist the good bacteria in your gut.

2. **Detoxification supplements**—To help eliminate from your body anything that is slowing down healing, such as parasites, bacteria, viruses, fungi, and heavy metals.

3. **Immune boosters**—To help bring vitamins and hormone levels within a normal range. These include supplements such as cannabis, mistletoe, vitamin $B_{12}$, vitamin C, vitamin D, fish oil, melatonin, mushrooms, and trace minerals.

Remember to always consult a health professional before embarking on a supplement regimen to ensure you maximize your healing and avoid any negative interactions with your current medications or other supplements. Here are some additional ideas to help you get started with herbs and supplements.

## Expand Your Healing Team

Your primary doctor will be able to test your basic vitamin and mineral levels with a simple blood test, but to determine your full supplement needs, you will need to see a practitioner who specializes in looking at your body holistically, conducts thorough testing, and has extensive training in the use of supplements. Here is a partial list of various specialists who have such training, along with their professional organizations, so that you may find a practitioner to work with locally (or remotely via video conferencing):

- Functional medicine doctors — Institute of Functional Medicine — ifm.org

- Naturopaths — The American Association of Naturopathic Physicians — naturopathic.org

- Nutritionists — Academy of Nutrition and Dietetics — eatright.org

- Homeopaths — Society of Homeopaths — homeopathy-soh.org

- Traditional Chinese herbalists — National Certification Commission for Acupuncture and Oriental Medicine — nccaom.org

- Cannabis dispensaries — Marijuana Doctors — marijuanadoctors.com

- Trained mistletoe practitioners — BelieveBig.org

## Get Tested for Toxins

When you find a qualified health professional to guide you in taking personalized supplements, you will want to do some testing with them first to see exactly which supplements your body needs. Here is a partial list of conditions that many radical remission survivors get tested for before they start taking supplements:

- heavy metals (via a blood or urine test, or hair analysis)
- parasites (via a blood, stool, and/or urine test)
- leaky gut (via a blood, stool, and/or urine test complemented by genetic testing)
- overgrowth of *Candida* or other fungi (via a blood, stool, and/or urine test)
- bacterial and viral infections (via a blood, urine, and/or stool test)
- vitamin deficiencies (via a blood test complemented by genetic testing)

## Try Some DIY Detoxing

In addition to taking detoxifying supplements from a qualified health professional, here are some other ways you can help detoxify your body while at home:

- Exercise until you build up a good sweat to flush out impurities.
- Take a hot bath, either with Epsom salt or baking soda for extra detoxification.
- Drink a lot of water, ideally half your body weight in ounces (e.g., a 150-pound person should try to drink at least 75 ounces of water per day).

- Do an at-home enema, either with filtered water or with organic coffee made with filtered water.

- Spend 20 minutes per day in a one-person, at-home infrared sauna, which generally costs less than $200.

## Learn about Cannabis in Your State

Given the rapidly changing laws from state to state regarding the legality of cannabis for medical and/or recreational use, you will need to investigate your options for using cannabis in your state. You may need to visit a certified medical marijuana doctor to get a medical marijuana card (see marijuanadoctors.com). Look for consumer reviews of nearby dispensaries to learn about the quality of that particular location's cannabis. If possible, purchase only cannabis that has been grown organically, without the use of pesticides.

If taking one or two specific supplements would help your body to overcome cancer, this chapter would have been a lot simpler, and we as a society would be that much closer to finding a single cure for cancer. However, the fact that radical remission survivors take various supplements depending on their individual body's needs at a particular point in time is more realistic. Scientists know for a fact that different cancers are caused by a variety of factors—toxins, viruses, bacteria, mitochondrial failure, genetic mutation—therefore, it makes sense that the supplements a cancer patient should take will also depend on a variety of factors. The main thing to remember is that everyone's body is different, which means you will need individual testing with a qualified health professional to determine which supplements are right for you.

## CHAPTER 9

# HAVING STRONG REASONS FOR LIVING

## Alex's Story

*He who has a "why" to live can bear almost any "how."*
— FRIEDRICH NIETZSCHE

What gets you out of bed in the morning? Do you know why you want to live another day on this earth? Maybe you have a bucket list, or an unfinished project, or you simply want to spend one more day with your children or grandchildren. According to radical remission survivors, it does not matter what the reason is. The important thing is that you have one. In their opinion, your reasons for living are critical to the healing process.

For some people, figuring out their reasons for living can be a difficult task, especially if they have recently gotten divorced, been fired, retired, or lost a loved one. For others who have young children, the reason is often obvious. For those who are children themselves, like Alex in our featured healing story, life itself—and the chance to experience it—is the reason for living.

In this chapter, we will explain why this factor is so critical for healing, review new trends and research, and share with you the inspiring story of Alex, whose strong will to live after being diagnosed with aggressive cancer at age 12 helped him blossom into a thriving college student. As always, we will conclude with simple action steps to help you find your own strong reasons for living.

As I began interviewing survivors during my initial radical remission research, I came to understand that "having a strong reason for living" is very different from "not wanting to die." Some of the people I studied were afraid of death, while others had accepted the possibility, but the one thing they all had in common was a strong commitment to life.

Radical remission survivors and their healers emphasize that a person's desire to live must be a firm conviction that comes from deep within. This leads to a very different emotional state than when someone is fighting off their cancer or fighting off death. As we have discussed, the fighting mentality puts your body into fight-or-flight mode, which increases cortisol (the "stress hormone") and suppresses the immune system. Alternatively, when you focus on your reasons for living, you feel joy, purpose, and happiness, which leads to immune-boosting hormonal changes throughout the body.

Put simply, the body listens to what the mind is saying. If your mind is focused on living, your brain will flood your bloodstream with so-called happy (and immune-boosting) hormones, including serotonin, oxytocin, and dopamine. According to many holistic healers, having strong reasons for living infuses your body with life-giving chi, or life force energy. The opposite is also true. If your mind is hopeless and you have given up on life, then your blood test results would show low levels of those immune-boosting hormones, and an acupuncturist who analyzed your pulse would tell you that your chi levels were too low.

Radical remission survivors all report that becoming focused on living required discovering—or, in some cases, rediscovering— the true sources of joy and purpose in their lives. For many, their cancer diagnoses prompted them to focus on aspects of their lives that had previously made them feel joyful, such as their professional goals, friendships, family, spirituality, creativity, community, or long-forgotten hobbies.

Your reasons for living will likely change during your lifetime. Think about the person you were at 20, and then try to imagine who you will be at 80. Do you think these two versions of yourself have the exact same priorities? Now add in an unexpected diagnosis such as cancer. How might that change things? For most people, the diagnosis of any serious disease or condition forces them to reevaluate their priorities and view their lives through a different lens. Over and over again, radical remission survivors report that their diagnosis was a wake-up call that prompted them to redefine their life purpose.

# Recent Developments

These days, there are a variety of apps to help you find your purpose, not to mention books by renowned authors such as Jack Canfield, Louise Hay, and Iyanla Vanzant. There are online videos on this topic as well by self-help experts such as Joe Dispenza, Elizabeth Gilbert, and Brené Brown, as well as many podcasts from leaders like Oprah and Lewis Howes. Aaron Teich, an energy healer and spiritual counselor who works with many cancer patients, offers this advice regarding finding your purpose:

> We don't have a purpose. We have and will have many. We are not one thing; we are multidimensional: physical, mental, emotional, creative, playful, relational. And we each play many roles—friend, partner, parent, child, sibling, colleague, student, mentor, etc. Each of these requires engagement and expression. As we grow and change through the phases of our lives, our interests and relationships will change, spawning new avenues of purpose and meaning. When we search for meaning in just one thing, such as our profession, we feel lost. When we recognize and honor our multiplicity, we find many paths.

## Research Says: Find Your Purpose

Intangible healing factors like having strong reasons for living may seem too "out there" for those who are more scientifically minded.

However, a large body of research shows that living with purpose is associated with better mental and physical health and long life. There are more than 60 years of scientific evidence on the topic of depression which demonstrate that depression—whose definition includes not having strong reasons for living—suppresses the immune system and leads to significantly shorter survival time for cancer patients.[1]

On the positive side, innovative researchers and medical doctors have demonstrated that living a purposeful life is associated with longevity and improved mental and physical health. One of them is Abdul Kadir Slocum, M.D., who is from the United States originally but grew up in Istanbul, Turkey, where he now treats cancer using both conventional (e.g., low-dose chemotherapy) and integrative treatments. He founded his own integrative cancer clinic, Chemothermia, with his colleagues Bülent Berkarda, M.D., and Mehmet Salih İyikesici, M.D. Dr. Slocum states:

*After many years of experience treating mostly stage 4 cancer patients, I have seen that the primary factor in a person's ability to overcome cancer is their will to live. When this is in place, the second most important element is [having] a trusting relationship with your health care provider. When these two conditions have been fulfilled, we have found it is important to take a disciplined approach of [following] the health care provider's treatment protocol while maintaining positive thoughts as part of an emotional-spiritual discipline, and following a dietary discipline based on the awareness that food is medicine. All this being said, I must reiterate that the will to live is the first and foremost condition for healing.*

Recent research backs up Dr. Slocum's assertion, showing that having a strong sense of purpose in life is associated with lower mortality and decreased risk of disease, disability, and cognitive impairment.[2] One study showed that children of centenarians (people who live to be 100 years old) have a significantly higher purpose in life (PIL) as compared to their spouses and people their same age.[3] These researchers concluded that having higher PIL may "play a role in the ability to delay age-associated illnesses"—and to delay the inflammation and immunity conditions that lead to cancer.[4]

A recent study out of the University of Michigan found that having a strong sense of PIL leads to improvements in both physical and mental health and enhances your overall quality of life. The researchers studied almost 7,000 people who were over age 50, and discovered that those who had the highest PIL scores were 2.5 times less likely to die than those who had the lowest PIL scores.[5]

Other studies from Japan have shown that having a strong *ikigai*—a subjective sense of well-being—is associated with reduced risk of cardiovascular disease, while not having a strong sense of *ikigai* is associated with higher mortality.[6]

Having strong reasons for living has also been associated with a significantly longer life span. A study that reviewed 10 prospective studies on the topic of life purpose, which in total analyzed more than 136,000 individuals, concluded that having a strong sense of life purpose is associated with a reduced risk of all-cause mortality.[7]

Another study following adults over a 10-year period found that having a greater life purpose predicted lower levels of allostatic load, that is, the wear and tear on one's body due to chronic stress. It is measured through both urine and blood tests, which analyze biomarkers associated with the neuroendocrine, cardiovascular, immune, and metabolic systems. This study is unique in that it is one of the first studies to show conclusively that having strong reasons for living in your mind leads to long-term, positive biological benefits in your body.[8]

## The Search for Meaning

Radical remission survivors show us that there is no one-size-fits-all approach to finding strong reasons for living. Some people are goal-oriented and prefer to keep their focus on the future. Some people find goals stressful, and instead focus on the joy to be found in each new day.

Because of the rising popularity of self-love, self-care, and the importance of increasing one's happiness, we have witnessed an explosion of new ways to explore this healing factor. Some credit millennials for this trend, given their alleged desire to find happiness in their daily lives and meaning in their work. However, the trend may be even broader than that. Perhaps society at large has finally realized that overworking, overscheduling, and overdosing on screen time may not actually lead to a fulfilling life.

Radical remission survivors who are more goal-focused like to have long-term aspirations to keep them going during their healing journeys (and to keep their blood, oxygen, and chi flowing strongly). Like some radical remission survivors, you might want to walk your daughter down the aisle on her wedding day, finish the novel you have always wanted to write, witness the birth of your first grandchild, or travel to 50 more countries before you die.

One radical remission survivor who focused on her long-term goals during her healing journey is Cindy Handler, who was diagnosed in 2015 at age 44 with a grade 3 anaplastic soft-tissue sarcoma, an aggressive meningeal tumor in the brain. Cindy recalls:

> *There is really no way to prepare for receiving a life-threatening diagnosis or the shock and terror that follows. We discovered my brain tumor three weeks into a new school year, when my girls were 7, 10, and 14 years old. We had also recently purchased our first home and were busily settling in and actualizing our dream of living by the ocean. When I imagined all the major developmental transitions coming up in our family, my heart knew how deeply my girls would need my nurturing and guidance. My family became my motivation for waking up every day and for actively transforming my life. I was willing to do anything necessary to be here to witness my kids blossom and grow up.*

By combining the best of conventional and integrative medicine, including brain surgery and all 10 radical remission factors, Cindy overcame tremendous odds and has no evidence of disease five years later. Her healing journey has given her new reasons for living and she now coaches others with life-threatening illnesses to rediscover their innate sense of well-being through mind-body connections and lifestyle changes. Cindy is also a certified Radical Remission workshop instructor. She and her husband recently celebrated a major milestone when they dropped their oldest daughter off for her freshman year of college.

While some radical remission survivors, like Cindy, choose to focus on long-term goals, others shy away from future-oriented hopes and instead try to rediscover the joys of everyday life. For these radical remission survivors, their reasons for living center on improving their day-to-day lives, and include things like watching the sunrise or sunset, going for walks in nature, or spending quality time with friends and family.

One radical remission survivor who focused on the joys of daily life is Kate. In 2009, Kate was living with her husband in rural Colorado when she was diagnosed with aggressive stage 3c ovarian cancer. Given their remote location and decision not to have children, Kate found herself quite isolated and lonely during her medical treatment. Thankfully, one of her dogs, Jasper, proved to be an unexpected source of support and inspiration.

*Jasper didn't leave my side the entire time I was sick. I was on the couch one day when I realized that life had been kind of hard up until then. I asked myself, Is it going to be worth it? Do I really want to do this? It occurred to me that I could probably decide I just didn't want to [live] and my body would comply. Then I looked at Jasper, who was looking at me like she could hear this conversation going on in my head, and I thought,* Don't worry, I'm not leaving you behind. *So then I started focusing on what I wanted to do when I got better. . . . I just started daydreaming about going up in the mountains with the dogs and the horse and camping in the forest. I didn't think about how miserable things were in the moment. I thought about what I had to look forward to once I got through all of this.*

Like many radical remission survivors, Kate made the decision to focus on her personal reasons for living rather than dwelling on the discomfort of her treatment or the possibility of dying. This strategy helped her get through the treatment, which included using both conventional medicine (surgery and chemotherapy) and all 10 radical remission healing factors. Despite being given only one year to live by her doctors, Kate is alive and well more than 10 years later, happily enjoying a nature-filled, high-quality daily life with her husband and dogs.

## Using Play to Find Purpose

One of the ways radical remission survivors get in touch with their reasons for living, whether they be future goals or daily joys, is by being playful. Play is not just for children; it has become a recognized source of relaxation, stimulation, and health for adults as well.[9] Adult play is a time to forget about your work, responsibilities, or even your illness while allowing your brain something that it sorely lacks in today's busy culture: unstructured, creative time. Playtime creates a healthier immune system by reducing stress, improving your sense of connectedness, and boosting your creativity.[10] By giving yourself permission to play with the joyful abandon you had in childhood, you will increase your positive emotions, and may find that everyday joy can become your strong reason for living. And, of course, your body will reap the many physiological and psychological benefits of play.[11]

The adult play trend has gone global, which makes it easier for cancer patients to include play as part of their treatment. For example, adult coloring books consistently top the best-seller lists, and many cancer centers have added them to their chemotherapy suites. Coloring provides an outlet for creative expression, reduces your stress,[12] and enhances your ability to live in the moment, as opposed to worrying about an uncertain future. In addition, adult board games and game nights are increasing in popularity. Good old-fashioned board games, card games like poker, or modern game nights with new twists (e.g., "escape rooms") help increase your social connections as well as exercise your laughter muscles.[13]

Adult art and craft options can be explored either alone or in a group. For instance, at a paint-and-sip, you bring a bottle of wine (or kombucha) and potentially a group of friends to a local art studio, and you paint the same scene on your own canvas under the guidance of a professional artist. Painting is not your only option. You can find themed nights for making wood signs, stained glass, floral arrangements, or homemade sushi. In addition, local community centers now host playful activities for adults, such as dodgeball, zip lining, nature hikes, and talent shows. Some vacation resorts and summer camps have caught on to this adult play trend and now offer summer camps for adults and families.

It is never too late to develop or remember your playful side. Don't forget that as a child you were naturally playful and did not worry about other people's reactions or about "more important" things that needed to get done. As we covered in Chapter 4, laughter is literally medicine for the body. Being playful will help you to release positive endorphins, rediscover everyday joy, and maybe even understand your reason for living. You can start to reclaim your inner child by setting aside time for regular, unstructured play. For many radical remission survivors, learning to fully enjoy each moment—whether through playful fun or peaceful gratitude—became their strong reason for living.

One radical remission survivor who never questioned his reason to live is Alex, who was diagnosed with a rare form of bone cancer at the young age of 12. His love of life, nature, and especially birds gave Alex strong reasons to never give up hope.

# Alex's Story

Alex grew up in a happy home in Connecticut with his mother, father, and two younger sisters. His early and middle childhood years were, in Alex's opinion, "wonderful"—filled with home-cooked family dinners, lots of baseball, and fun vacations. Although there were harder times, such as when Alex lost both of his grandmothers to cancer, overall he had a great life.

In spring 2009, Alex was 12 years old, finishing up the sixth grade, and enjoying two of his biggest passions in life: baseball and bird-watching. That season, he had been struggling to hit the ball well and get on base, and then one day he began having trouble throwing the baseball overhand. He adjusted by throwing the ball sidearm, but still, he got benched a lot. This was a new experience because he had previously been a valuable member of the team. As baseball became more and more of a challenge, Alex spent more time in nature birding and eventually decided that maybe he was not meant to play baseball.

At the end of the summer, Alex and his family were at the beach for their annual family vacation when he started feeling pain and swelling in his right upper arm. The pain continued for a week, so his parents took him to see a pediatrician, who diagnosed Alex with tendinitis and told him to put ice on his arm, although that did nothing to relieve the pain. After a week of futile icing, the pain became so severe one night that Alex told his parents he wanted to cut off his arm, so they knew something was very wrong.

First thing the next morning, Alex's dad took him to the local hospital where an X-ray revealed a grapefruit-sized tumor in Alex's right shoulder. The hospital doctor wanted to admit Alex immediately, but Alex's dad had a close friend who was an oncologist, so instead, they grabbed Alex's X-ray and the whole family jumped in the car and drove back home, including Alex's sisters, who were eleven and six at the time.

The abrupt departure frightened Alex. Their family had *never* left a vacation early. When they got home, their oncologist friend took one look at the X-ray and said it looked like osteosarcoma, the most common type of bone cancer. This friend immediately referred Alex to an orthopedic surgeon at Memorial Sloan Kettering Cancer Center (MSKCC) in New York City, who ordered scans and then performed a biopsy on the tumor.

The biopsy confirmed it: Alex indeed had osteosarcoma. A cancer diagnosis is traumatic for anyone, but it is especially difficult for a 12-year-old boy and his parents. Alex recalls:

> *I remember the exact room at Memorial Sloan Kettering Cancer Center. I was with my folks. We were pretty sure what he was going to say, but I remember verbatim the first words out of the surgeon's mouth. He looked me in the eye and said, "You're going to be fine, but you have osteosarcoma." And my mom started crying.*

Osteosarcoma accounts for about 3 percent of cancers in children,[14] and it most commonly affects teenage boys who are having a growth spurt.[15] After the official diagnosis, Alex's care shifted from the surgeon to an oncologist. The plan was three months of chemotherapy, followed by surgery to remove as much of the cancer as possible, and then six more months of chemo. At this point, Alex's case was very typical for osteosarcoma. It had been caught before it had spread, which meant he had a 60–80 percent chance of surviving for five years (with all the recommended conventional treatment). His doctors told him—and Alex agreed—that in 10 months, he was "going to be good."

Instead of starting seventh grade that September, Alex took an extended leave from school and began chemo while his parents and teachers worked out a home-school curriculum. After a few weeks of treatment, Alex lost all his hair.

> *In addition to having a really supportive core group of family and friends, the main thing that got me through treatment was my love of birds and birding. When I'd be in the hospital,*

*I'd constantly be thinking about getting out of the hospital, going birding, planning trips, and seeing new birds. I also had the hope of getting past treatment very soon—I kept thinking that by May, it's going to be all over.*

Unfortunately, things did not work out that way. In late November, his scans showed that the tumor had actually grown and that the cancer had spread to both his lungs. In short, the chemotherapy was not working. Alex's doctors immediately added an immunotherapy regimen to his chemotherapy. That December, he had a 14-hour surgery to remove most of his right upper-arm bone and replace it with a bone transplant. His doctors also removed Alex's entire right rotator cuff and right deltoid muscle, which permanently limited his range of motion in that arm. He would never again throw a baseball the way he had before.

Based on the "terrible" pathology report that came back after the surgery, Alex's doctors decided they needed to switch to a new chemotherapy while still continuing the immunotherapy. That spring Alex had two more surgeries, one on each lung, to remove the cancerous nodules that had appeared while he was on the first type of chemotherapy. To everyone's utter relief, the surgeries led to some good news: The pathology report showed a high rate of cell death within the nodules, suggesting that the new chemotherapy/immunotherapy combo was working. Alex and his family were thrilled. At this point, Alex and his parents realized his treatments would not end in May as they had hoped, but—forever an optimist—Alex just said to himself, *Alright, now it's going to be October.*

By the time summer rolled around, after being on both chemotherapy and immunotherapy for close to nine months, Alex's body began to wear down. His blood cell counts no longer rebounded as quickly after each treatment, which meant his doctors had to slow his treatment schedule. Making matters worse, Alex and his family were now facing the fact that there were significant health risks associated with continuing the harsh treatments.

*We became cognizant that there was a trade-off here. Essentially, it was just a cost-benefit analysis. Either we continued on the chemo and increased the [future] leukemia risk, or we stopped [the chemo] and would take our chances.*

Alex and his family decided to continue the chemotherapy and immunotherapy for a few more months, until that fall, when he was finally done with treatment. He reentered school, having learned enough seventh-grade material to keep up with his classmates. In October 2010, Alex turned 14, and it was a very happy birthday indeed.

*I went birding, of course—like I did on most of my birthdays back then. And I just slid right into eighth grade. In math, I was kind of confused for the first month. I didn't really understand the whole algebra thing. I was like, "Why is the 'x' there? Why are things disappearing here?" But after that, I was fine.*

Besides getting check-up scans every three months and not being able to move his right arm like he used to, Alex almost felt like a normal kid again. However, shortly after his eighth-grade graduation, his check-up scan showed new nodules on his right lung. They were not yet large enough to operate, so his doctors monitored him over the summer with monthly scans. The shadow of cancer loomed large.

From there, things continued to spiral downhill. In September, Alex learned that the nodules on his lung had grown even further, which meant that the chemotherapy/immunotherapy combo from the previous year had not worked. As a last-ditch effort, his doctors enrolled him in a clinical trial that used a new, untested immunotherapy. Through all of this, Alex struggled.

*That fall was weird because I was starting a new high school and at the same time this cancer was hanging over me. This thing that had been growing all summer was still there. And now that nebulous, broad world of clinical trials was open to me. I learned that the [clinical trial] treatments were easier for me and didn't feel as awful [as chemo], but we were also just kind of clutching at straws.*

The academics at Alex's new high school were intense and rigorous. He struggled to keep his grades strong while dealing with his new cancer treatment. Thankfully, Alex had extra support.

*The head adviser in my class was my never-ending advocate and support throughout all of this treatment. She was so incredible at talking to faculty: updating them on my situation, figuring out how to get me through my classes, accommodating my needs, moving things around, being more flexible.*

Despite all of this support, by December Alex began having terrible pains in his stomach. He and his parents met with a gastroenterologist who performed an endoscopy, a procedure in which a small camera is threaded down your esophagus to examine your stomach. They learned that his stomach was actually healthy, which meant the pain was most likely caused by stress. The doctor prescribed an antacid and antianxiety medication to ease his symptoms, and his parents immediately pulled him out of school. Alex continued to see the psychologist he had been seeing since before his diagnosis. However, he found the most relief from being outdoors, even though it was winter.

*Birding was definitely a huge thing for me at that time. After my normal outdoor passions—baseball and tennis—were taken away from me, I had to find other activities. Birding is like hiking, it's just walking most of the time. I also discovered soccer, which you're not supposed to use your arms for anyway, so that was great.*

In January, Alex had a fourth surgery to remove the new tumors on his lungs. In March, he was hospitalized for severe colitis—an unfortunate side effect from the clinical trial immunotherapy treatment—and he was not allowed to eat or drink for two weeks (IV fluids and nutrition only). As a result of this severe reaction, Alex's doctors took him off the immunotherapy clinical trial. By June, new lung nodules had grown, which meant he had to undergo yet another surgery.

That summer, Alex was invited to join a birding and ornithology summer program at Cornell University, which brought him great joy. He and his dad also took a special father-and-son birding trip to California.

*My parents were incredibly supportive of me, my hobbies, and my passions throughout all of my treatment. They really tried to keep a positive mind-set around my illness. My parents were always there, supporting my favorite interests and taking me on some wonderful trips. I have no doubt that they, too, were suffering. Remarkably, they were able to hide their suffering incredibly well during those times, and helped keep me positive and excited. I am so grateful for them.*

Alex always understood that his cancer could be fatal, but he never dwelled on his mortality.

*I never let go of the increasingly fantastical notion that one day I could live free of osteosarcoma. I was 15 years old and I had things I wanted to do! I didn't ruminate on death—I'm not sure how I was able to resist doing that, but I was. Even in the midst of treatment, the notion that birds had saved my life was never far from my mind. Mere months into my treatment, I had determined that since birds had done so much to save my life, I would work to help save theirs. I soon developed an unremitting passion for the planet we live on and I consider the Earth to be my greatest love.*

That August, Alex's doctors started him on a different immunotherapy clinical trial. This drug, 3F8, was very painful because it affected his nerve cells. Nevertheless, Alex soldiered on and returned to school as a sophomore that September. A month later, he celebrated his 16th birthday.

In November, the family received disheartening news. Alex's routine CT scan showed more new cancerous nodules on his left lung, so Alex underwent two more surgeries in December. The first was to remove the nodules, and the second, just four days later, was to remove a hemothorax (a collection of blood in the space between the chest wall and the lung), which was a side effect of his very first surgery. A silver lining appeared when the pathology report came back after the surgery and showed some necrosis (dead cancer cells) within the nodules. This news led Alex to continue with school and with the second clinical trial treatment.

After his February 2013 scan, Alex got a bit of a reprieve. No new nodules had grown since his surgery, and he and his parents felt like they could take a breath. It was around this time that Alex and his parents started looking into complementary therapies and began a kitchen sink approach, meaning they threw everything they could think of at Alex's health and wellness. One of the first things they did was visit a well-known medical intuitive who recommended that Alex begin taking a variety of supplements, one of which was cat's claw tincture. Feeling like he had nothing to lose, Alex began taking the supplements.

Unfortunately, just three months later, in May 2013, Alex's follow-up CT scan found a new tumor on his left shoulder blade. Alex's left side had taken over the bulk of the lifting and moving ever since Alex's first surgery when his right scapula was removed. To remove the new tumor on his left scapula, Alex had yet another surgery, this one to remove his left shoulder blade and one-third of his left rotator cuff (the muscles around the shoulder joint). Thankfully, Alex was still able to use his left arm normally after this difficult surgery.

Given the new tumor growth, Alex and his parents decided to stop the immunotherapy clinical trial. Alex was understandably depressed that summer, but he and his family still did not give up hope. He stopped taking the cat's claw tincture and instead tried hemp oils (THC and CBD). Unfortunately, these oils were not effective for Alex, although they are for many others.

In fall 2013, Alex turned 17, became a junior in high school, and felt a new lump on his rib. A CT scan showed that it was an additional metastasis, so that October, he underwent additional surgery to remove the cancer-infected rib. As Alex healed, his teachers worked to give him a reduced workload at school.

At this point, Alex had undergone nine surgeries in four years, endured endless rounds of chemotherapy and immunotherapy, and still, the cancer just kept coming back. Nevertheless, his will to live was incredibly strong.

*I very much wanted to live and attack the cancer head-on with as many different weapons as possible. My parents and I quickly realized that the myopic path of conventional therapy was not going to work for me any longer. I didn't take the words of my conventional team as being directly sent from the man above [God], but sought out other methods when theirs failed to stem the tide of my disease. I wanted to survive and I would do whatever it took to do so. It was that path that ultimately made the difference in my life.*

Alex and his family decided to take charge of his health care by adding a naturopathic doctor, Mark Bricca, N.D., to Alex's medical team. Dr. Bricca is a protégé of Dwight McKee, M.D.—a board-certified oncologist and pioneer of integrative oncology. As a naturopath, Dr. Bricca believes in treating the whole patient. After thorough testing with Dr. Bricca, Alex began a regimen of personalized herbs and supplements to rebuild his immune system. Dr. Bricca helped Alex create a healthy foundation for his life with regular exercise, a healthy diet, and daily meditation.

As part of their new, take-charge approach, Alex and his parents arranged to send samples of his cancerous scapula to both Rational Therapeutics and Champions Oncology for cytometric cancer profiling. This new form of testing, which falls under the umbrella of personalized medicine, takes a sample of your cancer cells and tests those cells (in petri dishes or in mice) against a variety of chemotherapy and immunotherapy agents before you start any treatment.[16] Instead of determining which chemotherapy you should use based on the results of a clinical trial conducted on a group of strangers, these personalized tests are intended to find the most effective therapy for *your unique* cancer cells.[17] Such a personalized approach excited Alex and his family because, after being disappointed by so many different chemotherapies and immunotherapy agents over the years, he now had the chance to find the exact agent or agents that could help his particular cancer. They also sent his cancerous tissue in to Foundation Medicine for genomic sequencing of his cancer cells.

The results of the cytometric cancer profiling came back in October, and surprisingly, the chemotherapy that Alex's cancer cells responded to best in the petri dish was cabazitaxel, a chemotherapy primarily used for prostate cancer patients, not sarcoma patients. As fate would have it, a clinical trial was just starting for cabazitaxel and Alex qualified for it.

> *Finally, we weren't just picking random clinical trials! We were actually going to try therapies that worked with my disease, which is what my mom wanted to do at the beginning, in 2009, because she knew about Champions Oncology back then. But my conventional team at Sloan [MSKCC] refused.*

Alex's mother and his maternal grandfather had believed in the power of complementary treatments from the very beginning of Alex's journey, and had tried to work with his conventional doctors early on to incorporate therapies such as high-dose vitamin C infusions into his care. Unfortunately, Alex's conventional doctors flat-out rejected doing anything beyond the standard of care and said to his mother, "You know, broccoli is not going to cure him." Because of their skepticism, Alex has still never told his conventional doctors that he started working with a naturopath.

Dr. Bricca prescribed Alex a large number of personalized supplements, including green tea extract, Power Adapt, CV-Res-Q, Immucare II, Ther-biotic Complete, Botanical Treasures, and others that were appropriate for Alex's body at that time. Alex is especially grateful to his mother, who sorted all of his supplements into daily containers and set timers on his phone so that he would remember to take them every few hours.

In terms of diet, Alex's mother had always been steadfast in providing her children with fresh, organic, whole foods, so

Dr. Bricca did not have many changes to suggest when it came to improving Alex's diet. Alex says he was "extremely fortunate to have a mother whose mind-set was, 'If you're going to spend money on anything, spend it on food.'" Alex's mother was already cooking her family homemade meals every night that included healthy sources of protein, lots of fresh vegetables, and small portions of healthy carbohydrates, such as brown rice or quinoa. "Cheat foods" for Alex included organic orange juice, Clif bars, organic white bread, or—during stressful periods at school—chocolate chip cookies.

Prior experience had shown Alex that his cancer would usually grow back within three to six months after any given surgery. However, since his last surgery, Alex had started on the new clinical trial of cabazitaxel, thanks to the cytometric profiling test. He had also begun Dr. Bricca's lifestyle changes, including personalized supplements, regular exercise, a healthier diet, and meditation. Alex and his parents prayed that these new tactics would help, and hoped that Alex's January 2014 scan would show no new cancer growth.

Their prayers were answered when the scan results came back. Although he still had small nodules on his lungs, they had not grown since his last surgery, and, more important, no new cancer had appeared anywhere else. They attributed this success equally to the new, personalized chemotherapy (cabazitaxel) and also to Dr. Bricca's personalized supplements and lifestyle changes. Alex was able to dive fully into the second half of his junior year, and his health continued to improve that spring and into the summer, with his three-month scans showing no new growth. By taking a more holistic approach to his treatment, Alex felt he was strengthening his immune system to better deal with the cancer.

By September 2014, Alex confidently entered his senior year of high school and turned 18 one month later. By this time, he had his routine down: He would miss one week of school for chemotherapy treatment, then spend two weeks attending school as usual, and then it was back for more chemo. He took his supplements throughout and continued to exercise and meditate regularly. Throughout this entire year, Alex kept up with a full course load of classes, which meant he was able to graduate high school in four years.

After a very celebratory high school graduation in June 2015, Alex decided to take a gap year before going to college. After almost five years of surgeries, difficult cancer treatments, and rigorous academics, he needed a break. He spent that summer working a low-stress job, enjoying time at the beach with his family, and, of course, birding. That fall, Alex's CT scan once again showed that his osteosarcoma was stable. The nodules on his lungs, which had been there since October 2013, had not changed for two whole years—a major feat with metastatic osteosarcoma.[18] He soon started applying to colleges.

Midway through his gap year, in January 2016, Alex went on one of the best trips of his life: a birding adventure to Australia with a longtime friend. He was in absolute heaven seeing birds he had only ever read about in books, spending time with his friend, traveling halfway across the world, and knowing his cancer was stable. When he returned from that trip, Alex got even more good news: He had been accepted into Brown University, a prestigious Ivy League university in Rhode Island.

As Alex's high school friends came home from their freshman years at college that summer, they started playing baseball together. Alex had to learn how to play with his left arm, but he adapted quickly. During one summer game, Alex hit a home run at his first at bat and the crowd went wild. As a result, the pitcher did not take it as easy on him the next time Alex stepped up to the plate. He swung as hard as he could, missed the ball, and broke his right upper-arm bone (the allograft, or donor's bone) in the process. Yet another surgery followed in July to replace his elbow and to reinforce the upper part of the allograft with a steel rod.

As summer wore on and Alex recovered from the arm surgery, he began to worry.

*I was going to start Brown [University] in September. At the same time, I was starting my 43rd cycle of cabazitaxel and was thinking, I can't do this. This is college. This is a hard school. The cabazitaxel was also starting to have a real impact on my mental health because the side effects of the treatment were getting worse. I was having bad thrush, dry mouth, chemo brain, and my taste was all messed up after [each] treatment. I also had some PTSD, after 43 bloody cycles, that was starting to weigh on me. And so I just couldn't continue [with chemotherapy]. It was a scary decision, but I decided to give it a go without treatment.*

So in fall 2016, Alex voluntarily stopped the chemotherapy and left home to attend Brown University. Treatment-free for the first time since his diagnosis seven years earlier, Alex was nervous that his cancer might return, so he asked Dr. Bricca to expand his holistic healing protocol. One of the things Dr. Bricca added was a copper chelating agent to reduce the amount of copper in Alex's body (which has been shown to increase tumor growth in certain patients).[19]

Alex left for college while still trying to process his years of cancer treatment, which unfortunately led him to struggle with depression, anxiety, and PTSD. To help with these struggles, Alex continues to see a psychologist and meditate regularly. He specifically enjoys meditating with the Calm app and reading the teachings of Byron Katie, Steve Mattus, and others. Lastly, he makes sure to stay active—to exercise even when he does not feel like it—and to force himself to be social whenever he is feeling down.

*It is not an understatement to say that this experience has been traumatizing. It's deeply impacted me physically, emotionally, and psychologically from the beginning. Even now, I have a range of issues like PTSD, anxiety, depression, apathy, and memory loss. All of these are inexorably linked to my diagnosis. Seeking help from psychologists is not easy, but it has helped me a lot. In addition, Dr. Bricca is like a healer, Buddhist teacher, and friend all at the same time.*

Alex continued with only holistic healing methods throughout his first, second, and third years at Brown—and, as of this writing, he has not had any recurrences. At first, Alex was monitored every three months by his medical team at MSKCC, then every six months, and now once a year. His CT scans have remained stable for the past six years. While he has not done any further chemotherapy treatment since 2016, he still works closely with his naturopath, Dr. Bricca, who carefully monitors Alex's blood and adjusts his supplements, diet, and lifestyle recommendations accordingly. Not surprisingly, Alex chose to major in biology, with a focus on ecology and evolution, and he hopes to enjoy a career studying avian evolution and conservation.

Skeptics may argue that it was the introduction of personalized chemotherapy, namely cabazitaxel, that led to Alex's remission. However, given the statistically high rate of osteosarcoma recurrence in general, as well as Alex's personal experience with frequent recurrences before he added holistic protocols to his treatment, Alex believes that the holistic treatments and lifestyle changes played an absolutely critical role in his healing.

> *As a scientist, you look for cause and effect. We eliminated conventional treatment three years ago [in 2016], and I'm still here and still stable. So if you think this alternative stuff is all fluff, [then] these last three years are a really great demonstration otherwise. My conventional doctors have no explanation for why I've survived. They just see this kid who did treatments, surgeries, got on cabazitaxel, and it worked. Now I'm just sitting with stable nodules in my lungs. But osteosarcoma is an aggressive, fast-growing disease. The nodules have not been stable for three years just by the grace of God. They're stable because we've pursued these alternative therapies.*

As of this writing, Alex is halfway through his senior year at Brown, 10 years after his initial diagnosis and six years after his cancer stabilized thanks to personalized chemotherapy, supplements, and diet and lifestyle changes. Even though the two (stable) nodules in his lungs serve as a constant reminder of his cancer, he is, for the most part, a typical college senior focused on what will happen after graduation. His love of nature has not waned in the slightest.

*Every time I'm out birding or read reports on climate change, I'm called to action for the original reason I was called to action as a 12-year-old. Nature is something that always straightened me out.*

Alex was just a 12-year-old boy when he was diagnosed with osteosarcoma. While he was aware that he could die, his strong will to live—fueled by his deep love of life, family, and nature—helped him to endure multiple surgeries and endless rounds of chemotherapy, all of which, unfortunately, did not stop his cancer. Once Alex and his family took control of the healing process and added both personalized chemotherapy and holistic healing methods into his regimen, he was able to achieve a six-year (and counting!) remission from a very aggressive form of cancer.

Looking back on his journey, Alex is extremely grateful to every member of his healing team for their support, especially to his parents, his conventional and integrative doctors, and his friends and family. He believes it is crucial for patients to be open to healing not just the body, but the mind and spirit as well. These days, when he is not working on maintaining his own health, you will likely find him working to maintain the health of our planet—especially its birds.

## Action Steps

In *Radical Remission*, I suggested a few simple writing exercises to make your life feel more vibrant and meaningful. To summarize: Grab a pen, find a quiet spot, and dig into these exercises that seek to uncover your life's meaning.

- Write down how old you want to be when you die (e.g., 100).

- Write your ideal obituary.

- Make a simple list of all your current reasons for living.

- Imagine you have $300 billion dollars, perfect health, and guaranteed success. What would you do? Then imagine your doctors tell you that you will die suddenly in 18 months without experiencing any prior symptoms. What would you do with your remaining time? Now compare your two answers. Where do they match up, and what does this tell you about your reasons for living, regardless of circumstances?

We love these writing exercises because they are quick ways to jump-start your thinking about your reasons for living. Remember that not everyone will be goal-oriented in their reasons. For some people, the joy to be found in everyday life is purpose enough. Below are a few more ideas to help you explore your reasons for living. (Note: If you are very sick and finding a life purpose seems overwhelming, then focus on today, and perhaps tomorrow. What joy will you find today?)

- **Don't presume that your passion should be your job.**

  You do not need to quit your day job in order to find your life's purpose. All you need are windows of time to be spontaneous, set aside your inhibitions, try something fun, and enjoy a change of pace. Block out some meaningful time for an afternoon or evening. Start by turning off your phone, TV, computer, and other devices, and then give yourself permission to do whatever you want for the time you have allotted.

- **Find the experts.**

  Read books, listen to podcasts, or watch online videos to help you identify your own unique reasons for living. Some of the most popular experts on this topic include Jack Canfield, Iyanla Vanzant, Elizabeth Gilbert, Michael Beckwith, Martha Beck, Louise Hay, and Joe Dispenza.

- **Connect to your inner child.**

  What games, sports, art, and/or activities did you enjoy as a child? Did you like riding your bike? Fixing things? Playing a certain sport? Painting? Dancing? Writing stories? When did you experience the greatest joy in your life? Think back to the activities you enjoyed most, write them down, and brainstorm how you might incorporate them into your life now.

- **Play with children.**

  Children know how to play. If you have nieces or nephews (biological or honorary), or children or grandchildren of your own, make time to play with them. Observe their ability to live in the moment, and practice being playful with them. Sometimes our reason for living can be as simple as having fun and enjoying each day as much as possible. Children can show you how to do just that.

- **Create a life purpose statement.**

  Take a few minutes and write down a description of what your life would look like if everything were

"perfect" from your unique point of view. Write in
the present tense. What are you and those around
you doing? How do you feel? What does it mean and
look like to have everything you want? Combine
these thoughts into one statement, and you will have
a clearer idea of your life purpose.

- **Volunteer for a charity that interests you.**

  When you give of yourself to help others,
  it fills your soul and gives meaning to your life.
  Volunteering for a nonprofit organization in your
  community—ideally in person, as opposed to
  online—will not only make you feel good, but will
  also help others and help you to live according to
  your values.

For human beings, it is a gift to start each day with hope—to feel
eager about seeing what happens next. As Alex's story shows—and
the research supports—having purpose and finding joy in your life
is essential to healing and health.

What have you always wanted to do in life? We give you a
permission slip to go and do it! What would you look back and
regret *not* doing if you knew your time was limited? Having strong
reasons for living provides a sense of purpose that can support
your healing and ensure that you spend your time doing what
matters most.

## CHAPTER 10

# INCREASING SOCIAL SUPPORT

## Sally's Story

*Be with people who make you feel good.*

— Louise Hay

One of the biggest flaws of modern society is how the notion "I can do it on my own" is revered. While independence is an important human trait, we need to remember that humans are social creatures who have survived over millennia together, living in groups whose members depended on one another for survival, health, and happiness.

People diagnosed with cancer or another serious illness typically experience a deluge of emotions, including shock, disbelief, fear, anxiety, anger, frustration, grief, guilt, and despair. These emotions are too overwhelming to deal with by yourself. For this reason, radical remission survivors have reported that finding the right social support from their friends, family, and healing teams was essential for their healing.

In this chapter, we will explain why and how building a social support network benefits your healing and will discuss new and easy ways to find your community, as well as some of the pitfalls that modern technology presents. We will share a heartwarming story about Sally, a courageous woman who used all the radical remission healing factors, including social support, to reverse Alzheimer's disease. Finally, we will conclude the chapter with some practical action steps that can help you build your own social support network.

My research on radical remissions reinforces what we all instinctively understand: At a fundamental level, humans need each other in order to survive. Humans depend on each other throughout their lives, from birth until death. Over the course of human history, banding together has improved our chances of survival. The formation of agrarian societies has allowed humans to live in ever-larger groups and to reap the benefits of specialization. Today we are more interconnected than ever, and few of us possess the skills to survive alone in the wilderness.

Receiving love from others when we are healthy helps us to fight off infection, and when we are sick, it actually helps our bodies heal. When we are surrounded by loved ones, including pets, the feeling of being loved releases a flood of healing hormones into the bloodstream.[1] This makes us feel better emotionally while also strengthening our immune systems.[2]

Over the long term, researchers have found that people with strong social connections live significantly longer and have lower cancer rates than people with weak social connections.[3,4] And in a recent study, researchers found that higher levels of social support were associated with improved cognitive health.[5] Surprisingly, social connections can be more beneficial to your health than exercise, a healthy diet, or avoiding smoking and alcohol.[6] When you look at the science behind social connections, these findings begin to make sense. For example, when you receive love, support, or comforting human contact,[7] your brain increases its output of healing hormones, such as dopamine, oxytocin, serotonin, and endorphins,[8] all of which boost your immune system by decreasing inflammation, increasing blood and oxygen circulation, and increasing your number of white blood cells, red blood cells, helper T cells, and natural killer cells.[9]

While social connection is a powerful immune booster, its opposite—loneliness—can be a silent killer. In one recent study, cardiac patients who reported feeling lonely had a significantly higher risk of death.[10]

Radical remission survivors report that it does not matter how you get your social support, whether it be from three close friends, 30 acquaintances, or one life partner. Rather, they claim—and researchers agree—the only thing that matters is that you feel supported.[11] Your social support network can be made up of anyone in your life who offers you support, love, inspiration, or guidance. For many people, this includes family, friends, pets, co-workers, clergy, healers, doctors, and teachers. Beyond the comfort of family, the nonfamilial communities we consciously create throughout our lives have the ability to restore, heal, and uplift us. Finally, pets also qualify as sources of support. They offer unconditional love and companionship, which causes a release of the same healing hormones. As a result, studies have shown that pet owners live significantly longer than people who don't have pets.[12]

We know that many people feel awkward asking for help because they do not want to be a burden on others. Perhaps you have always prided yourself on being independent and self-reliant. However, radical remission survivors have found that their friends and family truly wanted to help them, even if they did not know exactly how to help. Fortunately, there are many new and exciting ways to connect with others these days, which we will discuss later in this chapter.

Ian Gawler is a radical remission survivor of osteosarcoma (bone cancer) who became a prominent advocate of mind-body medicine, meditation, and social support for cancer healing. When he was diagnosed in 1975, Dr. Gawler had his right leg surgically amputated to remove the cancer. Unfortunately, the cancer returned swiftly. To overcome his dire prognosis, Dr. Gawler embarked on an intensive health regimen that included anticancer nutrition, a positive attitude, regular meditation, and the acceptance of loving support. Based on his own healing experience, Dr. Gawler went on to establish Australia's first cancer support group and write several best-selling books about healing. Here is what Dr. Gawler has to say:

*From a practical point of view, we all recognize that having [social] support can help us maintain a positive mental state, reduce stress, and adopt better coping practices. Social isolation, on the other hand, predisposes us to a whole range of illnesses, including cancer, and is associated with a higher mortality rate. The lack of a relationship and adequate support has been shown to undermine the body's immune system and therefore our capacity to heal.*

Today, more than 45 years after being diagnosed with an aggressive form of cancer, Dr. Gawler is alive and well. The nonprofit he founded, The Gawler Cancer Foundation, continues to offer retreats for people affected by cancer where the focus is on training the mind, increasing social support, reducing stress, eating a healthy diet, and meditation.

# Recent Developments

## Loneliness Research

Put simply, not having enough social support can be harmful to your health. In fact, loneliness is nearing the point of becoming a public health crisis. According to a recent study, nearly half of all Americans feel alone, isolated, or left out at least some of the time,[13] and 10 percent of Americans say they feel lonely all or most of the time.[14] This may not seem like a public health crisis until you understand that the effects of loneliness shorten your life span as much as smoking 15 cigarettes a day, being obese, or being an alcoholic does.[15]

Being lonely can harm our health by causing us to engage in unhealthy behaviors. One study found that socially isolated participants were less likely to report doing moderate-to-vigorous exercise each week or to be eating five servings of fruits and vegetables each day. However, they *were* more likely to smoke cigarettes, and among those who smoked regularly, being lonely decreased their chances of quitting successfully.[16]

Another recent study looked at more than 10,000 individuals in Finland, Poland, and Spain and found that loneliness was the one variable most strongly correlated with poor health.[17] In fact, loneliness contributed more strongly to poor health than any other component of the participants' social network (e.g., number of friends). Researchers found that some consequences of loneliness included impairments in attention and cognition, negative changes to gene expression and hormone levels, and negative modifications to the nervous and immune systems.[18] These negative effects contributed to adverse health outcomes, such as whether a participant was diagnosed with a serious disease and/or died during the course of the study.

Interestingly, the researchers found that the *frequency* of social contact was the only component of one's social network that was correlated with improved health, while the size and quality of one's social network did not affect the level of loneliness in participants.[19] Therefore, regardless of whether you have 200 friends or only a few quality friendships, the only factor that actually makes you feel less lonely is seeing your friends more often.

Another study out of the United Kingdom looked at the effects of loneliness across different neighborhoods. The researchers found that loneliness was highest among those who had limited contact with family or neighbors and had no other sources of practical or emotional support.[20] These feelings of loneliness were associated with long-term problems with stress, anxiety, and depression.[21]

This study suggests that neighborly behaviors (such as friendly interactions in parks or local shopping areas) and being an active acquaintance with your neighbors (as opposed to someone they just recognize) are important for protecting against loneliness.[22] The researchers concluded that three mechanisms may link loneliness to poor health: First, loneliness itself is a stressor on the body; second, lonely people do not respond as well to other stressors in their lives; and third, being lonely means that you do not reap the benefit of having friends to help you in a time of crisis.[23]

## Building Your Own Community

Over the past few years, there has been a growing awareness of so-called toxic relationships and their negative impact on mental and physical health. Even if you have always thought your social support network was strong, there is nothing like a serious diagnosis to shake things up and reveal the true nature of your relationships. Therefore, radical remission survivors report that it is important to meet new people and welcome new resources into one's life after a diagnosis. As they often said in our interviews, "Your new friends may not look like your old ones."

Many radical remission survivors found their long-held beliefs thrown into disarray after diagnosis. Many were confused about treatment. Some were disappointed by friends they thought they could count on but who let them down, and others were happily surprised by strangers who unexpectedly stepped up to show support. Regardless of their situation, radical remission survivors found that as they faced their fears, doubts, blame, guilt, and mortality, it helped tremendously to have support from friends, family, and healers to hold them steady.

One such survivor is Debra Nozik, who has used conventional medicine plus the 10 radical remission healing factors to manage stage 4 breast cancer for more than 20 years. Deb discovered the radical remission healing factors on her own, and she felt especially uplifted by the support she received from others, including her loved ones, her dog, a local breast cancer support group, and even strangers. However, receiving love and support did not always come easily for Deb. Rather, it was something she had to learn and practice—a refrain that many other radical remission survivors echo. As Deb describes it:

> When I was diagnosed with metastatic breast cancer in 1999, one of the most profound lessons I learned was how to

*become a receiver as well as a giver. As a wife, mother, daughter, sister, friend, and therapist, I was an expert at giving help, support, and love. The crisis of such a life-threatening illness gave me the opportunity to learn how to accept and ask for the same from others. I even received prayers from people I did not know. I became a member of a local breast cancer support group, which enabled me to navigate my way through all of the challenges cancer sent my way. And the unconditional love of my dog, Daisy, was my daily oxytocin surge! Within a few years, my cancer totally reversed. I am a true believer that love heals!*

These days, Deb has learned to balance her giving and receiving. She currently gives support to cancer patients as a certified Radical Remission workshop instructor, and also receives love and support from her family, friends, and fellow workshop instructors.

Radical remission survivors like Deb report that they tried to surround themselves with people who supported their healing choices and provided new knowledge, perspective, or ideas. They also looked for positive people who believed healing was possible, people to hold them accountable for their new healthy lifestyle changes, and people who would let them feel whatever they were feeling without changing the subject or telling them everything would be all right. For radical remission survivors, a strong social support network includes nonjudgmental friends who let them cry, scream, or laugh as needed.

Radical remission survivors report that being diagnosed forced them to reevaluate every area of their lives, including their existing social support networks. Sometimes they saw a harsh reality. As the radical remission survivors began to explore unconventional treatment options, some members of their existing support network felt threatened by these new ideas with respect to their own set of deeply held beliefs.

This happened to Andrea Sexton, a five-year radical remission survivor of ovarian cancer who is also a certified Radical Remission workshop instructor. In 2014, Andrea had recently moved away from her longtime home in New Jersey when she received her grim cancer diagnosis. The diagnosis combined with the isolation was crushing, and she intuitively felt she would not survive the recommended chemotherapy, especially given that she did not have any local social support. Therefore, she made the personal decision to go through with the recommended surgery but to refuse chemotherapy and instead receive alternative treatment at the Klinik Marinus am Stein in Germany.

*I was sure that all of my friends would see that I had made a well-thought-out, well-researched choice. I was so naive. Some friends were unconditionally supportive; others thought I was being reckless with my health. I realized that cancer terrified them—they could only support my treatment choice if it was one that they would feel comfortable with. So I drew an imaginary circle around myself and decided who would get inside the circle, and who wouldn't. I got very good at recognizing people who were outside the circle. They were the ones who always changed the subject, wouldn't look me in the eye, or became silent when I mentioned anything about my cancer experience. That's fine. The ones inside the circle are more than enough.*

Another interesting revelation radical remission survivors report is that the more confidently they embraced their treatment decisions, the more their friends and family were willing to accept those decisions. Any friends they did lose from their inner circle after announcing their treatment decisions were often replaced by an even stronger, more supportive group of new friends—even if that new group was smaller in size.

## Social Support Research

Researchers have discovered that social support helps to reduce your anxiety, even if you are pessimistic about your prognosis.[24] One study of people with advanced cancer showed that those who had higher levels of perceived social support had a significantly higher quality of life.[25] And even for those cancer patients in this study who had low levels of optimism about their health situation, higher levels of social support were still associated with lower anxiety levels.

Similarly, a recent study in Germany wanted to measure the impact of psychological stress on women who were told to have chemotherapy to shrink their breast cancer tumors before they had surgery.[26] The researchers hypothesized that these women were in an especially stressful situation, because they not only had to deal with the shock of their diagnosis, but also with the fact that their malignant tumor would be removed after weeks of chemotherapy instead of immediately. The researchers felt this situation was unusually stressful and might require additional personal strength.

Not surprisingly, the researchers found that patients who had a poor psychosocial adjustment to their situation also exhibited poor social coping strategies. Their coping behavior was characterized by resignation and by making no attempts to seek social support. This behavior was found to significantly increase their overall risk of cancer recurrence as well as their risk of developing another type of cancer during the three- to five-year follow-up period.[27]

There is some good news, though. These researchers also found that patients who found a way to *strengthen* and *improve* their coping strategies—such as reaching out for more social support—were able to cope significantly better with their cancer treatment as compared to those who made no effort to improve their coping strategies or social support network.

## Finding Your People Online

Social media and technology offer many new ways to connect with like-minded people around the globe. In 2018, approximately 3.8 billion people—51 percent of the global population—were connected to the Internet.[28] This means we can now find people around the world who share our interests, diagnoses, and passions, rather than just interacting with people who happen to live in our neighborhood or local community. With the use of apps, video conferencing, and virtual meet-ups, we now have access to millions of people at any hour of the day or night. In addition, this technology allows us to reconnect with people with whom we have lost touch, such as old friends from elementary or high school.

Radical remission survivors use technology to build a stronger social support network by joining online support groups for their specific cancer type or by finding an online cancer mentor. For example, radical remission survivor Bob Granata, whom you met in Chapter 3, had a rare appendiceal cancer that affects only about nine in a million cancer patients. Due to its rarity, his doctors could not connect him with former patients who shared the same diagnosis, so instead, Bob searched online for other survivors of his rare cancer. Other radical remission survivors have used the Internet to discover local support groups or fun group activities. In addition, technology has allowed radical remission survivors to connect with people at any time of day, which is good news for anyone suffering from treatment-related insomnia.

Despite these benefits, social media and technology also have their drawbacks. For one thing, connecting online lacks the energy of an in-person connection. Studies have shown that humans need real, physical touch for psychological and physical well-being, from infancy through adulthood.[29] When we substitute digital connection for in-person connection, we deny ourselves the healing benefits that physical proximity and face-to-face interactions provide.

We all know we should not be checking our phones while watching our children or at lunch with our friends since such "digital moments" cause us to lose out on moments of true, in-person social connection. We need to beware of technology addiction that leaves us feeling depressed and, ironically, less socially supported. For instance, in our need to feel liked and accepted in some online communities, we might post only good news or idealized images of our lives. The craving for likes can leave us feeling deflated or even depressed when we don't get them.[30] Radical remission survivors try to find online communities where they can be authentic, flaws and all, on good days and bad.

Lastly, while it is wonderful to have a distraction at 3 A.M. when you are awake with chemotherapy-induced nausea, the Internet can lead you down a time-sucking rabbit hole. This will disrupt your sleep patterns and circadian rhythms, both of which are essential for healing. Therefore, it is important to use technology and social media for limited amounts of time each day, and only in ways that leave you feeling uplifted and more connected.

## Inflammation and Fight-or-Flight

Breast cancer survivors feel more quickly threatened than healthy people, which makes sense. Cancer survivors are more on edge than the general population, given that they are survivors of trauma from their cancer diagnosis and treatment and may constantly be worried about a cancer recurrence. As we have discussed, inflammation and the stress of being in chronic fight-or-flight mode create conditions in which cancer cells thrive, and these states are associated with increased risk of cancer recurrence and mortality among breast cancer survivors.[31] In a recent study across University of California institutions, researchers set out to assess the relationship between social support, inflammatory markers, and amygdala reactivity (an indicator of fight-or-flight mode) in breast cancer survivors as compared to healthy people who had never had cancer. The researchers looked at inflammatory markers in blood samples and images from functional MRI (fMRI) scans, which assessed activity in the amygdala after showing the subjects images of a perceived threat. After these tests, participants also self-reported their levels of social support.[32]

The researchers found that the breast cancer survivor group's inflammation levels and amygdala activity increased sharply after being shown the perceived threat, while the healthy control group's levels did not. However, the breast cancer survivors who had a higher level of social support had *lower* levels of inflamma-tion and amygdala reactivity.[33] This study reiterates that cancer patients need social support even more so than the general pop-ulation, due to their easily triggered fight-or-flight responses in the brain.[34]

More broadly, your level of social support may help determine whether you get sick in the first place or how severe that sick-ness becomes. In a recent study, researchers reviewed more than 40 studies on social support and inflammation, which altogether looked at more than 73,000 subjects,[35] and found that higher social support was significantly associated with lower levels of inflamma-tion. The researchers boldly stated that "inflammation is at least one important biological mechanism linking social support and social integration to the development and course of disease."

Another study out of Ohio State University investigated the association between social relationships and inflammation in black women, a population with higher rates of cardiovascular disease.[36] The researchers looked at almost 2,000 young black women ages 24–34 with various social relationships, such as marriage/cohabitation, church attendance, volunteerism, and close friendships.[37] The women's inflammation was measured via a blood test to determine if they had high hs-CRP (high-sensitivity C-reactive protein) levels, a well-known marker of inflammation in the body.[38]

The researchers found that stronger social integration and a higher quality of specific social relationships, such as a spouse or mother figure, were significantly associated with lower inflamma-tion levels, and they concluded that strengthening social support is key for young black women's health, especially given that can-cer rates for that population are on the rise.[39] Also, while the cor-relation between high hs-CRP levels and cardiovascular disease is well-known, recent studies show that high hs-CRP levels are also indicative of an increased cancer risk.[40]

## Vulnerability and Authenticity

Part of the backlash against the picture-perfect lives we see on social media is a movement away from being fake, filtered, rehearsed, polished, or showing only your best days, and a movement toward being more authentic, vulnerable, and honest. This is not only good news for humanity, but also for cancer patients, who may not have as many good days to share on social media.

World-renowned sociologist Brené Brown, Ph.D., has spent decades studying and interviewing people about deep emotions such as vulnerability, courage, worthiness, and shame. Brown's TED Talk on "The Power of Vulnerability" has been viewed more than 40 million times, she has written several *New York Times* best-sellers on these topics, and is credited with starting a global conversation around the need for vulnerability and connection in our lives. Dr. Brown says:

> *Connection is why we're here. It's what gives purpose and meaning to our lives, and "belonging" is in our DNA. . . . We are biologically, cognitively, physically, and spiritually wired to love, be loved, and to belong. When those needs are not met, we don't function as we're meant to be. We break. We fall apart. People love you not despite your imperfections and vulnerability, but because of your imperfections and vulnerability.*

There is no more vulnerable time than the period following a life-threatening diagnosis. Brown's research findings echo the feedback we get from radical remission survivors who emphasize the importance of building an authentic support network. As vulnerability becomes more socially acceptable, we hope you will surround yourself with people who can be vulnerable and authentic alongside you. Openness to vulnerability plays a large role in cancer support groups, whose members are increasingly encouraged to be raw and honest.

## Financial Support

Cancer patients often find it hard to ask for financial help. In our society, particularly in the United States, we believe that it is our responsibility to pay our own way in life, including for expensive cancer treatment. Thirty percent of cancer survivors report experiencing financial hardship,[41] and cancer patients have bankruptcy rates that are two and a half times higher than those without cancer.[42] Even patients with adequate health insurance are not immune. A recent Duke University study found that more than one-third of insured cancer patients faced greater out-of-pocket medical costs than they expected for their treatment, including some patients who were spending almost one-third of their income on health care–related costs.[43]

Many radical remission survivors reported that receiving financial assistance from their community, church, friends, family, or even strangers was one of the most humbling and helpful forms of social support they received during their healing journey.

Thankfully, in recent years, crowdfunding websites like GoFundMe and Kickstarter have made it easier for cancer patients to ask for financial assistance in a streamlined, efficient way. In fact, GoFundMe reports that one-third of its site's donations go toward medical fund-raising campaigns to help cover medical bills and related health care costs.[44]

Recent trends and scientific research continue to demonstrate that social support is critical in maintaining one's physical and emotional health, especially during times of crisis, including the diagnosis of cancer or serious illness. One of our goals in writing *Radical Hope* was to feature stories of people who have had radical remissions from diseases other than cancer. Ever since *Radical Remission* was published, we have received e-mails from people around the world who have said they used the radical remission healing factors to cure themselves—but not from cancer. Instead, they have gone into remission from multiple sclerosis (MS), Lyme disease, lupus, heart disease, diabetes, and more.

For this reason, we reconfigured our database at RadicalRemission.com so that it can accept healing stories about illnesses other than cancer. In Chapter 5, we shared with you Palmer's story about healing from MS, the first non-cancer healing story we received in our database. In this chapter, as we explore how social support can enable physical healing, we are excited to introduce you to Sally, a fiery woman from the southern United States who used all 10 radical remission factors, including incredible support from her husband, to overcome Alzheimer's disease.

Today, 5.8 million Americans are living with Alzheimer's disease,[45] and it is the third leading cause of death in the United States.[46] One-third of all U.S. citizens older than 65 will die of Alzheimer's or dementia, which means it kills more seniors than breast and prostate cancer combined.[47]

While most of us have met someone who has overcome cancer, very few of us have met anyone who has reversed Alzheimer's. However, one pioneering doctor—UCLA researcher Dale Bredesen, M.D.—has developed a specialized healing protocol that happens to incorporate almost all the 10 radical remission healing factors. His protocol has helped hundreds of people achieve complete remissions from Alzheimer's. Sally is one such survivor.

## Sally's Story

Sally is a retired nurse and doting grandmother of six grandchildren with a warm presence and boisterous laugh. Her generous nature and Southern charm are immediately apparent to anyone she meets. Sharp intellect and natural leadership qualities led her to having a very successful career in nursing and health research, for which she received many accolades and awards at the local, state, and national levels.

Like many older adults, Sally would rather die from anything other than Alzheimer's. Four of her aunts and uncles (on both sides of her family) have died from the disease, so Sally understands all too well the pain it can cause. She has also always suspected that her family history might put her at heightened genetic risk. However, when she started to experience mental confusion, she rationalized her symptoms and denied the truth for a long time.

Sally spent the early years of her nursing career in geriatric care, so she has a much better sense of early Alzheimer's symptoms than most people, who tend to associate the disease only with its advanced symptoms (e.g., forgetting loved ones' names, personality changes, not being able to carry out basic activities like getting dressed). But there are earlier warning signs.

Sally's symptoms began to appear as early as 2000, when she (then age 53) and her husband, Martin, moved to a different state for her exciting, yet stressful, new job. Making a beautiful 50-year-old house their new home, they had no reason to suspect mold in the basement insulation or the carpet padding. Nor did they realize that their proximity to the busy interstate would cause Sally's eyes to burn from the fumes during the evenings. When she began to experience mental confusion, Sally attributed it to stress and depression due to the move and new job.

Back in the 1980s, Sally had taught her gerontology students that confusion was a common side effect of depression and that treating the depression usually cured the confusion. So Sally began to take an antidepressant. Thankfully, this eased her depression somewhat and resolved her confusion.

In 2005, Sally and her husband moved once again, this time to work at another university in a different state, where she recalls:

> I would mix up words, saying an incorrect but similar word instead of the one I thought I was saying. I told my nursing students and colleagues, family, and friends that I had developed dyslexia in speech as I aged. To an outsider—and to myself—I did not appear to have any real symptoms of Alzheimer's disease. In retrospect, though, I believe I had subjective cognitive impairment, but didn't recognize it. And indeed, the term

*subjective cognitive impairment had not even been developed at this time.*

Also known as subjective memory disorder or subjective cognitive decline, subjective cognitive impairment can have many different causes. It occurs when a patient reports a worsening of their thinking abilities, including memory, before the changes can be detected using assessments of cognitive function.[48,49] By itself, this symptom is not sufficient to diagnose Alzheimer's. It is, however, one of the earliest warning signs.[50]

Three years later, when she was 61, Sally and her husband excitedly retired and moved back to her home state to be close to her son and his family, including three young granddaughters. Sally believed that her ongoing symptoms could be attributed to normal aging. But two more years later, she began to notice an intermittent worsening of her symptoms. She had trouble remembering the correct day of the month and figuring out when to leave home for appointments, sometimes forgetting appointments entirely. Her "dyslexia" deteriorated to the point that her speech would confuse listeners during conversation. She experienced three near-miss car accidents that would have been her fault had a wreck actually occurred. Remembering where she put things, using the computer, and spelling became frustrating endeavors. This was alarming, to say the least.

*I would try to think of the next sentence I wanted to say, but then I would think and it wouldn't connect. It's like your thought would hit a brick wall, and you knew there was something on the other side that you wanted to think of, but it wouldn't connect.*

A year later, Sally struggled to lead a group activity—decorating gingerbread cookies with her granddaughter's class at school— even though she had done this without difficulty many times before. When she confused the minute and hour hands on the clock, Sally finally had to confront the truth: These symptoms could not be attributed to normal aging.

*I had a dose of reality when I forgot to pick up my grand-
children, whom I would never purposely forget, twice in four
weeks. That's when I thought,* Sally, denial isn't working anymore. Forget denial. You have to deal with this. *I decided,*
Sally, you've got it [Alzheimer's]. You might as well tell
people, so they can help you and so you can get support
and not hide it.

Sally's first step was to review the published research on
Alzheimer's, in hopes of finding clinical trials that she could join
as a patient. She even made an appointment to be assessed at Duke
University's Alzheimer's center, but canceled it after deciding to
enroll in a different, nationwide research study whose goal was to
treat Alzheimer's by removing beta-amyloid plaques. She was 67
years old.

As part of her initial assessment in the research study, Sally
underwent a PET scan. The results confirmed her worst fears:
There were beta-amyloid plaques in her brain.

*When I was told I was positive for Alzheimer's, I remember
the physician wanted to keep talking. I said, "Wait, you've gotta
give me a minute!" I hugged my husband. I was so depressed—I
didn't want to live. Both [of my adult] children had known for
a long time that I didn't want to be treated if I couldn't call the
grandchildren [by] their correct names.*

At the time, Sally was told that a positive scan for beta-amyloid
plaques was a definitive indicator of future Alzheimer's disease.
Since then, studies have shown that the presence of plaque does
not always lead to Alzheimer's, and new research is demonstrating
that mild cognitive impairment can be reversed.[51]

Sally remained under treatment in the trial for nine months,
stopping when the side effects (irritability and increased confusion that lasted several days after each infusion) became a cause
for concern. Three months later, she formally withdrew from
the trial.

After the PET scan forced Sally to face her worst fears, she decided to take a more empowered role. In addition to participating in the clinical trial, Sally asked her husband to administer the Montreal Cognitive Assessment (MoCA) Test.[52] She wanted a baseline measure of cognition that she could use to assess changes over time. MoCA scores range from 1 to 30. A score above 25 is considered normal, while a score between 18 and 25 indicates mild cognitive impairment (MCI), between 10 and 17 indicates moderate cognitive impairment, and any score below 10 indicates severe cognitive impairment.

Sally scored 24.5 on her MoCA, yet another data point confirming that her difficulties were not simply "normal aging changes." Common symptoms of MCI—all too familiar to Sally—include forgetting scheduled appointments, mixing up words, stopping in the middle of a sentence, having trouble remembering where you put your wallet or keys, and poor spatial awareness, which makes driving difficult.[53]

Around this time, Martin happened to hear Dr. Dale Bredesen speak about Alzheimer's on a national radio show. Dr. Bredesen is a UCLA professor, an internationally recognized expert in the mechanisms of neurodegenerative diseases, and one of the first physicians to successfully reverse Alzheimer's Disease. His treatment protocol, named ReCODE (for Reversal of Cognitive Decline), is based on his decades of lab and clinical research in the area of dementia.

Both Sally and Martin were highly intrigued when they read Dr. Bredesen's 2014 journal article describing successful reversal of Alzheimer's symptoms in 9 of the first 10 patients to adopt his formal ReCODE protocol.[54] Sally immediately implemented two of the recommended lifestyle changes related to sleep and meditation.

Alzheimer's patients, like radical remission cancer survivors, vary widely and have highly personalized needs. Dr. Bredesen has identified three types of Alzheimer's: type 1, associated with inflammation and common viruses; type 2, associated with hormonal or metabolic imbalances or deficiencies; and type 3, associated with enhanced sensitivity to inhalational biotoxins, like mold or other mycotoxins.[55,56] For Dr. Bredesen, a patient's treatment plan depends on his or her individual test results and the type of Alzheimer's he or she has.

Shortly after her PET scan, Sally asked a local doctor friend and former research colleague to be her primary care provider as she attempted to treat her Alzheimer's disease. He agreed since he, too, was intrigued by Dr. Bredesen's ReCODE protocol.

Sally e-mailed Dr. Bredesen and asked to participate in his research studies, only to learn that it would not be possible. His research studies at that time required patients to be based in California. However, Dr. Bredesen generously offered to share his ReCODE program with her and her local physician.

The first step was for Sally to obtain a *cognoscopy*, Dr. Bredesen's term for a detailed assessment of her health, including blood labs, genetic tests, and other factors.[57] Many of the laboratory tests were new to Sally, her physician, and even to the commercial labs that were asked to conduct the tests, and the process took four months to complete. Of the 36 tests, every single one showed a problem that needed to be corrected, which meant that Sally had all three types of Alzheimer's. Dr. Bredesen's resulting 12-page ReCODE report recommended specific lifestyle changes, interventions, and supplements.

At first Sally was overwhelmed, but she was also a strong, resilient woman who had overcome many challenges. She thought, *I can look at this as "Oh, no!" or I can tell myself, "If I have all three causes of Alzheimer's, it sure helps to know about it. This way, I can do something about it."*

Sally had always assumed that she would test positive for the Alzheimer's gene (apolipoprotein E, or APoe4), and it turns out, she did. However, she was relieved to learn that she had only one copy of the gene rather than two. Her single copy increased her lifetime risk of Alzheimer's from 10–15 percent to 20–25 percent. Having two copies would have increased her lifetime risk to somewhere between 30 and 55 percent.[58,59] She also had a genetic variant that made it difficult for her to metabolize B vitamins and folate, and another variant that prevented her body from clearing toxins effectively following exposure.

Sally knew from her own research that changing your behavior is hard but that you can make it easier by creating specific cues for the new behavior.[60] With this in mind, Sally posted reminder notes where she would readily see them each day—the refrigerator door, kitchen cabinet doors, and the bathroom mirror. She set alarms on her phone to remind her to take specific supplements at specific times. She also made check marks on a printed monthly calendar to document her progress. Each of these cues to behavior helped her form new habits that have now become part of her daily life.[61]

Under the ReCODE protocol, lifestyle changes like sleep, physical exercise, mental exercise, nutrition, stress reduction, and dental hygiene are recommended for people with all three types of Alzheimer's.[62] Sally had not prioritized sleep before her Alzheimer's diagnosis. Raised with a strong work ethic, she had always prided herself on getting up daily at 6 A.M., usually after about six hours of sleep. But after reading Dr. Bredesen's journal article, months before her own cognoscopy, Sally had already set the goal of sleeping at least eight hours each night.

Sleep has enormous benefits for those who have Alzheimer's, cancer, or other diseases, as research has shown that it plays a vital role in brain, immune, cardiovascular, and neurocognitive function.[63,64] A 2013 study showed that during non-REM sleep, toxins like beta-amyloid are cleared away.[65] This new understanding of "brain washing"—or a cleaning of the brain during sleep—opens up new avenues for research and, potentially, a cure for Alzheimer's disease.[66]

As a result, Sally now schedules only afternoon or late-morning appointments. She began (and continues) to take a small dose of melatonin six days a week to enhance sleep. She skips melatonin one day a week (per the ReCODE protocol), to remind her body to continue its own natural production of melatonin.

The ReCODE protocol also emphasizes stress reduction. Sally had already begun a meditation practice, but she had more work to do in this area. In order to better manage her stress response, she first had to understand it, and for that she needed to look to her childhood.

Sally did not have an easy childhood. Her father died when she was five years old and her mother had to be institutionalized after becoming mentally ill. As a result, Sally attended boarding schools. Sally describes the theme of her childhood as being "one without a permanent home."

At the beginning of seventh grade, Sally and her two siblings were taken in by several of their aunts and uncles, to whom they will always be grateful for loving and caring for them. Each of them provided living examples of how to live a positive and meaningful life.

Sally's new family life was complicated by her cousin's recurring major health problems, deepening her feelings of not having a permanent home. Moreover, a strong sense of responsibility, combined with an acute awareness of the feelings of everyone around her, tended to make Sally feel responsible for difficult emotional situations that were entirely beyond her control. She developed excellent people skills, but they came at a price.

As an adult, Sally found herself divorced after 13 years of marriage to her first husband, with a seven-year-old son and five-year old daughter. Three years after she met Martin, her current husband, they married and merged their families. Each had custody of two children from their first marriages, and combining the two families was a challenge for all of them, particularly the kids.

Sally also took on a series of professional challenges that added to her overall stress load. She believes that these multiple sources of stress had an overall negative effect on her immune system, and that this, along with her Alzheimer's gene, contributed to her developing Alzheimer's.

Today Sally's stress reduction program is multifaceted. Dr. Bredesen emphasizes that finding joy and relaxation is critical to reducing brain-damaging stress,[67] and Sally's regular meditation practice provides a level of peace and joy she had not previously experienced.

> *As a nurse with a Ph.D., I really enjoy seeing all the research that supports meditation. But I'm also strongly spiritual. There are lots of Bible verses that support the benefit of talking and listening to God. And one of the things I do now is try to listen quietly, rather than just making requests. This involves calming my brain down, and the meditation really helps with that. I do a combination of prayer, silent meditation, guided meditation, and mindfulness-based stress reduction.*

After just one month of daily meditation practice, Sally noticed that she was making far fewer word substitutions and could subtract sevens from 100 (a somewhat tricky mental exercise that Dr. Bredesen recommends) more rapidly than before. In addition to meditation, Sally has worked on increasing positive emotions. She has become a jokester who enjoys both hearing and telling jokes, and has chosen to stop listening to and reading the news. At first, this led to challenges with her husband.

> *I will claim what I need for my brain. In the past, it caused a lot of conflict because my husband liked to express his concern about the news. But it's the "New Sally" now, not the "Old Sally," who would listen to him for his sake. I need more positive emotions, so I assert myself. I tell him, "That's not good for my brain," and I ask him to go talk to his friends instead of me. And if I'm around two people disagreeing, I say, "That's bad for my brain. I can't hear that," or I withdraw myself from the situation.*

When it comes to the healing factor of exercise, it was easy for Sally to implement Dr. Bredesen's exercise recommendation.

*I think in retrospect that I delayed my Alzheimer's for 15 years because I was hiking the Appalachian Trail every summer, which involved hiking for eight hours a day for two or more weeks at a time. When I first started Dr. Bredesen's protocol, I would exercise up to two hours a day. My cognition was better with the two hours [of exercise] a day. I've always done more than the recommended 30 minutes a day because I've always liked [exercise]. I do all types of exercise that gets me into nature—I walk, swim, bicycle, hike, kayak.*

Sally also exercised her brain with the computer game BrainHQ from Posit Science,[68] which has extensive documented research behind it. She plays the game three to five days a week for 10–45 minutes at a time.

The easiest nutritional change for Sally was the implementation of ReCODE's version of intermittent fasting, which suggests at least 12 hours of fasting between dinner and breakfast, and three hours before bedtime.[69] Sally was already eating a fairly healthy diet. Her nursing research, starting in the 1980s, had inspired her to start eating what was then considered a cancer-prevention diet, including four cups of green tea a day, lots of green vegetables, and little meat. Luckily for Sally, these were all aspects of the ReCODE diet. Sally found it hard at first to eliminate sugar and gluten from her diet, but now it's part of her daily routine. She follows a ketogenic diet that is high in vegetables and foods with a glycemic index lower than 35.[70]

Sally's ReCODE report included the recommendation that she add or adjust dosages of 20 specific supplements. Because of her gene variant, which makes it difficult for her to metabolize B vitamins and folate, she also needs to take methylated supplements. As a nurse, Sally was wary of side effects that can occur when patients start new medications, so she began to add one new supplement to her regimen every two to four weeks, in order to detect any side effects and identify their cause. She researched each supplement carefully ahead of time, learning its method of action and its possible side effects, and kept notes on what she found.

With her type 1 Alzheimer's, Sally needed to reduce inflammation, bring her viral infections under control, and heal her intestinal permeability (leaky gut). Her low albumin levels indicated the need for more healthy protein. To heal her gut, Sally eliminated sugar from her diet and started taking several supplements to promote intestinal healing. Cone beam computed tomography (a 3-D dental X-ray) revealed that she had abscesses in five teeth due to bacterial infection. Also, her 45-year history of mouth sores from the virus HSV-1 (herpes simplex virus 1) was contributing to her inflammation, so she increased her daily dosage of lysine in order to decrease the frequency and severity of the sores.

Due to her type 2 Alzheimer's, Sally's cognoscopy revealed abnormal or suboptimal values of her thyroid hormone, TSH, and female sex hormones, including elevated estrogen and progesterone levels and very low levels of T3 (triiodothyronine). Because her thyroid had been removed in 2007, Sally will always need to closely monitor her T3, T4, and TSH levels. After her physician replaced her thyroid supplement with a different formulation, Sally noticed increased energy and improved cognition. He also adjusted dosages of her bioidentical estrogen and progesterone.

In retrospect, Sally could see that her earliest symptoms of type 3 Alzheimer's coincided with her five years of exposure to a mold-filled home. In addition to her genetic susceptibility to toxins, Sally's ReCODE report showed several blood values indicative of type 3 Alzheimer's, including low magnesium and zinc as well as abnormal C4a and TGF-beta 1. She had developed chronic inflammatory response syndrome (CIRS), also known as biotoxin illness, which heightened her sensitivity to toxins.[71]

Dr. Bredesen recommended that Sally follow Dr. Ritchie Shoemaker's method for treating CIRS, which involves 13 progressive steps in sequence, each tailored to the patient's physiology, as determined by various blood and nasal swab tests.[72] With the help of her local physician, Sally is now in the final stages of the Shoemaker protocol and most of her CIRS symptoms have disappeared. However, she realizes that her rare and highly susceptible genetic profile means that she will always need to pay close attention to her strong negative reactions to biotoxins.[73] Her ongoing brain health depends on it.

While social support is not an official part of Dr. Bredesen's ReCODE protocol, it is one of the common healing factors among radical remission survivors. Sally looks to her family and friends for social support. Frequent phone calls and visits from family bring her great joy. Bimonthly visits with Bible study friends create spiritual connection. And walking and kayaking for daily exercise is a lot more enjoyable with her friends.

In Sally's case, her husband's daily involvement, love, help, and support were absolutely essential to her recovery. Martin actually joined our interview with Sally to help elaborate certain points, and the mutual love and respect they feel for each other was immediately apparent. Martin says:

> For Alzheimer's, if your spouse or partner is only half-heartedly with you, your road is going to be 10 times harder. I cannot emphasize that [point] enough, and I'd also extend that to friends and family. Most people are really glad to hear when you're doing well, but the details don't matter to them. People want the positive summary. They don't want to hear the struggles. If you're really in it for the long haul, and you're really committed to each other, and you really love each other—then you're going to do whatever it takes.

After Martin proudly rattled off a long list of Sally's professional accomplishments, he said succinctly, "She's my hero," to which a blushing Sally replied, "He has been a wonderful help. I can't brag about him enough!" Both concur that they grew closer because of Sally's diagnosis and because of Martin's willingness to support her, and that they are closer now than they have ever been.

Perhaps most of all, Sally deeply appreciates that Martin was willing to make so many of the lifestyle changes along with her—a sentiment we hear often from radical remission survivors. Because Sally's Alzheimer's symptoms are easily triggered by environmental toxins, Martin had to make personal changes that included changing his bath time to the evenings, washing his towel every night, and running a fan to dry out the shower so there would be no mold-friendly moisture in the bathroom. In addition, Martin has joined Sally in making dietary changes, and often joins her in both physical and mental exercises.

Dr. Bredesen's ReCODE protocol notes that anger is a toxic emotion for your brain. Therefore, both Sally and Martin took an anger management course and proactively work to find ways to support each other, taking into account their different communication styles. Sally describes it this way:

> In a discussion, what my husband saw as [his] expressing frustration or making a request, I perceived as attacking. It is just two different opinions, but he has changed his way of talking, and I've changed my way of reacting. I have learned to withdraw from the situation when I react negatively, and my husband has learned to talk more gently.

Sally and her husband also discovered that touch therapy was crucial to Sally's healing. The couple started snuggling more often, as touch calmed Sally quickly and effectively. A new nighttime ritual was established when Martin, who would often read or play computer games in the evenings, would stop what he was doing at 9 o'clock in order to snuggle with Sally until she fell asleep. The two would then snuggle again in the morning before starting their day. They have found that this kind of touch therapy has been therapeutic in ways that words are not.

As we hear from so many radical remission survivors, learning how to accept such tremendous love and support was challenging for Sally at first.

*One of the hardest things for me to deal with is learning to focus on myself, not others. As a nurse, I was always the one who was listening sympathetically and knew just the right thing to say. I also grew up in a boarding school and with different relatives, so thinking of others before myself became my usual behavior. But ReCODE takes so much [of my] energy and time, and my big adjustment was putting myself first rather than others. If my husband wants something or needs me to stop and listen, and I need to do something for my mind and health, then I've got to first focus on me and my mind. And I didn't use to do that.*

By following Dr. Bredesen's ReCODE protocol religiously, and incorporating the remaining radical remission healing factors including social support, Sally has been able to fully reverse her Alzheimer's symptoms. Seventeen months after her initial diagnosis, Sally's MoCA score increased from 24 to 30, which is considered normal. A brain scan revealed that her hippocampal volume increased from the 14th to the 28th percentile for women her age, which means she experienced an improvement in her memory.[74] Sally's ability to spell words returned, her speech improved markedly, and her ability to drive and work on the computer all improved significantly.

Today, Sally is an advocate for Alzheimer's patients and speaks readily about her experiences. Dr. Bredesen calls Sally's case a reversal of Alzheimer's, but it can also be called a remission, because she has experienced a regression of her symptoms and has remained stable. However, Sally will always need to be vigilant.

*My cognitive ability changes constantly based on my inhalation of toxins. Fatigue and stress also negatively affect my cognition. My mind gives me constant reminders of the need to practice positive and healthy behaviors daily. . . . Alzheimer's is now part of me, and reversing Alzheimer's is now part of my life. I mean, I only have one brain. I can't get a brain transplant. I have to accept that my brain has plaque in it. At first, I didn't accept it and just fought it. But now I can think lovingly toward my brain, including my beta-amyloid plaques. It's a gradual process, but the transition [to acceptance] is critical.*

Sally continues to meditate every evening because she sleeps better and feels calmer the next day. She spends as much time in nature as possible, because the fresh air helps to clear her brain. Sally continues to eat a vegetable-rich ketogenic diet and takes an array of personalized supplements to support her sleep, hormone balance, and overall wellness. And while Sally loves to exercise, she is down to 60 minutes a day (from two hours), simply because she is doing so many other things right now.

When Sally and Martin are not spending time with their children or grandchildren or in nature, they enjoy reading and visiting with friends. Both are eager to discuss Alzheimer's and the many things that one can do to prevent or reverse it. Martin says:

*I see a real purpose to Sally's continued existence, and [to] my work giving her support. How many people over 70 years old get a chance to influence millions of lives, however small a part? I just don't even have words to say how powerful that is to my life's meaning.*

Sally's story demonstrates that you should never give up hope, even when faced with an "incurable" disease. At first, Sally felt like she would rather die than live with Alzheimer's, but her background in research led her to look for answers. Thanks to the cutting-edge protocol developed by Dr. Bredesen, Sally has found a way to keep her Alzheimer's in remission. Dr. Bredesen and many other forward-thinking health practitioners are shifting the health paradigm from a sickness model to a wellness model, where a healthier lifestyle can have incredible positive effects on your quality of life—and perhaps even reverse diseases that were once considered incurable.

# Action Steps

We hope Sally's profound healing story, along with the latest trends and research, have inspired you to strengthen your social support network. In *Radical Remission*, I made the following suggestions to increase your social support, which are still applicable and useful. If you're someone who is dealing with a health challenge, try reaching out to someone you love to make a connection; sign up for a gentle group exercise class, support group, or group activity to connect with like-minded people; and do not be afraid to ask for help.

If you love someone who is going through a health challenge, what is most important is showing up for them and showing you care. This may include calling them to let them know you are thinking of them, dropping off healthy meals, running errands, helping with chores, or planning a day of pampering. Here are a few more ideas to get you started on finding the right social support for you:

- **Make a four-legged friend.**

  Getting your social support in the form of unconditional love from a pet has proven to be just as beneficial as human social support. If the idea of having a pet resonates with you, many communities have either an animal shelter or a no-kill animal care center filled with animals who are looking for a loving home. In addition, many pet-finding websites and apps can help you find your perfect pet, including hypoallergenic ones.

- **Become a surrogate support.**

  Have you always wanted grandkids but never had kids, or have your adult children chosen to live far away? Or would you love a cat to cuddle, but your apartment does not allow pets? Good news! New "surrogate support" offerings allow you to spend time with children, pets, or nonprofits on a temporary basis. For instance, thanks to surrogate grandparent websites, you can become a surrogate grandparent (or aunt/uncle) by volunteering to spend time with a child near you.[75] And in cities around the globe, you can pop into a cat or dog café where the café owners have an assortment of cuddly pets for you to play with while you dine or drink.[76] Similarly, volunteer-matching organizations allow you to volunteer at a single event, rather than making a longer commitment to a specific organization.

- **Build your community.**

  As you begin to build your own network of supportive friends and family, look for people who provide a safe space for you to be yourself and who allow you to share your true thoughts and feelings without the worry of being judged. The people you surround yourself with often mirror your beliefs, language, and actions, so be choosy. Your community will likely be comprised of optimists who believe in you and your goals, and will help you when you get stuck in any one emotion (e.g., fear, depression, grief) for too long of a time.

  Your local hospital, library, and/or community center may offer emotional support or activity-oriented groups or classes. Social media sites offer specialized groups that can help you connect with other people who have the same diagnosis. Also, you can follow @RadicalRemission on social media for inspiring posts from our online community, and on our website—RadicalRemission.com—you can search through our ever-expanding database of healing stories to make a connection.

- **Get a massage or energy work for human touch.**

  You may not have a partner, child, or loved one who is able to provide you with oxytocin-releasing cuddles, but this does not mean you do not have access to human touch. Physical touch is essential to healing, so consider getting a massage or working with an energy healer to ensure that your body gets all the oxytocin it needs. If you are concerned about cost, ask whether the practitioner or clinic offers a sliding scale for cancer patients.

- **Start a crowdfunding campaign.**

  Whether it is a stack of hospital bills or the high price of organic food and supplements, the cost of medical treatment often causes financial stress for patients. If you are in this situation, you may want to consider starting an online fund-raising campaign through free sites such as GoFundMe or Kickstarter. One radical remission survivor, Ryan Luelf, raised more than $100,000 for his treatment and is so convinced that crowdsourcing is essential to healing that he developed an online course—Freely Funded (freelyfunded.com)—to help teach people how to run a successful online fund-raising campaign.

- **Practice asking for help.**

  Try to remember how you felt the last time a friend reached out to you for help. Did you feel grateful to be able to help them, or did you feel they were a burden? People who care about you truly want to help you, but often do not know how. Therefore, get specific in your requests to friends and practice asking questions such as, "I really need your help. Can you please babysit for me? Take me to my doctor's appointment? Pick up the groceries on this list?" It may feel uncomfortable at first, but remember that your friends and family really do want to help you.

We hope this chapter has convinced you that receiving love and support is as essential to your health as eating a vegetable-rich diet, exercising, or taking supplements. Spending time with friends and family can distract you from your stressors while also strengthening your immune system, thanks to the healing hormones that are released when you are with them. In addition, seeking out other people who are going through, or who have successfully gone through, whatever challenge you may be facing can help alleviate your fears, provide hope, and inspire new solutions along your path.

Try asking yourself at the end of each day: Did I give love today? Did I allow myself to receive love? If you can answer affirmatively to both these questions each day, you will go a long way in increasing your social support and strengthening your immune system.

# CONCLUSION

*What is called genius is the abundance of life and health.*
— Henry David Thoreau

Every journey must come to an end, or, more accurately, a transition point. Although this book is now coming to a close, we hope it will spark the continuation of your own healing journey, whether that path includes conventional medical treatment, alternative options, or a combination of the two.

We have explored the 10 radical remission healing factors by reviewing the recent societal trends, analyzing the latest research, and sharing in-depth healing stories from 10 new radical remission survivors. We also introduced you to the 10th common healing factor among radical remission survivors: exercise/movement, which has the ability to improve nearly every aspect of your body-mind-spirit, including your immune, cardiovascular, lymphatic, and nervous systems, as well as your mental, emotional, and spiritual states.

Along with the other non-cancer radical remission cases that have come into our website over the years, Sally's recovery from Alzheimer's disease and Palmer's recovery from advanced multiple sclerosis tentatively imply that the 10 healing factors may not only be helpful for cancer recovery and prevention, but also for the recovery and prevention of other diseases. In fact, many radical remission survivors have told us that they view the 10 factors as a "way to live a healthy and meaningful life," as opposed to a temporary treatment plan.

The multitude of research studies that have come out recently regarding the power of lifestyle—how you choose to eat, drink, think, feel, move, sleep, and spend your time—to improve your immune system is incredibly empowering. The research studies on this topic are so numerous and compelling that the American Institute for Cancer Research recently announced that "nearly half of all U.S. cancer cases could be prevented by changing our everyday habits," and such habits include, but are not limited to, diet, exercise, sun protection, and smoking cessation.[1]

Finally, the fact that radical remission cases have continued to be submitted to our website week after week, year after year, shows us that these 10 lifestyle changes may do more than simply prevent cancer. At least for the group of people who experience radical remissions, the 10 healing factors appear to be powerful enough to actually reverse cancer and other serious diseases and bring them into remission. We plan to continue our research—which already includes a pilot study with Harvard University and will hopefully one day include a randomized controlled trial—until we are able to understand more fully for whom exactly the 10 radical remission healing factors are effective.

## The Big Picture

When we step back and review the content of this book, we are struck by a few things. First, there is so much you can do for your health. Even though our society prefers simple lists of three and the medical field prefers one solution, pill, or surgery for each disease, researchers are not allowed to condense their findings simply out of convenience. The path that radical remission survivors take is a complex one, involving the complete transformation of 10 areas of their lives, with some of those areas being worlds of possibilities unto themselves.

Instead of feeling overwhelmed by all that can be done for our health, we choose to focus on the abundance of lifestyle changes that can strengthen our immune systems, letting that range of possibilities empower us as opposed to burden us. It is also comforting to know, as we saw in the in-depth healing stories, that radical remission survivors rarely engage all 10 healing factors at the same time. Rather, they tend to start with the specific factors that need their personal, immediate attention and then add the other factors one by one until they have reached a state of health and balance. Radical remission survivors don't become new people overnight.

The second thing that we are struck by is the fact that the exact causes of and cure for cancer remain elusive to conventional medicine. Researchers have learned in the past 100 years how cancer can be caused by a range of factors, including toxins, bacteria, viruses, genetic mutations, epigenetic changes, and mitochondrial failure. Despite this range of causes, researchers are still unclear as to exactly what causes some of the most prevalent cancers, such as breast cancer or prostate cancer, and other aggressive cancers, such as lung cancer in nonsmokers or pancreatic cancer.

Third, in the absence of clear causes (and therefore clear solutions to those causes), radical remission survivors have little choice but to take a more general approach to healing. What this means is that they do everything they can via the 10 healing factors to improve their immune systems. This, in turn, allows their immune systems to do what they were *designed* to do: identify and remove cancer cells. Our bodies contain incredible immune cells called natural killer (NK) cells—or what radical remission survivor Shin Terayama chooses to call "natural hugging cells"—whose primary function is to find and remove viruses and cancer cells.[2] We find it reassuring simply knowing that humans are born with these wonderful, cancer-fighting cells right inside our bodies.

At the Radical Remission Project, we are currently helping biotech companies study the blood and genetics of radical remission survivors in the hope that, someday, new immunotherapies will be developed that will allow *all* cancer patients to have a radical remission. However, until that day comes, the people we study practice "old-school" immunotherapy. That is, they boost their immune systems the old-fashioned way by fully bringing the 10 radical remission healing factors into their day-to-day lives. It may not be easy to overhaul so many physical, emotional, and spiritual aspects of your life, but the end results of a supercharged immune system and higher quality of life are undoubtedly worth the effort.

## Continuing the Journey

If you don't want your journey with the Radical Remission Project to end just yet, there are many ways to get involved, stay inspired, and support our ongoing research. First, feel free to share this book with a friend who may need it, or a doctor who may be open to it, or consider donating a copy to your local library. Also, let us know your thoughts on the book by writing an online review or giving us a shout-out on social media (tag @radicalremission with the hashtag #radicalhope).

## Healing Database

Please help us expand our research database by submitting your story at RadicalRemission.com. Current patients, survivors of cancer and other diseases, health practitioners and companies, wellness-seekers, and friends and family can all create free profiles on our site. Our list of research questions takes as little as 10 minutes to answer, and you can maintain your privacy by choosing a nondescript username, if you wish.

While you are on our website, feel free to search our database for other inspiring healing stories to read. From the launch of our site, we made the decision to keep our ever-growing database free and online because we wanted cancer patients and those facing other health challenges to be able to read about others who have dealt with their same diagnosis and hopefully find inspiration in their stories.

## Research Studies

In terms of our academic research, check out our nonprofit foundation's website at RadicalRemissionFoundation.org to learn about our current research studies, as well as how you can make a tax-deductible donation to support our ongoing research efforts. Our goal is to eventually conduct a prospective, randomized, controlled trial looking at the effects of the 10 radical remission healing factors on cancer patients. Every donation, regardless of how small, gets us closer to achieving that goal.

## Docuseries and Feature Film

If you're looking for visual and emotional inspiration, I filmed a 10-part docuseries on the topic of radical remission. You will find a link to it on our website, RadicalRemission.com. In this docuseries, we show you in-depth interviews with 20 radical remission survivors, including some survivors from *Radical Remission* and *Radical Hope*. We also bring you insights from more than 20 doctors and researchers who are on the forefront of integrative cancer treatment and radical remission research. These experts help explain the science behind why and how the 10 radical remission healing factors strengthen the immune system.

We are currently working on making a feature film about a woman who experiences a radical remission, inspired by the true cases in *Radical Remission* and *Radical Hope*. This project is near and dear to my heart, since it combines my love of screenwriting and visual storytelling with my love of radical remission stories. The film's current title is *Open-Ended Ticket*, and I hope to be able to share it with you soon, either in theaters and/or on your TV screen. You can learn more at RadicalRemission.com.

## Workshops and Courses

If you want to work on bringing the 10 radical remission healing factors into your own life in order to strengthen your immune system as much as possible, we have created a variety of offerings in response to our readers' requests. First, we offer our signature Radical Remission workshop, which is an in-person event offered either over one weekend or eight weeks (meeting two hours per week). These workshops are led by our wonderful certified Radical Remission instructors, many of whom have experienced a radical remission themselves. You can search for an upcoming workshop or find an instructor near you on our website, RadicalRemission.com.

If you are too sick to attend an in-person workshop, or if there is not one offered in your area, we also offer an online version, which you can take at your own pace from the comfort of your own home (or hospital room). Finally, many of our workshop attendees have requested one-on-one coaching after their workshops have ended so they can receive personalized guidance in integrating the 10 healing factors into their lives. In response to this request, we now have a wonderful group of certified Radical Remission health coaches who have been thoroughly trained in our research findings and in one-on-one coaching.

Our mission is to serve cancer patients, patients of other diseases, and their friends and family by providing resources that both educate and uplift. If you have other ideas about how we can serve this mission, please contact us via our website, RadicalRemission.com.

It has been a privilege to write this book and be able to share with you the continued research on radical remissions, the immune system, and the power of making healthy lifestyle changes. We hope you enjoyed getting to know Mary, Bailey, Bob, Di, Palmer, Alison, Jeremiah, Tom, Alex, and Sally as much as we enjoyed interviewing them. May this book and all the resources on the Radical Remission Project website inspire you to live your best life, take nothing for granted, and always find reasons to have radical hope.

# AFTERWORD

This book is dedicated to my dear friend and co-author Tracy White. I welcomed the chance to have Tracy help me write this book because she knew firsthand what it felt like to receive a cancer diagnosis. In February 2016, she was diagnosed with aggressive, recurrent cervical cancer and given just 15 months to live. Her doctor told her, "You will have chemo until you can't and then you will die." With an eight-year-old son and loving husband to live for, she wanted to do everything in her power to extend that timeline.

Four years prior, Tracy had been diagnosed with stage 1B cervical cancer. She had received a radical hysterectomy, after which her doctors told her she would be fine and to "get on with her life." So, she did—until the recurrence. After the recurrence, she immediately jumped into all the conventional treatments her doctors recommended, namely a strong chemotherapy regimen of Taxol, cisplatin, and Avastin once every three weeks. She quickly lost 30 pounds, all her hair, and almost all her energy.

In October 2016, Tracy was forced to stop chemotherapy because her body could not withstand any more conventional treatment. She was incredibly underweight and frail at this point, and her immune system was virtually non-existent. Her doctors believed her time had come, but Tracy was determined to live longer. During this time, she embarked on a transformative journey in which she ultimately changed every aspect of her life: she quit her stressful corporate job, moved to a new house, switched from the standard American diet to a vegan and then ketogenic one, built a strong team of healers and supportive friends and family, and removed every toxin she could find from her life.

Amazingly, Tracy went on to live another three, high-quality years, during which time she utilized many complementary healing modalities and dedicated her time to helping others.

Her new path involved writing, teaching, and health coaching. This is when I met Tracy. I knew from the moment we met that she and I had a strong connection. What I didn't realize was that the connection would be in the form of this book. Tracy's deepest professional dream had always been to be a writer, and although I didn't have enough space in my schedule to carve out the long chunks of time needed to write another book, Tracy did. She ultimately convinced me that together we could take on the challenge of writing a follow-up book to *Radical Remission*.

Tracy and I both knew she was dealing with an aggressive cancer recurrence even before we began typing the first words of *Radical Hope*. Nevertheless, writing this book was one of her strong reasons for living (after her son and husband), and that was enough reason for me to agree to take on this hefty project with her. We planned ahead for what might happen if she ever needed to stop writing and focus fully on her health, and that moment eventually came. Tracy passed away in December 2019— two and a half years after her doctors had told her she would die— surrounded by her close friends and family.

Although she never got to hold this book in her hands, you are holding her words, which means you are also holding her heart— and her heart was as big as they come. Tracy, I miss you every day. You became the author you always wanted to be, and I know your energy, passion, and words will inspire so many. Thank you for touching my life—and all our lives—through this book.

*— KAT*

# ENDNOTES

## CHAPTER 1

1. U.S. Centers for Disease Control and Prevention. *A Report of the Surgeon General Physical Activity and Health At-A-Glance.* 1996.

2. Office of Disease Prevention and Health Promotion, U.S. Department of Health and Human Services. *2008 Physical Activity Guidelines for Americans.* https://health.gov/paguidelines/2008/pdf/paguide.pdf.

3. Office of Disease Prevention and Health Promotion, U.S. Department of Health and Human Services. *Physical Activity Guidelines for Americans, 2nd edition.* February 2018. https://health.gov/paguidelines/second-edition/pdf/Physical_Activity_Guidelines_2nd_edition.pdf.

4. Ibid.

5. World Health Organization. "Obesity and Overweight." Last modified February 16, 2018. https://www.who.int/en/news-room/fact-sheets/detail/obesity-and-overweight.

6. "Cleveland Clinic Study Finds Obesity as Top Cause of Preventable Life-Years Lost." *Consult QD.* Last modified May 2, 2017. https://consultqd.clevelandclinic.org/cleveland-clinic-study-finds-obesity-top-cause-preventable-life-years-lost/.

7. Nimptsch, K., and T. Pischon. "Obesity Biomarkers, Metabolism and Risk of Cancer: An Epidemiological Perspective." *Recent Results in Cancer Research.* 208 (2016): 199–217. doi: 10.1007/978-3-319-42542-9_11.

8. "Cleveland Clinic Study." See note 6 above.

9. U.S. CDC. See note 1 above.

10. Booth, F. W., et al. "Lack of Exercise Is a Major Cause of Chronic Diseases." *Comprehensive Physiology.* 2, no. 2 (April 2012): 1143–1211. doi: 10.1002/cphy.c110025.

11. Li, Y., et al. "Impact of Healthy Lifestyle Factors on Life Expectancies in the US Population." *Circulation.* 138, no. 4 (July 24, 2018): 345–355. doi: 10.1161/CIRCULATIONAHA.117.032047.

12. Ekelund, U., et al. "Does physical activity attenuate, or even eliminate, the detrimental association of sitting time with mortality? A harmonised meta-analysis of data from more than 1 million men and women." *Lancet.* 388, no. 10051 (September 24, 2016): 1302–10. doi: 10.1016/S0140-6736(16)30370-1.

13. Hart, N., and R. Newton. "Exercise is Medicine for Cancer: The Evolution and Role of Exercise Oncology." *Sports Health.* 36, no. 2 (2018): 6–11.

14. Schmitz, K. H., et al, and the American College of Sports Medicine. "American College of Sports Medicine roundtable on exercise guidelines for cancer survivors." *Medicine & Science in Sports & Exercise.* 42, no. 7 (July 2010): 1409–26. doi: 10.1249/MSS.0b013e3181e0c112.

15. Ashcraft, K. A., et al. "Exercise as Adjunct Therapy in Cancer." *Seminars in Radiation Oncology.* 29, no. 1 (January 2019): 16–24. doi: 10.1016/j.semradonc.2018.10.001.

16. Schmitz, K. H., et al. "Exercise Is Medicine in Oncology: Engaging Clinicians to Help Patients Move through Cancer." *CA: A Cancer Journal for Clinicians.* 69, no. 6 (November 2019): 468–484. doi: 10.3322/caac.21579.

17. Galvão, D. A., et al. "Combined resistance and aerobic exercise program reverses muscle loss in men undergoing androgen suppression therapy for prostate cancer without bone metastases: A randomized controlled trial." *Journal of Clinical Oncology.* 28, no. 2 (January 10, 2010): 340–7. doi: 10.1200/JCO.2009.23.2488.

18. Backman, M., et al. "A randomized pilot study with daily walking during adjuvant chemotherapy for patients with breast and colorectal cancer." *Acta Oncologica.* 53, no. 4 (April 2014): 510–20. doi: 10.3109/0284186X.2013.873820.

19. Ashcraft, K. A., et al. See note 15 above.

20. Mishra, S. I., et al. "Exercise interventions on health-related quality of life for cancer survivors." *Cochrane Database of Systematic Reviews.* 2012, no. 8 (August 15, 2012): doi: 10.1002/14651858.CD007566.pub2.

21. Fong, D. Y., et al. "Physical activity for cancer survivors: meta-analysis of randomised controlled trials." *BMJ.* 2012, no. 344 (January 30, 2012): e70. doi: 10.1136/bmj.e70.

22. "Physical Activity and Cancer." National Cancer Institute. Last modified January 27, 2017. https://www.cancer.gov/about-cancer/causes-prevention/risk/obesity/physical-activity-fact-sheet.

23. Ashcraft, K. A., et al. See note 15 above.

24. Ashcraft, K. A., et al. See note 15 above.

25. Brown, J. C., et al. "Cancer, Physical Activity, and Exercise." *Comprehensive Physiology.* 2, no. 4 (October 2012): 2775–809. doi: 10.1002/cphy.c120005.

26. Kenfield, S. A., et al. "Physical activity and survival after prostate cancer diagnosis in the health professionals follow-up study." *Journal of Clinical Oncology.* 29, no. 6 (February 20, 2011): 726–32. doi: 10.1200/JCO.2010.31.5226.

27. Holick C.N., et al. "Physical activity and survival after diagnosis of invasive breast cancer." *Cancer Epidemiology, Biomarkers & Prevention.* 17, no. 2 (February 2008): 379–86. doi:10.1158/1055-9965.EPI-07-0771; "Can Exercise Reduce the Risk of Cancer Recurrence?" https://blog.dana-farber.org/insight/2018/02/can-exercise-reduce-risk-cancer-recurrence/. Date of publication: February 7, 2018. Date accessed: December 11, 2019.

28. Arem, H., et al. "Pre- and postdiagnosis physical activity, television viewing, and mortality among patients with colorectal cancer in the National Institutes of Health-AARP Diet and Health Study." *Journal of Clinical Oncology.* 33, no. 2 (January 10, 2015): 180–8. doi: 10.1200/JCO.2014.58.1355.

29. Ashcraft, K. A., et al. See note 15 above.

30. Lu, M., et al. "Exercise inhibits tumor growth and central carbon metabolism in patient-derived xenograft models of colorectal cancer." *Cancer & Metabolism.* 2018, no. 6 (November 15, 2018): 14. doi: 10.1186/s40170-018-0190-7.

31. Pedersen, L., et al. "Voluntary Running Suppresses Tumor Growth through Epinephrine- and IL-6-Dependent NK Cell Mobilization and Redistribution." *Cell Metabolism.* 23, no. 3 (March 8, 2016): 554–62. doi: 10.1016/j.cmet.2016.01.011.

32. Hart, N., and R. Newton. See note 13 above.

33. AKTIV Against Cancer, c/o WCPG, 207 Front Street, 3rd Floor, New York, NY 10038. http://www.aktivagainstcancer.org/.

34. "Aerobic Exercise." Cleveland Clinic. Last modified July 16, 2019. https://my.clevelandclinic.org/health/articles/7050-aerobic-exercise.

35. Padilha, C. S., et al. "Evaluation of resistance training to improve muscular strength and body composition in cancer patients undergoing neoadjuvant and adjuvant therapy: a meta-analysis." *Journal of Cancer Survivorship.* 11, no. 3 (June 11, 2017): 339–349. doi: 10.1007/s11764-016-0592-x.

36. Ibid.

37. Cormie, P., et al. "The Impact of Exercise on Cancer Mortality, Recurrence, and Treatment-Related Adverse Effects." *Epidemiologic Reviews.* 39, no. 1 (January 1, 2017): 71–92. doi: 10.1093/epirev/mxx007.

38. Milanović, Z., et al. "Effectiveness of High-Intensity Interval Training (HIT) and Continuous Endurance Training for VO2max Improvements: A Systematic Review and Meta-Analysis of Controlled Trials." *Sports Medicine.* 45, no. 10 (October 2015): 1469–1481. doi: 10.1007/s40279-015-0365-0.

39. Toohey, K., et al. "A pilot study examining the effects of low-volume high-intensity interval training and continuous low to moderate intensity training on quality of life, functional capacity and cardiovascular risk factors in cancer survivors." *PeerJ—the Journal of Life and Environmental Sciences.* 2016, no. 4 (October 20, 2016): e2613. doi: 10.7717/peerj.2613.

40. Devin, J. L., et al. "The influence of high-intensity compared with moderate-intensity exercise training on cardiorespiratory fitness and body composition in colorectal cancer survivors: a randomised controlled trial." *Journal of Cancer Survivorship.* 10, no. 3 (June 2016): 467–79. doi: 10.1007/s11764-015-0490-7.

41. "The lymphatic system and cancer." Cancer Research UK. Last modified December 13, 2017. https://www.cancerresearchuk.org/what-is-cancer/ body-systems-and-cancer/the-lymphatic-system-and-cancer.

42. Aberdour, S. "The Lymphatic System: It's Life-Supporting." *Alive.* Last modified April 24, 2015. https://www.alive.com/health/the-lymphatic-system/.

43. Lane K., et al. "Exercise and the lymphatic system: Implications for breast-cancer survivors." *Sports Medicine.* 35, no. 6. (2005): 461–71. doi: 10.2165/00007256-200535060-00001.

44. Franchi, M. V., et al. "Bouncing Back! Counteracting Muscle Aging with Plyometric Muscle Loading." *Frontiers in Physiology.* 2019, no. 10 (March 5, 2019): 178. doi: 10.3389/fphys.2019.00178.

45. Cugusi, L., et al. "Effects of a mini-trampoline rebounding exercise program on functional parameters, body composition and quality of life in overweight women." *Journal of Sports Medicine and Physical Fitness.* 58, no. 3 (March 2018): 287–294. doi: 10.23736/S0022-4707.16.06588-9.

46. Požgain, I., et al. "Placebo and Nocebo Effect: A Mini-Review." *Psychiatria Danubina.* 26, no. 2 (June 2014): 100–7.

47. Diamond, S. A. "Essential Secrets of Psychotherapy: What is the 'Shadow'?" *Psychology Today.* April 20, 2012.

48. Rock, C. L., et al. "Nutrition and physical activity guidelines for cancer survivors." *CA: A Cancer Journal for Clinicians.* 62, no. 4 (July–August 2012): 243–74. doi: 10.3322/caac.21142.

49. "A Healthy Salute to New Year's Resolutions." The Nielsen Company. Last modified January 20, 2016. https://www.nielsen.com/us/en/insights/news/2016/ a-healthy-salute-to-new-years-resolutions.htm.

## CHAPTER 2

1. *Why Americans Go (and Don't Go) to Religious Services.* (Washington, D.C.: Pew Research Center, 2018).

2. Lipka, M., and C. Gecewicz. "More Americans now say they're spiritual but not religious." Pew Research Center. Last modified September 6, 2017. https://www.pewresearch.org/fact-tank/2017/09/06/ more-americans-now-say-theyre-spiritual-but-not-religious/.

3. Pew Research Center. "Attendance at Religious Services." Date accessed: December 11, 2019. https://www.pewforum.org/religious-landscape-study/ attendance-at-religious-services/.

4. "More adults and children are using yoga and meditation." National Center for Complementary and Integrative Health. Last modified November 13, 2018. https://nccih.nih.gov/news/press/ More-adults-and-children-are-using-yoga-and-meditation.

5. "2016 Yoga in America Study Conducted by Yoga Journal and Yoga Alliance." *Yoga Journal* and Yoga Alliance. January 13, 2016. https://www.yogajournal.com/page/ yogainamericastudy.

6. Brodesser-Akner, T. "The Big Business of Being Gwyneth Paltrow," *New York Times Sunday Magazine.* (July 29, 2018): 22.

7. Jacobs, T. L., et al. "Intensive meditation training, immune cell telomerase activity, and psychological change." *Psychoneuroendocrinology.* 36, no. 5 (June 2011): 664–68. doi: 10.1016/j.psyneuen.2010.09.010.

8. Shammas, M. A. "Telomeres, lifestyle, cancer, and aging." *Current Opinion in Clinical Nutrition and Metabolic Care.* 14, no. 1 (January 2011): 28–34. doi: 10.1097/MCO.0b013e32834121b1.

9. Rosenkranz, M. A., et al. "Reduced stress and inflammatory responsiveness in experienced meditators compared to a matched healthy control group." *Psychoneuroendocrinology.* 68 (June 2016): 117–125. doi: 10.1016/j.psyneuen .2016.02.013.

10. Heid, M. "How Stress Affects Cancer Risk." MD Anderson Cancer Center. Last modified December 2014. https://www.mdanderson.org/publications/focused-on -health/how-stress-affects-cancer-risk.h21-1589046.html.

11. Tadi Uppala, P. P., et al. "Stress, spiritual wellbeing and cancer risk among diverse racial faith-based communities: Elevated levels of stress proteomic biomarkers in breast cancer patients." *Cancer Research.* 2017, no. 77, suppl. 13 (July 1, 2017): 4999. doi: 10.1158/1538-7445.AM2017-4999.

12. Bhasin, M. K., et al. "Relaxation Response Induces Temporal Transcriptome Changes in Energy Metabolism, Insulin Secretion and Inflammatory Pathways." *PLOS ONE.* 8, no. 5 (May 1, 2013): e62817. doi: 10.1371/journal.pone.0062817.

13. Buric, I., et al. "What Is the Molecular Signature of Mind–Body Interventions? A Systematic Review of Gene Expression Changes Induced by Meditation and Related Practices." *Frontiers in Immunology.* 2017, no. 8:670. doi: 10.3389/fimmu.2017.00670

14. "What is Coley's toxins treatment for cancer?" Cancer Research UK. Last modified August 22, 2012. https://www.cancerresearchuk.org/about-cancer/cancer-in -general/treatment/complementary-alternative-therapies/individual-therapies/ coleys-toxins-cancer-treatment.

15. Gerson Institute. Accessed November 11, 2019. https://gerson.org/gerpress/ about-us/.

16. U.S. National Institutes of Health, National Cancer Institute. "Laetrile/Amygdalin (PDQ)–Patient Version." Last modified April 5, 2018. https://www.cancer.gov/ about-cancer/treatment/cam/patient/laetrile-pdq.

17. Brouwer, B. "YouTube Now Gets Over 400 Hours of Content Uploaded Every Minute." TubeFilter. Last modified July 26, 2015. https://www.tubefilter.com/ 2015/07/26/youtube-400-hours-content-every-minute/.

CHAPTER 3

1. Wu, X., et al. "Ultraviolet blood irradiation: Is it time to remember 'the cure that time forgot'?" *Journal of Photochemistry and Photobiology B: Biology.* 157 (April 2016): 89–96. doi: 10.1016/j.jphotobiol.2016.02.007.

2. Heynsbergh, N., et al. "Feasibility, useability and acceptability of technology-based interventions for informal cancer carers: a systematic review." *BMC Cancer.* 18, no. 1, art. no. 244 (March 2, 2018). doi: 10.1186/s12885-018-4160-9.

3. Chida, Y., et al. "Do stress-related psychosocial factors contribute to cancer incidence and survival?" *Nature Reviews Clinical Oncology.* 5, no. 8 (August 2008): 466–75. doi: 10.1038/ncponc1134.

4. Paek, M. S., et al. "Longitudinal Reciprocal Relationships Between Quality of Life and Coping Strategies Among Women with Breast Cancer." *Annals of Behavioral Medicine.* 50, no. 5 (October 2016): 775-783. doi: 10.1007/s12160-016-9803-y.

5. Cheng, C. T., et al. "Cancer-coping profile predicts long-term psychological functions and quality of life in cancer survivors." *Supportive Care in Cancer.* 27, no. 3 (March 2019): 933–941. doi: 10.1007/s00520-018-4382-z.

6. White, L. L., et al. "Perceived Self-Efficacy: A Concept Analysis for Symptom Management in Patients With Cancer." *Clinical Journal of Oncology Nursing.* 21, no. 6 (December 1, 2017): E272–E279. doi: 10.1188/17.CJON.E272-E279.

7. Mirrione, M. M., et al. "Increased metabolic activity in the septum and habenula during stress is linked to subsequent expression of learned helplessness behavior." *Frontiers in Human Neuroscience.* 8 (February 3, 2014): 29. doi: 10.3389/ fnhum.2014.00029.

8. Schou Bredal, I., et al. "Effects of a psychoeducational versus a support group intervention in patients with early-stage breast cancer: results of a randomized controlled trial." *Cancer Nursing.* 37, no. 3 (May–June 2014): 198–207. doi: 10.1097/NCC.0b013e31829879a3.

9. Harvey, A., et al. "Factors Influencing Treatment Decisions Among Cancer Patients: Results from National Patient Education Workshops." Presented at the 2015 World Congress of Pyscho-Oncology, July 28–August 1, 2015, Washington, D.C. P1–61. Accessed November 11, 2019. https://www.cancersupportcommunity. org/sites/default/files/uploads/our-research/presentations/treatment-decision -making/2014_biennial_cer_scp_poster.pdf.

# Endnotes

10. Conners, A. "Does Patient Empowerment Lead to Better Cancer Treatment Outcomes?" Patient Empowerment Network. Last modified August 10, 2015. https://powerfulpatients.org/2015/08/10/does-patient-empowerment-lead-to-better-cancer-treatment-outcomes/.

11. Price, M. A., et al. "Helplessness/hopelessness, minimization and optimism predict survival in women with invasive ovarian cancer: a role for targeted support during initial treatment decision-making?" *Supportive Care in Cancer*. 24, no. 6 (June 2016): 2627–34. doi: 10.1007/s00520-015-3070-5.

12. Marmor, S., et al. "The Rise in Appendiceal Cancer Incidence: 2000–2009." *Journal of Gastrointestinal Surgery*. 19, no. 4 (April 2015): 743–750. doi: 10.1007/s11605-014-2726-7.

13. "What Is HIPEC and How Does It Work?" Accessed November 11, 2019. https://hipectreatment.com/the-hipec-procedure/; Chalikonda, S. (online chat). "What Is HIPEC and Is it Right for Me?" Cleveland Clinic. Last modified November 8, 2011. https://my.clevelandclinic.org/health/transcripts/1301_hipec.

## CHAPTER 4

1. U.S. Department of Health and Human Services, Centers for Disease Prevention and Control. "Suicide rates rising across the U.S." Last modified June 7, 2018. https://www.cdc.gov/media/releases/2018/p0607-suicide-prevention.html.

2. World Health Organization. "Depression: Key Facts." Last modified March 22, 2018. https://www.who.int/news-room/fact-sheets/detail/depression.

3. Zaorsky, N. G., et al. "Suicide among cancer patients." *Nature Communications*. 10 (2019): 207. doi: 10.1038/s41467-018-08170-1.

4. Salimpoor, V. N., et al. "Anatomically Distinct Dopamine Release During Anticipation and Experience of Peak Emotion to Music," *Nature Neuroscience*. 14, no. 2 (February 2011): 257–62. doi: 10.1038/nn.2726; Burgdorf, J., and J. Pankseep. "The Neurobiology of Positive Emotions," *Neuroscience and Biobehavioral Reviews*. 30, no. 2 (2006): 173–87. doi: 10.1016/j.neubiorev.2005.06.001; Benarroch, E. E., "Oxytocin and Vaspressin: Social Neuropeptides with Complex Neuromodulatory Functions," *Neurology*. 80, no. 16 (April 16, 2013): 1521–28. doi: 10.1212/WNL.0b013e31828cfb15.

5. Sarkar, D. K., et al. "Regulation of cancer progression by *β*-endorphin neuron." *Cancer Research*. 72, no. 4 (February 15, 2012): 836–40. doi: 10.1158/0008-5472. CAN-11-3292.

6. Zaninotto, P., et al. "Sustained enjoyment of life and mortality at older ages: analysis of the English Longitudinal Study of Ageing." *BMJ*. 355, no. 8086 (2016): i6267. doi: 10.1136/bmj.i6267.

7. Helliwell, J., et al., eds. *World Happiness Report 2019*. New York: United Nations Sustainable Development Solutions Network, 2019. Central Intelligence Agency. "Country Comparison: Life Expectancy at Birth (2017)." *The World Fact Book*. https://www.cia.gov/library/publications/the-world-factbook/rankorder/2102rank.html.

8. GNH Centre Bhutan. Accessed November 11, 2019. http://www.gnhcentrebhutan.org/about/; Wyss, J. "Happy by Decree: Ecuador's Chief of 'Good Living' Tries to Raise National Contentment," *Miami Herald*. July 17, 2015 (updated July 18, 2015). Accessed November 11, 2019. https://www.miamiherald.com/news/nation-world/world/americas/article27536497.html; Burgess, K. "ACT Government to Introduce Wellbeing Index," *The Canberra Times*. January 16, 2019.

9. A connected society: A strategy for tackling loneliness–laying the foundations for change. London: United Kingdom Department for Digital, Culture, Media and Sport, 2018. "Her Excellency Ohoud Bint Khalfan al Roumi, Minister of State for Happiness and Wellbeing." United Arab Emirates, The Cabinet. Accessed November 11, 2019. https://uaecabinet.ae/en/details/cabinet-members/her-excellency-ohoud-bint-khalfan-al-roumi.

10. Cunha, L. F., et al. "Positive Psychology and Gratitude Interventions: A Randomized Clinical Trial." *Frontiers in Psychology.* 10 (March 21, 2019): 584. doi: 10.3389/fpsyg.2019.00584.

11. Emmons, R. A., and M. E. McCullough. "Counting blessings versus burdens: An experimental investigation of gratitude and subjective well-being in daily life." *Journal of Personality and Social Psychology.* 84, no. 2 (2003): 377-389. doi: 10.1037//0022-3514.84.2.377.

12. Algoe, S. B., et al. "Beyond reciprocity: gratitude and relationships in everyday life." *Emotion.* 8, no. 3 (June 2008): 425–429. doi: 10.1037/1528-3542.8.3.425; Emmons, R. A., and M. E. McCullough. See note 11 above; Wood, A. M., et al. "Gratitude influences sleep through the mechanism of pre-sleep cognitions." *Journal of Psychosomatic Research.* 66, no. 1 (January 2009): 43–8. doi: 10.1016/j.jpsychores.2008.09.002.

13. Hill, P. L., et al. "Examining the Pathways between Gratitude and Self-Rated Physical Health across Adulthood." *Personality and Individual Differences.* 54, no. 1 (January 2013): 92–96. doi: 10.1016/j.paid.2012.08.011.

14. Cash, H., et al. "Internet Addiction: A Brief Summary of Research and Practice." *Current Psychiatry Reviews.* 8, no. 4 (November 2012): 292–298. doi: 10.2174/157340012803520513; Montag, C., et al. "Internet Communication Disorder and the Structure of the Human Brain: Initial Insights on WeChat Addiction." *Scientific Reports.* 8, no. 1 (February 1, 2018): 2155. doi: 10.1038/s41598-018-19904-y.

15. "Global mobile consumer trends, 2nd edition: Mobile continues its global reach into all aspects of consumers' lives." Deloitte Touche Tohmatsu Limited. 2017. https://www2.deloitte.com/us/en/pages/technology-media-and-telecommunications/articles/global-mobile-consumer-trends.html.

16. Ibid.

17. Cash, H., et al. See note 14 above.

18. Montag, C., et al. See note 14 above.

19. Montag, C., et al. See note 14 above; Alexander, G. E., et al. "Parallel Organization of Functionally Segregated Circuits Linking Basal Ganglia and Cortex." *Annual Review of Neuroscience.* 9, no. 1 (March 1, 1986): 357–381. doi: 10.1146/annurev.ne.09.030186.002041.

20. Miller, A. B., et al. "Cancer epidemiology update, following the 2011 IARC evaluation of radiofrequency electromagnetic fields (Monograph 102)." *Environmental Research.* 167 (November 2018): 673–683. doi: 10.1016/j.envres.2018.06.043.

21. Ibid.

22. Smith-Roe, S. L., et al. "Evaluation of the genotoxicity of cell phone radiofrequency radiation in male and female rats and mice following subchronic exposure." *Environmental and Molecular Mutagenesis.* October 21, 2019 (epub ahead of print). doi: 10.1002/em.22343.

23. Miller, A. B., et al. See note 20 above.

24. Tausk, F., et al. "Psychoneuroimmunology." *Dermatologic Therapy.* 21, no. 1 (January–February 2008): 22–31. doi: 10.1111/j.1529-8019.2008.00166.x.

25. Moraes, L. J., et al. "A systematic review of psychoneuroimmunology-based interventions." *Psychology, Health & Medicine.* 23, no. 6 (July 2018): 635–652. doi: 10.1080/13548506.2017.1417607.

26. Chacin-Fernández, J., et al. "Psychological intervention based on psychoneuroimmunology improves clinical evolution, quality of life, and immunity of children with leukemia: A preliminary study." *Health Psychology Open.* 6, no. 1 (April 1, 2019). doi: 10.1177/2055102919838902.

# Endnotes

27. Ben-Shaanan, T. L., et al. "Modulation of Anti-Tumor Immunity by the Brain's Reward System." *Nature Communications.* 9, no. 1 (July 13, 2018): 2723. doi: 10.1038/s41467-018-05283-5.

28. Dinan, T.G., et al. "Psychobiotics: A Novel Class of Psychotropic." *Biological Psychiatry.* 74, no. 10 (November 15, 2013): 720–6. doi: 10.1016/j.biopsych.2013.05.001.

29. Rajagopala, S. V., et al. "The Human Microbiome and Cancer." *Cancer Prevention Research.* 10, no. 4 (April 2017): 226–234. doi: 10.1158/1940-6207.CAPR-16-0249.

30. Sarkar, A., et al. "Psychobiotics and the Manipulation of Bacteria-Gut-Brain Signals." *Trends in Neurosciences.* 39, no. 11 (November 2016): 763–781. doi: 10.1016/j.tins.2016.09.002.

31. Kurokawa, S., et al. "The effect of fecal microbiota transplantation on psychiatric symptoms among patients with irritable bowel syndrome, functional diarrhea and functional constipation: An open-label observational study." *Journal of Affective Disorders.* 235 (August 1, 2018): 506–512. doi: 10.1016/j.jad.2018.04.038.

32. Lerman, B., et al. "Oxytocin and Cancer: An Emerging Link." *World Journal of Clinical Oncology.* 9, no. 4 (September 14, 2018): 74–82. doi: 10.5306/wjco .v9.i5.74.

33. Ibid.

34. Neumann, I. D. "Oxytocin: the neuropeptide of love reveals some of its secrets." *Cell Metabolism.* 5, no. 4 (April 2007): 231–3. doi: 10.1016/j.cmet.2007.03.008.

35. Misrani A., et al. "Oxytocin system in neuropsychiatric disorders: Old concept, new insights." *Acta Physiologica Sinica.* 69, no. 2 (April 25, 2017): 196–206. PMID: 28435979; Neumann, I. D., and D. A. Slattery. "Oxytocin in General Anxiety and Social Fear: A Translational Approach." *Biological Psychiatry.* 79, no. 3 (February 1, 2016): 213–221. doi: 10.1016/j.biopsych.2015.06.004.

36. Louie, D., et al. "The Laughter Prescription: A Tool for Lifestyle Medicine." *American Journal of Lifestyle Medicine.* 10, no. 4 (June 23, 2016): 262–267. doi: 10.1177/1559827614550279.

37. Ibid.

38. Fleishman, S. B., et al. "Beneficial effects of animal-assisted visits on quality of life during multimodal radiation-chemotherapy regimens." *Journal of Community and Supportive Oncology.* 13, no. 1 (January 2015): 22–6. doi: 10.12788/jcso.0102.

39. Ibid.

## CHAPTER 5

1. Liu, C., et al. "X-ray phase-contrast CT imaging of the acupoints based on synchrotron radiation." *Journal of Electron Spectroscopy and Related Phenomena.* 196 (October 2014): 80–84. doi: 10.1016/j.elspec.2013.12.005.

2. Jain, S., et al. "Clinical Studies of Biofield Therapies: Summary, Methodological Challenges, and Recommendations." *Global Advances in Health and Medicine.* 4, suppl. (November 2015): 58–66. doi: 10.7453/gahmj.2015.034.suppl.

3. Yang, P., et al. "Human Biofield Therapy and the Growth of Mouse Lung Carcinoma." *Integrative Cancer Therapies.* 18 (January–December 2019). doi: 10.1177/1534735419840797.

4. Liu, C., et al. See note 20 above.

5. Lu, W., et al. "The value of acupuncture in cancer care." *Hematology / Oncology Clinics of North America.* 22, no. 4 (August 2008): 631–48, viii. doi:10.1016/j. hoc.2008.04.005; Ohj, B., et al. "Acupuncture in Oncology: The Effectiveness of Acupuncture May Not Depend on Needle Retention Duration." *Integrative Cancer Therapies.* 17, no. 2 (June 2018): 458–466. doi: 10.1177/1534735417734912;

Potter, P. J. "Energy Therapies in Advanced Practice Oncology: An Evidence-Informed Practice Approach." *Journal of the Advanced Practitioner in Oncology.* 4, no. 3 (May 2013): 139–151. PMID: 25031994.

6.  Xu, Y., et al. "Acupuncture Alleviates Rheumatoid Arthritis by Immune-Network Modulation." *American Journal of Chinese Medicine.* 46, no. 5 (2018): 997–1019. doi: 10.1142/S0192415X18500520.

7.  Yang, P., et al. See note 3 above.

8.  Cuthbert, S. C., and A. L. Rosner. "Applied kinesiology methods for a 10-year-old child with headaches, neck pain, asthma, and reading disabilities." *Journal of Chiropractic Medicine.* 9, no. 3 (September 2010): 138–45. doi: 10.1016/j.jcm .2010.05.002.

9.  Cuthbert. S. C., and A. L. Rosner. "Conservative chiropractic management of urinary incontinence using applied kinesiology: a retrospective case-series report." *Journal of Chiropractic Medicine.* 11, no. 1 (March 2012): 49–57. doi: 10.1016/j.jcm .2011.10.002.

10. Moncayo, R., and H. Moncayo. "Evaluation of Applied Kinesiology meridian techniques by means of surface electromyography (sEMG): demonstration of the regulatory influence of antique acupuncture points." *Chinese Medicine.* 4 (May 29, 2009): 9. doi: 10.1186/1749-8546-4-9.

11. Molsberger, F., et al. "Yamamoto New Scalp Acupuncture, Applied Kinesiology, and Breathing Exercises for Facial Paralysis in a Young Boy Caused by Lyme Disease—A Case Report." *EXPLORE.* 12, no. 4 (July–August 2016): 250–255. doi:10.1016/j.explore.2016.02.001.

12. Scaer, R. *The Body Bears the Burden.* (New York: Routledge, 2014). doi: 10.4324/9780203081822.

13. Underwood, Emily. "Your gut is directly connected to your brain, by a newly discovered neuron circuit." *Science.* September 20, 2018. doi: 10.1126/science. aav4883.

14. Lufityanto, G., et al. "Measuring Intuition: Nonconscious Emotional Information Boosts Decision Accuracy and Confidence." *Psychological Science.* 27, no. 5 (May 2016): 622–34. doi: 10.1177/0956797616629403.

15. McCraty, R., and M. Atkinson. "Electrophysiology of Intuition: Pre-stimulus Responses in Group and Individual Participants Using a Roulette Paradigm." *Global Advances in Health and Medicine.* 3, no. 2 (March 2014): 16–27. doi: 10.7453/gahmj.2014.014.

16. Margittai, Z., et al. "Exogenous cortisol causes a shift from deliberative to intuitive thinking." *Psychoneuroendocrinology.* 64 (February 2016): 131–5. doi: 10.1016/ j.psyneuen.2015.11.018.

17. Liebowitz, J., et al., eds. *How Well Do Executives Trust Their Intuition.* 1st Edition. (Boca Raton: Auerbach Publications, 2018).

18. *PwC's Global Data and Analytics Survey 2016.* PwC. Accessed November 11, 2019. https://www.pwc.com/us/en/services/consulting/analytics/big-decision-survey .html.

19. Ibid.

20. Stolper, C. F., et al. "Family physicians' diagnostic gut feelings are measurable: construct validation of a questionnaire." *BMC Family Practice.* 14 (January 2, 2013): 1. doi: 10.1186/1471-2296-14-1.

21. "Uncovering the Mysteries of Multiple Sclerosis." *NIH Medline Plus Magazine.* 14, no. 2 (Summer 2018): 20–23.

22. U.S. Centers for Disease Control and Prevention. "Injury Prevention and Control: Adverse Childhood Experiences (ACES)." Accessed November 11, 2019. https://www.cdc.gov/injury/.

23. U.S. Centers for Disease Control and Prevention. "About the CDC-Kaiser ACE Study." Last modified April 2, 2019. https://www.cdc.gov/violenceprevention/childabuseandneglect/acestudy/about.html.

24. "Food sensitivities may affect gut barrier function." Mayo Clinic, Digestive Diseases. Last modified Nov. 12, 2016. https://www.mayoclinic.org/medical-professionals/digestive-diseases/news/food-sensitivities-may-affect-gut-barrier-function/mac-20429973.

25. Obrenovich, M.E.M. "Leaky Gut, Leaky Brain?" *Microorganisms.* 6, no. 4 (October 2018): pii: E107. doi: 10.3390/microorganisms6040107.

## CHAPTER 6

1. Roberts, A. L., et al. "Posttraumatic stress disorder (PTSD) is associated with increased risk of ovarian cancer: A prospective and retrospective longitudinal cohort study." *Cancer Research.* 79, no. 19 (October 2019): 5113–5120. doi: 10.1158/0008-5472.

2. Lengacher, C. A., et al. "Influence of mindfulness-based stress reduction (MBSR) on telomerase activity in women with breast cancer (BC)." *Biological Research for Nursing.* 16, no. 4 (October 2014): 438–447. doi: 10.1177/1099800413519495.

3. U.S. Centers for Disease Control and Prevention. "About the CDC-Kaiser ACE Study." Last modified April 2, 2019. https://www.cdc.gov/violenceprevention/childabuseandneglect/acestudy/about.html.

4. "Past trauma may haunt your future health: Adverse childhood experiences, in particular, are linked to chronic health conditions." Harvard Health Publishing, Harvard Medical School. Last modified February 2019. https://www.health.harvard.edu/diseases-and-conditions/past-trauma-may-haunt-your-future-health.

5. Chivers-Wilson, K.A. "Sexual assault and posttraumatic stress disorder: a review of the biological, psychological and sociological factors and treatments." *McGill Journal of Medicine.* 9, no. 2 (July 2006): 111–8. PMID: 18523613.

6. Smith, S. G., et al. *National Intimate Partner and Sexual Violence Survey: 2015 Data Brief – Updated Release.* Atlanta, GA: United States Centers for Disease Control and Prevention, National Center for Injury Prevention and Control, Division of Violence Prevention, November 2018.

7. Cash, H., et al. "Internet Addiction: A Brief Summary of Research and Practice." *Current Psychiatry Reviews.* 8, no. 4 (November 2012): 292–298. doi: 10.2174/157340012803520513; Montag, C., et al. "Internet Communication Disorder and the Structure of the Human Brain: Initial Insights on WeChat Addiction." Scientific Reports. 8, no. 1 (February 1, 2018): 2155. doi: 10.1038/s41598-018-19904-y.

8. U.S. Department of Veterans Affairs, National Center for Posttraumatic Stress Disorder. "How Common Is PTSD in Veterans?" Accessed November 11, 2019. https://www.ptsd.va.gov/understand/common/common_veterans.asp.

9. Kaster, T. S., et al. "Post-traumatic stress and cancer: Findings from a cross-sectional nationally representative sample." *Journal of Anxiety Disorders.* 65 (May 7, 2019): 11–18. doi: 10.1016/j.janxdis.2019.04.004.

10. Carletto, S., et al. "Neurobiological features and response to eye movement desensitization and reprocessing treatment of posttraumatic stress disorder in patients with breast cancer." *European Journal of Psychotraumatology.* 10, no. 1 (April 25, 2019). doi: 10.1080/20008198.2019.1600832.

11. Ibid.

12. Novo Navarro, P., et al. "25 years of Eye Movement Desensitization and Reprocessing (EMDR): The EMDR therapy protocol, hypotheses of its mechanism of action and a systematic review of its efficacy in the treatment of post-traumatic stress disorder." *Revista de Psiquiatria y salud mental.* 11, no. 2 (April–June 2018): 101–114. doi: 10.1016/j.rpsm.2015.12.002.

13. Carletto, S., et al. See note 10 above.

14. Borji, M., et al. "Efficacy of Implementing Home Care Using Eye Movement Desensitization and Reprocessing in Reducing Stress of Patients with Gastrointestinal Cancer." *Asian Pacific Journal of Cancer Prevention.* 20, no. 7 (July 1, 2019): 1967–1971. doi: 10.31557/APJCP.2019.20.7.1967.

15. "Tapping 101: What Is Tapping and How Can I Start Using It?" The Tapping Solution. Accessed November 11, 2019. https://www.thetappingsolution.com/tapping-101/.

16. Ortner, Nick. *The Tapping Solution: A Revolutionary System for Stress-Free Living.* (Carlsbad, CA: Hay House, Inc., 2013).

17. Clond, M. "Emotional Freedom Techniques for Anxiety: A Systematic Review with Meta-Analysis." *Journal of Nervous and Mental Disease.* 204, no. 5 (May 2016): 388–95. doi: 10.1097/NMD.0000000000000483.

18. Sebastian, B., and J. Nelms. "The Effectiveness of Emotional Freedom Techniques in the Treatment of Posttraumatic Stress Disorder: A Meta-Analysis." *Explore.* 13, no. 1 (January–February 2017): 16–25. doi: 10.1016/j.explore.2016.10.001.

19. Nelms, J. A., and L. Castel. "A Systematic Review and Meta-Analysis of Randomized and Nonrandomized Trials of Clinical Emotional Freedom Techniques (EFT) for the Treatment of Depression." *Explore.* 12, no. 6 (November–December 2016): 416–426. doi: 10.1016/j.explore.2016.08.001.

20. Bach, D., et al. "Clinical EFT (Emotional Freedom Techniques) Improves Multiple Physiological Markers of Health." *Journal of Evidence-Based Integrative Medicine.* 24 (January–December 2019). doi: 10.1177/2515690X18823691.

21. Ibid.

22. Church, D., et al. "Epigenetic Effects of PTSD Remediation in Veterans Using Clinical Emotional Freedom Techniques: A Randomized Controlled Pilot Study." *American Journal of Health Promotion.* 32, no. 1 (January 2018): 112–122. doi: 10.1177/0890117116661154.

23. Maharaj, M. E. "Differential Gene Expression after Emotional Freedom Techniques (EFT) Treatment: A Novel Pilot Protocol for Salivary mRNA Assessment." *Energy Psychology: Theory, Research, and Treatment.* 8, no. 1 (2016): 17–32. doi: 10.9769/EPJ.2016.6.8.1.MM.

24. Baker, B. S., and C. J. Hoffman. "Emotional Freedom Techniques (EFT) to reduce the side effects associated with tamoxifen and aromatase inhibitor use in women with breast cancer: A service evaluation." *European Journal of Integrative Medicine.* 7, no. 2 (April 2015): 136–142. doi: 10.1016/j.eujim.2014.10.004.

25. Stapleton, Peta. *The Science Behind Tapping: A Proven Stress Management Technique for the Mind and Body.* (Carlsbad, CA: Hay House, Inc., 2013).

26. Ortner, Nick. See note 16 above.

27. Fancourt, D., et al. "Effects of Group Drumming Interventions on Anxiety, Depression, Social Resilience and Inflammatory Immune Response among Mental Health Service Users." *PLOS One.* 11, no. 3 (March 14, 2016): e0151136. doi: 10.1371/journal.pone.0151136.

**CHAPTER 7**

1. Jankovic, N., et al. "Adherence to the WCRF/AICR Dietary Recommendations for Cancer Prevention and Risk of Cancer in Elderly from Europe and the United

# Endnotes

States: A Meta-Analysis within the CHANCES Project." *Cancer Epidemiology, Biomarkers, and Prevention.* 26, no. 1 (January 2017): 136–144. doi: 10.1158/1055 -9965.EPI-16-0428.

2. Ward, E., et al. "Annual Report to the Nation on the Status of Cancer, 1999-2015, Featuring Cancer in Men and Women ages 20-49." *Journal of the National Cancer Institute.* May 30, 2019 (epub ahead of print). doi: 10.1093/jnci/djz106.

3. Ibid.

4. Ibid.

5. Sung, H., et al. "Emerging cancer trends among young adults in the USA: Analysis of a population-based cancer registry." *Lancet Public Health.* 4, no. 3 (March 2019): e137–e147. doi: 10.1016/S2468-2667(18)30267-6.

6. Ward, E., et al. See note 2 above.

7. Ward, E., et al. See note 2 above.

8. Murray, C. J. L., et al. "The State of US health, 1990–2010: Burden of Diseases, Injuries, and Risk Factors." *JAMA.* 310, no. 6 (August 14, 2013): 591–608. doi: 10.1001/jama.2013.13805.

9. Adams, K., et al. "The State of Nutrition Education at US Medical Schools." *Journal of Biomedical Education.* 2015. doi: 10.1155/2015/357627.

10. Crowley, J., et al. "Nutrition in Medical Education: A Systematic Review." *The Lancet: Planetary Health.* 3, no. 9 (September 2019): e379–e389. doi: 10.1016/ S2542-5196(19)30171-8.

11. Adams, K. M., et al., "Nutrition Is Medicine: Nutrition Education for Medical Students and Residents," *Nutrition in Clinical Practice: Official Publication of the American Society for Parenteral and Enteral Nutrition.* 25, no. 5 (October 2010): 471– 80. doi: 10.1177/0884533610379606.

12. Danek, R. L., et al. "Perceptions of Nutrition Education in the Current Medical School Curriculum." *Family Medicine.* 49, no. 10 (November 2017): 803–806. PMID: 29190407.

13. Zhang, F. F., et al. "Preventable Cancer Burden Associated with Poor Diet in the United States." *JNCI Cancer Spectrum.* 3, no. 2 (May 2019). doi: 10.1093/jncics/ pkz034.

14. Ibid.

15. Jiao, L., et al. "Low-Fat Dietary Pattern and Pancreatic Cancer Risk in the Women's Health Initiative Dietary Modification Randomized Controlled Trial." *Journal of the National Cancer Institute.* 110, no. 1 (January 1, 2018): 49–56. doi: 10.1093/ jnci/djx117.

16. Muscaritoli, M., et al. "Prevalence of malnutrition in patients at first medical oncology visit: the PreMiO study." *Oncotarget.* 8, no. 45 (August 10, 2017): 79884– 79896. doi: 10.18632/oncotarget.20168.

17. Mourouti, N., et al. "Optimizing diet and nutrition for cancer survivors: A review." *Maturitas.* 105 (November 2017): 33–36. doi: 10.1016/j.maturitas.2017.05.012.

18. Grosso, G., et al. "Possible role of diet in cancer: systematic review and multiple meta-analyses of dietary patterns, lifestyle factors, and cancer risk." *Nutrition Reviews.* 75, no. 6 (June 1, 2017): 405–419. doi: 10.1093/nutrit/nux012.

19. Park, S. Y., et al. "High-Quality Diets Associate with Reduced Risk of Colorectal Cancer: Analyses of Diet Quality Indexes in the Multiethnic Cohort." *Gastroenterology.* 153, no. 2 (August 2017): 386–394. e2. doi: 10.1053/j.gastro .2017.04.004.

20. Ibid.

21. Toledo, E., et al. "Mediterranean Diet and Invasive Breast Cancer Risk among Women at High Cardiovascular Risk in the PREDIMED Trial: A Randomized Clinical Trial." *JAMA Internal Medicine*. 175, no. 11 (November 2015): 1752–1760. doi: 10.1001/jamainternmed.2015.4838.

22. Ibid.

23. Playdon, M. C., et al. "Pre-diagnosis diet and survival after a diagnosis of ovarian cancer." *British Journal of Cancer*. 116, no. 12 (June 6, 2017): 1627–1637. doi: 10.1038/bjc.2017.120.

24. Ibid.

25. Greenlee, H., et al. "Long-Term Diet and Biomarker Changes after a Short-Term Intervention among Hispanic Breast Cancer Survivors: The ¡Cocinar Para Su Salud! Randomized Controlled Trial." *Cancer Epidemiology, Biomarkers, and Prevention*. 25, no. 11 (November 2016): 1491–1502. doi: 10.1158/1055-9965.EPI-15-1334.

26. Reedy, J., et al. "Higher diet quality is associated with decreased risk of all-cause, cardiovascular disease, and cancer mortality among older adults." *Journal of Nutrition*. 144, no. 6 (June 2014): 881–889. doi: 10.3945/jn.113.189407.

27. Chen, Z., et al. "Dietary patterns and colorectal cancer: results from a Canadian population-based study." *Nutrition Journal*. 14 (January 15, 2015): 8. doi: 10.1186/1475-2891-14-8.

28. Government of Canada. "Eat a Variety of Healthy Foods Each Day." *Canada's Food Guide*. Last modified October 11, 2019. https://food-guide.canada.ca/en/.

29. Government of Canada. "Healthy Food Choices." *Canada's Food Guide*. Last modified July 16, 2019. https://food-guide.canada.ca/en/healthy-food-choices/.

30. "New food guide unveiled without food groups or recommended servings." CBS News, Health. Last modified January 22, 2019. https://www.cbc.ca/news/health/canada-food-guide-unveil-1.4987261.

31. Winter, S. F., et al. "Role of Ketogenic Metabolic Therapy in Malignant Glioma: A Systematic Review." *Critical Reviews in Oncology/Hematology*. 112 (April 2017): 41–58. doi: 10.1016/j.critrevonc.2017.02.016.

32. Weber, D. D., et al. "Ketogenic Diet in Cancer Therapy." *Aging*. 10, no. 2 (February 11, 2018): 164–165. doi: 10.18632/aging.101382.

33. Allen, B. G., et al. "Ketogenic diets as an adjuvant cancer therapy: History and potential mechanism." *Redox Biology*. 2 (2014): 963–970. doi: 10.1016/j.redox.2014.08.002.

34. Ibid.

35. Nebeling, L. C., et al. "Effects of a Ketogenic Diet on Tumor Metabolism and Nutritional Status in Pediatric Oncology Patients: Two Case Reports." *Journal of the American College of Nutrition*. 14, no. 2 (April 1995): 202–208. doi: 10.1080/07315724.1995.10718495.

36. Zuccoli, G., et al. "Metabolic Management of Glioblastoma Multiforme Using Standard Therapy Together with a Restricted Ketogenic Diet: Case Report." *Nutrition & Metabolism*. 7, no. 33 (April 22, 2010). doi:10.1186/1743-7075-7-33.

37. Hay, L. "18 Amazing Health Benefits oBone Broth." Accessed May 31, 2019. https://www.louisehay.com/18-amazing-health-benefits-bone-broth/.

38. Wheless, J. W. "History and Origin of the Ketogenic Diet." In: *Epilepsy and the Ketogenic Diet*, edited by C. E. Stafstrom and J. M. Rho, pp. 31–50. (Totowa, NJ: Humana Press, 2004).

39. Bischoff, S. C., et al. "Intestinal permeability—a new target for disease prevention and therapy." *BMC Gastroenterology*. 14, (November 18, 2014): 189. doi: 10.1186/s12876-014-0189-7.

40. Winters, N., and J. H. Kelley. *The Metabolic Approach to Cancer: Integrating Deep Nutrition, the Ketogenic Diet, and Nontoxic Bio-Individualized Therapies.* (White River Junction, VT: Chelsea Green Publishing, 2017).

41. Ibid.

42. Tinkum, K. L., et al. "Fasting protects mice from lethal DNA damage by promoting small intestinal epithelial stem cell survival." *Proceedings of the National Academies of Sciences of the United States of America.* 112, no. 51 (December 22, 2015): E7148–E7154. doi: 10.1073/pnas.1509249112.

43. Lee, C., et al. "Fasting cycles retard growth of tumors and sensitize a range of cancer cell types to chemotherapy." *Science Translational Medicine.* 4, no. 124 (March 7, 2012): 124ra27. doi: 10.1126/scitranslmed.3003293; Safdie, F. M., et al. "Fasting and cancer treatment in humans: a case series report." *Aging.* 1, no. 12 (December 31, 2009): 988–1007. doi: 10.18632/aging.100114.

44. Lee, C., et al. See note 42 above.

45. Marinac, C. R., et al. "Prolonged Nightly Fasting and Breast Cancer Prognosis." *JAMA Oncology.* 2, no. 8 (August 1, 2016): 1049–1055. doi: 10.1001/jamaoncol.2016.0164.

46. Wei, M., et al. "Fasting-mimicking diet and markers/risk factors for aging, diabetes, cancer, and cardiovascular disease." *Science Translational Medicine.* 9, no. 377 (February 15, 2017). doi: 10.1126/scitranslmed.aai8700.

47. Ibid.

48. Vighi, G., et al. "Allergy and the gastrointestinal system." *Clinical and Experimental Immunology.* 153, suppl. 1 (September 2008): 3–6. doi: 10.1111/j.1365-2249.2008.03713.x.

49. Hadrich, D. "Microbiome Research Is Becoming the Key to Better Understanding Health and Nutrition." *Frontiers in Genetics.* 9 (June 13, 2018): 212. doi: 10.3389/fgene.2018.00212.

50. Ibid.

51. Bischoff, S. C., et al. "Intestinal permeability—a new target for disease prevention and therapy." *BMC Gastroenterology.* 14 (November 18, 2014): 189. doi: 10.1186/s12876-014-0189-7.

52. Ibid.

53. Ibid.

54. Ibid.

55. Rajagopala, S. V., et al. "The Human Microbiome and Cancer." *Cancer Prevention Research.* 10, no. 4 (April 2017): 226–234. doi: 10.1158/1940-6207.

56. Bischoff, S. C., et al. See note 50 above.

57. Hadrich, D. See note 48 above.

58. Hadrich, D. See note 48 above.

59. Martin, C. R., et al. "The Brain-Gut-Microbiome Axis." *Cellular and Molecular Gastroenterology and Hepatology.* 6, no. 2 (April 12, 2018): 133–148. doi: 10.1016/j.jcmgh.2018.04.003.

60. Ibid.

61. Hadrich, D. See note 48 above.

62. Hadrich, D. See note 48 above.

63. Rajagopala, S. V., et al. See note 54 above.

64. Rajagopala, S. V., et al. See note 54 above.

65. Rajagopala, S. V., et al. See note 54 above.

66. Dinwiddie, M. T., et al. "Recent Evidence Regarding Triclosan and Cancer Risk." *International Journal of Environmental Research and Public Health.* 11, no. 2 (February 21, 2014): 2209–2217. doi: 10.3390/ijerph110202209.

67. Yang, J. J., et al. "Association of Dietary Fiber and Yogurt Consumption with Lung Cancer Risk: A Pooled Analysis." *JAMA Oncology.* October 24, 2019 (epub ahead of print). doi: 10.1001/jamaoncol.2019.4107.

68. Gopalakrishnan, V., et al. "Gut microbiome modulates response to anti–PD-1 immunotherapy in melanoma patients." *Science.* 359, no. 6371. (January 5, 2018): 97–103. doi: 10.1126/science.aan4236.

69. Reis Ferreira, M., et al. "Microbiota- and Radiotherapy-Induced Gastrointestinal Side-Effects (MARS) Study: A Large Pilot Study of the Microbiome in Acute and Late-Radiation Enteropathy." *Clinical Cancer Research.* 25, no. 21 (November 1, 2019): 6487–6500. doi: 10.1158/1078-0432.CCR-19-0960.

70. Senghor, B., et al. "Gut microbiota diversity according to dietary habits and geographical provenance." *Human Microbiome Journal.* 7–8 (April 2018): 1–9. doi: 10.1016/j.humic.2018.01.001.

**CHAPTER 8**

1. Jermini, M., et al. "A. Orcurto, L.E. Rothuizen. Complementary medicine use during cancer treatment and potential herb-drug interactions from a cross-sectional study in an academic centre." *Scientific Reports.* 9, no. 1 (March 25, 2019): 5078. doi: 10.1038/s41598-019-41532-3.

2. Ibid.

3. Guo, W., et al. "Magnesium deficiency in plants: An urgent problem." *The Crop Journal.* 4, no. 2 (April 2016): 83–91. doi: 10.1016/j.cj.2015.11.003.

4. Worldwatch Institute. "Crop yields expand, but nutrition is left behind." Environmental News Network. Accessed November 11, 2019. https://www.enn.com/articles/22903-crop-yields-expand,-but-nutrition-is-left-behind; Davis, D., "Declining fruit and vegetable nutrient composition: What is the evidence?" *Horticultural Science.* 44, no. 1 (February 2009): 15–19. doi: 10.21273/HORTSCI.44.1.15; Scheer, R., and D. Moss. "Dirt poor: Have fruits and vegetables become less nutritious?" *Scientific American.* April 27, 2011. Accessed November 11, 2019. https://www.scientificamerican.com/article/soil-depletion-and-nutrition-loss/.

5. Varshney, V. "Food Basket in Danger." *Down to Earth.* Last modified December 1, 2017. Accessed November 11, 2019. https://www.downtoearth.org.in/news/health/food-basket-in-danger-57079.

6. Daley, J. "Climate Change Could Lead to Nutrient Deficiency for Hundreds of Millions." *Smithsonian.* August 28, 2018. https://www.smithsonianmag.com/smart-news/climate-change-could-lead-nutrient-deficiency-hundreds-millions-180970149/.

7. Luo, K. W., et al. "EGCG inhibited bladder cancer SW780 cell proliferation and migration both in vitro and in vivo via down-regulation of NF-ϰB and MMP-9." *Journal of Nutritional Biochemistry.* 41 (March 2017): 56–64. doi: 10.1016/j.jnutbio.2016.12.004; Wang, J., et al. "A prodrug of green tea polyphenol (-)-epigallocatechin-3-gallate (Pro-EGCG) serves as a novel angiogenesis inhibitor in endometrial cancer." *Cancer Letters.* 412 (January 1, 2018): 10–20. doi: 10.1016/j.canlet.2017.09.054; Zan, L., et al. "Epigallocatechin gallate (EGCG) suppresses growth and tumorigenicity in breast cancer cells by downregulation of miR-25." *Bioengineered.* 10, no. 1 (December 2019): 374–382. doi: 10.1080/21655979.2019.1657327.

8.  Schuerger, N., et al. "Evaluating the Demand for Integrative Medicine Practices in Breast and Gynecological Cancer Patients." *Breast Care*. 14, no. 1 (March 2019): 35–40. doi: 10.1159/000492235.

9.  Tangen, J. M., et al. "Immunomodulatory effects of the Agaricus blazei Murrill-based mushroom extract AndoSan in patients with multiple myeloma undergoing high dose chemotherapy and autologous stem cell transplantation: a randomized, double blinded clinical study." *BioMed Research International*. 2015. doi: 10.1155/2015/718539.

10. Twardowski, P., et al. "A phase I trial of mushroom powder in patients with biochemically recurrent prostate cancer: Roles of cytokines and myeloid-derived suppressor cells for Agaricus bisporus-induced prostate-specific antigen responses." *Cancer*. 121, no. 17 (September 1, 2015): 2942–50. doi: 10.1002/cncr.29421.

11. Ghoneum, M., and J. Gimzewski. "Apoptotic effect of a novel kefir product, PFT, on multidrug-resistant myeloid leukemia cells via a hole-piercing mechanism." *International Journal of Oncology*. 44, no. 3 (March 2014): 830–7. doi: 10.3892/ijo.2014.2258.

12. Going, C. C., et al. "Vitamin D supplementation decreases serum 27-hydroxycholesterol in a pilot breast cancer trial." *Breast Cancer Research and Treatment*. 167, no. 3 (February 2018): 797–802. doi: 10.1007/s10549-017-4562-4.

13. Ma, J., et al. "Effect of ginseng polysaccharides and dendritic cells on the balance of Th1/Th2 T helper cells in patients with non-small cell lung cancer." *Journal of Traditional Chinese Medicine*. 34, no. 6 (December 2014): 641–5. doi: 10.1016/s0254-6272(15)30076-5.

14. Paur, I., et al. "Tomato-based randomized controlled trial in prostate cancer patients: Effect on PSA." *Clinical Nutrition*. 36, no. 3 (June 2017): 672–679. doi: 10.1016/j.clnu.2016.06.014.

15. Winters, N., and J. H. Kelley. *The Metabolic Approach to Cancer: Integrating Deep Nutrition, the Ketogenic Diet, and Nontoxic Bio-Individualized Therapies*. (White River Junction, VT: Chelsea Green Publishing, 2017).

16. World Health Organization, International Agency for Research on Cancer. "Agents Classified by the IARC Monographs, Volumes 1–124." Last modified September 23, 2019. https://monographs.iarc.fr/agents-classified-by-the-iarc/; Ma, X., et al. "Critical windows of exposure to household pesticides and risk of childhood leukemia." *Environmental Health Perspectives*. 110, no. 9 (September 2002): 955–960. doi: 10.1289/ehp.02110955.

17. McGinn, A. P. "POPs Culture." *World Watch*. 13, no. 2 (March–April 2000): 26–36. PMID: 12349645.

18. Alavanja, M. C. R., and M. R. Bonner. "Occupational pesticide exposures and cancer risk. A review." *Journal of Toxicology and Environmental Health, Part B: Critical Reviews*. 15, no. 4 (2012): 238–263. doi: 10.1080/10937404.2012.632358.

19. Winters, N., and J. Higgins Kelley. See note 15 above.

20. Winters, N., and J. Higgins Kelley. See note 15 above; Ma, J., et al. See note 13 above.

21. Evans, S., et al. "Cumulative risk analysis of carcinogenic contaminants in United States drinking water." *Heliyon*. 5, no. 9 (September 18, 2019). doi: 10.1016/j.heliyon.2019.e02314.

22. Tarazona, J. V., et al. "Glyphosate toxicity and carcinogenicity: a review of the scientific basis of the European Union assessment and its differences with IARC." *Archives of Toxicology*. 91, no. 8 (August 2017): 2723–2743. doi: 10.1007/s00204-017-1962-5.

23. Bayan, L., et al. "Garlic: A Review of Potential Therapeutic Effects." *Avicenna Journal of Phytomedicine*. 4, no. 1 (January–February 2014): 1–14. PMID: 25050296; Hudson, J. B. "Applications of the Phytomedicine *Echinacea purpurea* (Purple

Coneflower) in Infectious Diseases." *Journal of Biomedicine and Biotechnology*. (2012). doi: 10.1155/2012/769896.

24. Frenkel, M. "Is There a Role for Homeopathy in Cancer Care? Questions and Challenges." *Current Oncology Reports*. 17 (2015): 43. doi: 10.1007/s11912-015-0467-8.

25. Yadav, R., et al. "How homeopathic medicine works in cancer treatment: deep insight from clinical to experimental studies." *Journal of Experimental Therapeutics and Oncology*. 13, no. 1 (January 2019): 71–76. PMID: 30658031.

26. Gleiss, A., et al. "Re-analysis of survival data of cancer patients utilizing additive homeopathy." *Complementary Therapies in Medicine*. 27 (August 2016): 65–67. doi: 10.1016/j.ctim.2016.06.001.

27. Pathak, S., et al. "Ruta 6 selectively induces cell death in brain cancer cells but proliferation in normal peripheral blood lymphocytes: A novel treatment for human brain cancer." *International Journal of Oncology*. 23, no. 4 (October 2003): 975–982. doi: 10.3892/ijo.23.4.975.

28. Ibid.

29. Bridgeman, M. B., and D.T. Abazia. "Medicinal Cannabis: History, Pharmacology, and Implications for the Acute Care Setting." *Pharmacy and Therapeutics*. 42, no. 3 (March 2017): 180–188. PMID: 28250701.

30. Sidney, S. "Comparing cannabis with tobacco–again." *BMJ*. 327, no. 7416 (September 20, 2003): 635–636. doi: 10.1136/bmj.327.7416.635; Clark, P. A., et al. "Medical marijuana: medical necessity versus political agenda." *Medical Science Monitor*. 17, no. 12 (December 2011): RA249–61. doi: 10.12659/msm.882116.

31. "Annual Causes of Death in the United States." *Drug War Facts*. Accessed June 3, 2019. https://www.drugwarfacts.org/chapter/causes_of_death.

32. Gable, R. S., "The Toxicity of Recreational Drugs," *American Scientist*. 94, no. 3 (May–June 2006).

33. National Institutes of Health, National Institute on Drug Abuse. "Drug facts: is marijuana medicine?" December 2014. https://www.drugabuse.gov/sites/default/files/ismarijuanamedicine_12_2014.pdf; "Should marijuana be a medical option?" ProCon.org. Last modified September 20, 2019. https://medicalmarijuana.procon.org/; MacDonald, K., and K. Pappas. "Why Not Pot? A Review of the Brain-Based Risks of Cannabis." *Innovations in Clinical Neuroscience*. 13, no. 3–4 (March–April 2016): 13–22. PMID: 27354924.

34. Moreno, E., et al. "The Endocannabinoid System as a Target in Cancer Diseases: Are We There Yet?" *Frontiers in Pharmacology*. 10 (April 5, 2019): 339. doi: 10.3389/fphar.2019.003.

35. McCarthy, J. "Two in Three Americans Now Support Legalizing Marijuana." Gallup. October 22, 2018. https://news.gallup.com/poll/243908/two-three-americans-support-legalizing-marijuana.aspx.

36. Kisková, T., et al. "Future Aspects for Cannabinoids in Breast Cancer Therapy." *International Journal of Molecular Sciences*. 20, no. 7 (April 3, 2019): 1673. doi: 10.3390/ijms20071673.

37. Zias, J., et al. "Early medical use of cannabis." *Nature*. 363, no. 6426 (May 20, 1993): 215. doi: 10.1038/363215a0.

38. Hanus, L. O., et al. "Phytocannabinoids: A unified critical inventory." *Natural Product Reports*. 33, no. 12 (November 23, 2016): 1357–1392. doi: 10.1039/C6NP00074F.

39. Bridgeman, M. B., and D. T. Abazia. See note 29 above; Raypole, C. "A Simple Guide to the Endocannabinoid System." *Healthline*. Last modified May 17, 2019. https://www.healthline.com/health/endocannabinoid-system-2.

40. Bridgeman, M. B., and D. T. Abazia. See note 29 above; Wilson, R. I., and R. A. Nicoll. "Endocannabinoid signaling in the brain." *Science.* 296, no. 5568 (April 26, 2002): 678–82. doi: 10.1126/science.1063545; Klein, T. W. "Cannabinoid-based drugs as anti-inflammatory therapeutics." *Nature Reviews Immunology.* 5, no. 5 (May 2005): 400–11. doi: 10.1038/nri1602.

41. McPartland, J. M., et al. "Are cannabidiol and Δ9-tetrahydrocannabivarin negative modulators of the endocannabinoid system? A systematic review." *British Journal of Pharmacology.* 172, no. 3 (February 2015): 737–53. doi: 10.1111/bph.12944.

42. Moreno, E., et al. See note 34 above.

43. Moreno, E., et al. See note 34 above.

44. "Cannabidiol (compound of cannabis)." The World Health Organization. Last modified December 2017. https://www.who.int/features/qa/cannabidiol/en/.

45. Wang, T., et al. "Adverse effects of medical cannabinoids: a systematic review." *CMAJ.* 178, no. 13 (June 17, 2008): 1669–78. doi: 10.1503/cmaj.071178.

46. Ibid.

47. Ibid.

48. Lynch, M. E., and F. Campbell. "Cannabinoids for treatment of chronic noncancer pain: a systematic review of randomized trials." *British Journal of Clinical Pharmacology.* 72, no. 5 (November 2011): 735–44. doi: 10.1111/j.1365-2125.2011.03970.x.

49. Kisková, T., et al. See note 36 above.

50. Kisková, T., et al. See note 36 above.

51. Smith, L. A., et al. "Cannabinoids for nausea and vomiting in adults with cancer receiving chemotherapy." *Cochrane Database of Systematic Reviews.* No. 11 (November 12, 2015). doi: 10.1002/14651858.CD009464.pub2.

52. McAllister, S. D., et al. "The Antitumor Activity of Plant-Derived Non-Psychoactive Cannabinoids." *Journal of Neuroimmune Pharmacology.* 10, no. 2 (June 2015): 255–267. doi: 10.1007/s11481-015-9608-y.

53. Ramer, R., and B. Hinz. "Cannabinoids as anticancer drugs." *Advances in Pharmacology.* 80 (2017): 397–436. doi: 10.1016/bs.apha.2017.04.002.

54. "GW Pharmaceuticals Achieves Positive Results in Phase 2 Proof of Concept Study in Glioma." GW Pharmaceuticals, 2017 press release. ClinicalTrials.gov identifiers: NCT01812616, NCT01812603. https://www.gwpharm.com/about/news/gw-pharmaceuticals-achieves-positive-results-phase-2-proof-concept-study-glioma.

55. Ibid.

56. Manuzak, J. A., et al. "Heavy Cannabis Use Associated With Reduction in Activated and Inflammatory Immune Cell Frequencies in Antiretroviral Therapy–Treated Human Immunodeficiency Virus–Infected Individuals." *Clinical Infectious Diseases.* 66, no. 12 (June 15, 2018): 1872–1882. doi: 10.1093/cid/cix1116.

57. Ibid.

58. McAllister, S. D., et al. See note 52 above.

59. McAllister, S. D., et al. See note 52 above.

60. Takeda, S., et al. "Cannabidiolic acid as a selective cyclooxygenase-2 inhibitory component in cannabis." *Drug Metabolism and Disposition.* 36, no. 9. (September 2008): 1917–1921. doi: 10.1124/dmd.108.020909.

61. Kisková, T., et al. See note 36 above.

62. Ligresti, A., et al. "Antitumor activity of plant cannabinoids with emphasis on the effect of cannabidiol on human breast carcinoma." *Journal of Pharmacology and Experimental Therapeutics.* 318, no. 3 (September 2006): 1375–1387. doi: 10.1124/jpet.106.105247.

63. National Cancer Center, U.S. National Institutes of Health. "Mistletoe Extracts (PDQ)–Patient Version." Last modified April 25, 2019. https://www.cancer.gov/about-cancer/treatment/cam/patient/mistletoe-pdq.

64. Tröger, W., et al. "Viscum album [L.] extract therapy in patients with locally advanced or metastatic pancreatic cancer: A randomised clinical trial on overall survival." *European Journal of Cancer.* 49, no. 18 (December 2013): 3788–3797. doi: 10.1016/j.ejca.2013.06.043; National Cancer Center, U.S. NIH. "Mistletoe Extracts . . ." See note 63 above.

65. Kienle, G. S., et al. "Mistletoe in Cancer - A Systematic Review on Controlled Clinical Trials." *Database of Abstracts of Reviews of Effects (DARE): Quality-Assessed Reviews.* York (U.K.): Centre for Reviews and Dissemination (U.K.), 1995–. Available from: https://www.ncbi.nlm.nih.gov/books/NBK69731/; Kienle, G. S., and H. Kiene. "Complementary Cancer Therapy: A Systematic Review of Prospective Clinical Trials on Anthroposophic Mistletoe Extracts." *European Journal of Medical Research.* 12, no. 3 (March 26, 2007): 103–19. PMID: 17507307.

66. Rose, A., et al. "Mistletoe Plant Extract in Patients with Nonmuscle Invasive Bladder Cancer: Results of a Phase Ib/IIa Single Group Dose Escalation Study." *Journal of Urology.* 194, no. 4 (October 2015): 939–43. doi: 10.1016/j.juro.2015.04.073.

67. Han, S. Y., et al. "Anti-cancer effects of enteric-coated polymers containing mistletoe lectin in murine melanoma cells in vitro and in vivo." *Molecular and Cellular Biochemistry.* 408, no. 1–2 (October 2015): 73–87. doi: 10.1007/s11010-015-2484-1.

68. Liao, C., et al. "Chronomodulated chemotherapy versus conventional chemotherapy for advanced colorectal cancer: A meta-analysis of five randomized controlled trials." *International Journal of Colorectal Disease.* 25, no. 3 (March 2010): 343–50. doi: 10.1007/s00384-009-0838-4.

69. Mantovani, A. "Molecular pathways linking inflammation and cancer." *Current Molecular Medicine.* 10, no. 4 (June 2010): 369–73. doi: 10.2174/156652410791316968.

**CHAPTER 9**

1. Watson, M., et al. "Influence of Psychological Response on Survival in Breast Cancer: A Population-Based Cohort Study," *The Lancet.* 354, no. 9187 (October 16, 1999): 1331–36. doi: 10.1016/s0140-6736(98)11392-2; Pinquart, M., and P. R. Duberstein. "Depression and Cancer Mortality: A Meta-Analysis." *Psychological Medicine.* 40, no. 11 (November 2010): 1797–810. doi: 10.1017/S0033291709992285; Faller, H., and M. Schmidt. "Depression and Survival of Lung Cancer Patients," *Psycho-oncology.* 13, no. 5 (May 2004): 359–63. doi: 10.1002/pon.783; Goodwin, J. S., et al. "Effect of Depression on Diagnosis, Treatment, and Survival of Older Women with Breast Cancer." *Journal of the American Geriatrics Society.* 52, no. 1 (January 2004): 106–11. doi: 10.1111/j.1532-5415.2004.52018.x.

2. Cohen, R., et al. "Purpose in Life and Its Relationship to All-Cause Mortality and Cardiovascular Events: A Meta-Analysis." *Psychosomatic Medicine.* 78, no. 2 (February–March 2016): 122–133. doi: 10.1097/PSY.0000000000000274; Andersen, S. L., et al. "Health Span Approximates Life Span among Many Supercentenarians: Compression of Morbidity at the Approximate Limit of Life Span." *The Journals of Gerontology, Series A: Biological Sciences and Medical Sciences.* 67A, no. 4 (April 2012): 395–405. doi: 10.1093/gerona/glr223; Gellert, P., et al. "Centenarians Differ in Their Comorbidity Trends during the Six Years before Death Compared to Individuals Who Died in Their 80s or 90s." *The Journals of Gerontology, Series A: Biological Sciences and Medical Sciences.* 73, no. 10 (September 11, 2018): 1357–1362. doi: 10.1093/gerona/glx136; Ismail, K., et al. "Compression

# Endnotes

of Morbidity Is Observed across Cohorts with Exceptional Longevity." *Journal of the American Geriatrics Society.* 64, no. 8 (August 2016): 1583–1591. doi: 10.1111/jgs.14222; Sebastiani, P., et al. "Families Enriched for Exceptional Longevity Also Have Increased Health-Span: Findings from the Long Life Family Study." *Frontiers in Public Health.* 1 (September 30, 2013): 38. doi: 10.3389/fpubh.2013.00038; Terry, D. F., et al. "Disentangling the Roles of Disability and Morbidity in Survival to Exceptional Old Age." *Archives of Internal Medicine.* 168, no. 3 (2008): 277–283. doi: 10.1001/archinternmed.2007.75.

3.  Marone, S., et al. "Purpose in Life Among Centenarian Offspring." *The Journals of Gerontology, Series B: Psychological Sciences and Social Sciences.* March 7, 2018. doi: 10.1093/geronb/gby023.

4.  Friedman, E. M., et al. "Plasma interleukin-6 and soluble IL-6 receptors are associated with psychological well-being in aging women." *Health Psychology.* 26, no. 3 (May 2007): 305–313. doi: 10.1037/0278-6133.26.3.305; Thoma, M. V., et al. "Stronger hypothalamus-pituitary-adrenal axis habituation predicts lesser sensitization of inflammatory response to repeated acute stress exposures in healthy young adults." *Brain, Behavior, and Immunity.* 61 (March 2017): 228–235. doi: 10.1016/j.bbi.2016.11.030; Fogelman, N., and T. Canli. "'Purpose in Life' as a psychosocial resource in healthy aging: An examination of cortisol baseline levels and response to the Trier Social Stress Test." *NPJ Aging and Mechanisms of Disease.* 1 (September 28, 2015): 15006. doi: 10.1038/npjamd.2015.6.

5.  Alimujiang, A., et al. "Association between Life Purpose and Mortality among US Adults Older Than 50 Years." *JAMA Network Open.* 2, no. 5 (May 3, 2019): e194270. doi:10.1001/jamanetworkopen.2019.4270.

6.  Yasukawa, S., et al. "'Ikigai', Subjective Wellbeing, as a Modifier of the Parity-Cardiovascular Mortality Association—The Japan Collaborative Cohort Study." *Circulation Journal.* 82, no. 5 (April 25, 2018): 1302–1308. doi: 10.1253/circj.CJ-17-1201.

7.  Cohen, R., et al. See note 2 above.

8.  Zilioli, S., et al. "Purpose in life predicts allostatic load ten years later." *Journal of Psychosomatic Research.* 79, no. 5 (November 2015): 451–457. doi: 10.1016/j.jpsychores.2015.09.013.

9.  Proyer, R. T. "A multidisciplinary perspective on adult play and playfulness" *International Journal of Play.* 6, no. 3 (2017): 241–243. doi: 10.1080/21594937.2017.1384307.

10. Holland, E. "Adult Playtime: 6 Ways to Bring More Fun into Your Day." The Chopra Center. Last modified January 22, 2016. https://chopra.com/articles/adult-playtime-6-ways-to-bring-more-fun-into-your-day; Magnuson, C. D., and L. A. Barnett. "The Playful Advantage: How Playfulness Enhances Coping with Stress." *Leisure Sciences.* 35, no. 2 (2013): 129–144. doi: 10.1080/01490400.2013.761905.

11. Thiel, A., et al. "Have adults lost their sense of play? An observational study of the social dynamics of physical (in)activity in German and Hawaiian leisure settings." *BMC Public Health.* 16 (August 2, 2016): 689. doi: 10.1186/s12889-016-3392-3; Proyer, R. T. "The well-being of playful adults: Adult playfulness, subjective well-being, physical well-being, and the pursuit of enjoyable activities." *European Journal of Humour Research.* 1, no. 1 (2013): 84–98. doi: 10.7592/ejhr2013.1.1.proyer.

12. Krug, N. "Why Adults Coloring Books Are the Latest Trend." *Washington Post.* Last modified May 2, 2016. http://wapo.st/26KuQik.

13. Ajiboye, T. "Adults Need Recess Too. Here's Why You Should Make Time to Play." NBC News. Last modified July 7, 2018. https://www.nbcnews.com/better/health/adults-need-recess-too-here-s-why-you-should-make-ncna887396.

14. Sandler, E. S., ed. "Osteosarcoma." Kids Health from Nemours. Last modified January 2017. https://kidshealth.org/en/parents/cancer-osteosarcoma.html.

15. Ibid.

16. "Personalized Oncology." Champions Oncology. Accessed November 11, 2019. https://championsoncology.com/personalized-oncology-pdx-model/; "Personalized Cytometric Cancer Profiling Services." Weisenthal Cancer Group. Accessed November 11, 2019. https://www.weisenthalcancer.com/Services.html.

17. Ibid.

18. Wan, J., et al. "Strategies and developments of immunotherapies in osteosarcoma." *Oncology Letters.* 11, no. 1 (January 2016): 511–520. doi: 10.3892/ol.2015.3962.

19. Tornesello, A. L., et al. "New Insights in the Design of Bioactive Peptides and Chelating Agents for Imaging and Therapy in Oncology." *Molecules.* 22, no. 8 (August 2017): 1282. doi: 10.3390/molecules22081282.

CHAPTER 10

1. Ishak, W. W., et al. "Oxytocin Role in Enhancing Well-Being: A Literature Review." *Journal of Affective Disorders.* 130, nos. 1–2 (April 2011): 1–9. doi: 10.1016/j.jad .2010.06.001.

2. Steptoe, A., et al. "Positive Affect and Psychobiological Processes Relevant to Health." *Journal of Personality.* 77, no. 6 (December 2009): 1747–76. doi: 10.1111/j.1467-6494.2009.00599.x.

3. Berkman, L. F., and S. L. Syme. "Social Networks, Host Resistance, and Mortality: A Nine-Year Follow-Up Study of Alameda County Residents." *American Journal of Epidemiology.* 109, no. 2 (February 1979): 186–204. doi: 10.1093/oxfordjournals. aje.a112674; Glass, T. A., et al. "Population-Based Study of Social and Productive Activities as Predictors of Survival Among Elderly Americans." *BMJ.* 319 (August 21, 1999): 478–83. doi: 10.1136/bmj.319.7208.478; Giles, L. C., et al. "Effects of Social Networks on 10 Year Survival in Very Old Australians: The Australian Longitudinal Study of Aging." *Journal of Epidemiology & Community Health.* 59, no. 7 (July 2005): 574–79. doi: 10.1136/jech.2004.025429; House, J. S., et al. "The Association of Social Relationships and Activities with Mortality: Prospective Evidence from Tecumseh Community Health Study." *American Journal of Epidemiology.* 116, no 1 (July 1982): 123–40. doi: 10.1093/oxfordjournals.aje .a113387.

4. Reynolds, P., et al. "The Relationship Between Social Ties and Survival Among Black and White Breast Cancer Patients: National Cancer Institute Black/White Cancer Survival Study Group." *Cancer Epidemiology, Biomarkers, and Prevention.* 3, no. 3 (April–May 1994): 253–59. PMID: 8019376.

5. Zuelsdorff, M. L., et al. "Social support and verbal interaction are differentially associated with cognitive function in midlife and older age." *Neuropsychology, Development, and Cognition, Section B Aging Neuropsychology, and Cognition.* 26, no. 2 (March 2019): 144–160. doi: 10.1080/13825585.2017.1414769.

6. Berkman, L. F., and S. L. Syme. See note 3 above; Glass, T. A. , et al. See note 3 above; Wolf, S., and Bruhn, J. G. *The Power of Clan: The Influence of Human Relationships on Heart Disease.* (Piscataway, NJ: Transaction Publishers, 1998); Holahan, C.J., et al. "Late-Life Alcohol Consumption and Twenty-Year Mortality." *Alcoholism, Clinical and Experimental Research.* 34, no. 11 (November 2010): 1961–71. doi: 10.1111/j.1530-0277.2010.01286.x.

7. Steptoe, A. See note 2 above; Ader, R., ed., *Psychoneuroimmunology, 4th Edition.* (Burlington, MA: Elsevier Academic Press, 2011).

8. Uchino, B. N., et al. "The Relationship between Social Support and Physiological Processes: A Review with Emphasis on Underlying Mechanisms and Implications from Health." *Psychological Bulletin.* 119, no. 3 (May 1996): 488–531. doi: 10.1037/0033-2909.119.3.488; Uchino, B. N. "Social Support and Health: A Review of Physiological Processes Potentially Underlying Links to Disease Outcomes." *Journal of Behavioral Medicine.* 29, no. 4 (August 2006): 377–87. doi: 10.1007/s10865-006-9056-5.

9. Steptoe, A. See note 2 above; Ader, R., ed. See note 7 above.

# Endnotes

10. Christensen, A. V., et al. "Significantly Increased Risk of All-Cause Mortality among Cardiac Patients Feeling Lonely." *Heart*. November 4, 2019. doi: 10.1136/heartjnl-2019-315460.

11. Pinquart, M., and P. R. Duberstein. "Associations of Social Networks with Cancer Mortality: A Meta-Analysis." *Critical Reviews in Oncology/Hematology*. 75, no. 2 (August 2010): 122–37. doi: 10.1016/j.critrevonc.2009.06.003.

12. Friedmann, E., and S. A. Thoms. "Pet Ownership, Social Support, and One-Year Survival After Acute Myocardial Infarction in the Cardiac Arrhythmia Suppression Trial (CAST)." *American Journal of Cardiology*. 76, no. 17 (December 15, 1995): 1213–17. doi: 10.1016/s0002-9149(99)80343-9; McNicholas, J., et al. "Pet Ownership and Human Health: A Brief Review of Evidence and Issues." *BMJ*. 331, no. 7527 (November 26, 2005): 1252–54. doi: 10.1136/bmj.331.7527.1252; Steele, R. W., "Should Immunocompromised Patients Have Pets?" *Ochsner Journal*. 8, no. 3 (Fall 2008): 134–39. PMID: 21603465; Müllersdorf, M., et al. "Aspects of Health, Physical/Leisure Activities, Work and Socio-Demographics Associated with Pet Ownership in Sweden." *Scandinavian Journal of Public Health*. 38, no. 1 (February 2010): 53–63. doi: 10.1177/1403494809344358; Qureshi, A. I., et al. "Cat Ownership and the Risk of Fatal Cardiovascular Diseases: Results from the Second National Health and Nutrition Examination Study Mortality Follow-Up Study." *Journal of Vascular and Interventional Neurology*. 2, no. 1 (January 2009): 132–35. PMID: 22518240.

13. Cigna. *2018 Cigna U.S. Lonliness Index: Survey of 20,000 Americans Examining Behaviors Driving Loneliness in the United States.* Accessed November 11, 2019. https://www.multivu.com/players/English/8294451-cigna-us-loneliness-survey/.

14. Bialik, K. "Americans unhappy with family, social or financial life are more likely to say they feel lonely." Pew Research Center. Last modified December 3, 2018. https://www.pewresearch.org/fact-tank/2018/12/03/americans-unhappy-with-family-social-or-financial-life-are-more-likely-to-say-they-feel-lonely/.

15. Holt-Lunstad, J., et al. "Social Relationships and Mortality Risk: A Meta-Analytic Review." *PLOS Medicine*. 7, no. 7 (July 27, 2010): e1000316. doi: 10.1371/journal.pmed.1000316; Thomas, S. N. "Prescription for Living Longer: Spend Less Time Alone." *BYU News*. (2015). Last modified March 10, 2015. https://news.byu.edu/news/prescription-living-longer-spend-less-time-alone.

16. Kobayashi, L. C., and A. Steptoe. "Social Isolation, Loneliness, and Health Behaviors at Older Ages: Longitudinal Cohort Study. " *Annals of Behavioral Medicine*. 52, no. 7 (May 31, 2018): 582–593. doi: 10.1093/abm/kax033.

17. Rico-Uribe, L. A., et al. "Loneliness, Social Networks, and Health: A Cross-Sectional Study in Three Countries." *PLOS ONE*. 11, no. 1 (January 13, 2016): e0145264. doi: 10.1371/journal.pone.0145264.

18. Ibid.

19. Ibid.

20. Kearns, A., et al. "Loneliness, social relations and health and well-being in deprived communities." *Psychology, Health, and Medicine*. 20, no. 3 (2015): 332–344. doi: 10.1080/13548506.2014.940354.

21. Ibid.

22. Ibid.

23. Ibid.

24. Applebaum, A. J., et al. "Optimism, social support, and mental health outcomes in patients with advanced cancer." *Psychooncology*. 23, no. 3 (March 2014): 299–306. doi: 10.1002/pon.3418.

25. Ibid.

26. Tschuschke, V., et al. "Psychological Stress and Coping Resources during Primary Systemic Therapy for Breast Cancer. Results of a Prospective Study." *Geburtshilfe Frauenheilkd*. 77, no. 2 (February 2017): 158–168. doi: 10.1055/s-0043-101237.

27. Ibid.

28. Meeker, M. "Internet Trends 2019." *Bond*. Accessed November 11, 2019. https://www.bondcap.com/pdf/Internet_Trends_2019.pdf.

29. Jakubiak, B. K., and B. C. Feeney. "Affectionate Touch to Promote Relational, Psychological, and Physical Well-Being in Adulthood: A Theoretical Model and Review of the Research." *Personality and Social Psychology Review*. 21, no. 3 (August 2017): 228–252. doi: 10.1177/1088868316650307.

30. Shensa, A., et al. "Social Media Use and Depression and Anxiety Symptoms: A Cluster Analysis." *American Journal of Health Behavior*. 42, no. 2 (March 1, 2018): 116–128. doi: 10.5993/AJHB.42.2.11.

31. Muscatell, K. A., et al. "Links between inflammation, amygdala reactivity, and social support in breast cancer survivors." *Brain, Behavior, and Immunity*. 53 (March 2016): 34–38. doi: 10.1016/j.bbi.2015.09.008.

32. Ibid.

33. Ibid.

34. Ibid.

35. Uchino, B. N., et al. "Social support, social integration, and inflammatory cytokines: A meta-analysis." *Health Psychology*. 37, no. 5 (May 2018): 462–471. doi: 10.1037/hea0000594.

36. Ford, J., et al. "Social Integration and Quality of Social Relationships as Protective Factors for Inflammation in a Nationally Representative Sample of Black Women." *Journal of Urban Health*. 96, suppl. 1 (March 2019): 35. doi: 10.1007/s11524-018-00337-x.

37. Ibid.

38. Lee, S., et al. "High-sensitivity C-reactive protein and cancer." *Journal of Epidemiology*. 21, no. 3 (2011): 161–168. doi: 10.2188/jea.je20100128.

39. Ford, J., et al. See note 36 above.

40. Lee, S., et al. See note 38 above.

41. Banegas, M. P., et al. "For Working-Age Cancer Survivors, Medical Debt and Bankruptcy Create Financial Hardships." *Health Affairs*. 35, no. 1 (January 2016): 54–61. doi: 10.1377/hlthaff.2015.0830.

42. Ibid.

43. Chino, F., et al. "Out-of-Pocket Costs, Financial Distress, and Underinsurance in Cancer Care." *JAMA Oncology*. 3, no. 11 (November 1, 2017): 1582–1584. doi: 10.1001/jamaoncol.2017.2148.

44. Young, J. "Life and Debt: Stories from Inside America's GoFundMe Health Care System." *Huffpost*. Last updated June 19, 2019. https://www.huffpost.com/entry/gofundme-health-care-system_n_5ced9785e4b0ae6710584b27.

45. "2019 Alzheimer's Disease: Facts & Figures." *Alzheimer's & Dementia: The Journal of the Alzheimer's Association*. 15, no. 3 (March 2019): 321–387. doi: 10.1016/j.jalz.2019.01.010.

46. Bredesen, D. E., et al. "Reversal of cognitive decline in Alzheimer's disease." *Aging*. 8, no. 6 (June 2016): 1250–1258. doi: 10.18632/aging.100981.

47. "2019 Alzheimer's Disease: Facts & Figures." See note 45 above.

# Endnotes

48. U.S. Centers for Disease Control and Prevention, Division of Population Health, National Center for Chronic Disease Prevention and Health Promotion. "Subjective Cognitive Decline — A Public Health Issue." Last modified February 27, 2019. https://www.cdc.gov/aging/data/subjective-cognitive-decline-brief.html; "Subjective Cognitive Decline: The Earliest Sign of Alzheimer's Disease?" *Neurology Reviews*. 21, no. 9 (September 2013): 1, 33–37; Jessen, F., et al. "A conceptual framework for research on subjective cognitive decline in preclinical Alzheimer's disease." *Alzheimer's & Dementia: The Journal of the Alzheimer's Association*. 10, no. 6 (November 2014): 844–52. doi: 10.1016/j.jalz.2014.01.001.

49. Ibid.

50. Ibid.

51. Bredesen, D. E. *The End of Alzheimer's: The First Program to Prevent and Reverse Cognitive Decline*. (New York: Avery, 2017).

52. "About Us." MoCA: Montreal Cognitive Assessment. Accessed November 11, 2019. https://www.mocatest.org/about/.

53. "10 Early Signs and Symptoms of Alzheimer's." Alzheimer's Association. Accessed November 11, 2019. https://www.alz.org/alzheimers-dementia/10_signs.

54. Bredesen, D. E. "Reversal of cognitive decline: A novel therapeutic program." *Aging*. 6, no. 9 (September 2014): 707–17. doi: 10.18632/aging.100690.

55. Bredesen, D.E. "Metabolic profiling distinguishes three subtypes of Alzheimer's disease." *Aging*. 7, no. 8 (August 2015): 595–600. doi: 10.18632/aging.100801.

56. Bredesen, D. E. "Inhalational Alzheimer's disease: an unrecognized—and treatable—epidemic." *Aging*. 8, no. 2 (February 2016): 304–313. doi: 10.18632/aging.100896.

57. Bredesen, D. E. See note 51 above.

58. Qian, J., et al. "APOE-related risk of mild cognitive impairment and dementia for prevention trials: An analysis of four cohorts." *PLOS Medicine*. 14, no. 3 (March 21, 2017): e1002254. doi: 10.1371/journal.pmed.1002254.

59. Dacks, P. "What APOE Means for Your Health." *Cognitive Vitality*. November 26, 2016.

60. Nivens, A. S., et al. "Cues to participation in prostate cancer screening: a theory for practice." *Oncology Nursing Forum*. 28, no. 9 (October 2001): 1449–56. PMID: 11683314.

61. Ibid.

62. Bredesen, D.E. See note 51 above.

63. Medic, G., et al. "Short- and long-term health consequences of sleep disruption." *Nature and Science of Sleep*. 9 (2017): 151–161. doi: 10.2147/NSS.S134864.

64. Owens, R. L., et al. "Sleep and Breathing . . . and Cancer?" *Cancer Prevention Research*. 9, no. 11 (November 2016): 821–827. Published correction, 10, no. 1 (January 2017): 98. doi: 10.1158/1940-6207.CAPR-16-0092.

65. Xie, L., et al. "Sleep drives metabolite clearance from the adult brain." *Science*. 342, no. 6156 (October 18, 2013): 373–7. doi: 10.1126/science.1241224.

66. Fultz, N. E., et al. "Coupled electrophysiological, hemodynamic, and cerebrospinal fluid oscillations in human sleep." *Science*. 366, no. 6465 (November 1, 2019): 628–631. doi: 10.1126/science.aax5440.

67. Bredesen, D. E. See note 51 above.

68. Posit Science BrainHQ. Accessed November 11, 2019. https://www.brainhq.com/about.

69. Bredesen, D. E.. See note 51 above.

70. "Glycemic index for 60+ foods: Measuring carbohydrate effects can help glucose management." Harvard Health Publishing, Harvard Medical School. Last modified March 14, 2018. https://www.health.harvard.edu/diseases-and-conditions/ glycemic-index-and-glycemic-load-for-100-foods.

71. Berndtson, K. "Chronic Inflammatory Response Syndrome: Overview, Diagnosis, and Treatment." Accessed November 11, 2019. https://www.survivingmold.com/ docs/Berndtson_essay_2_CIRS.pdf.

72. Ibid.

73. Shoemaker, R. C., and D. E. House. "Sick building syndrome (SBS) and exposure to water-damaged buildings: time series study, clinical trial and mechanisms." *Neurotoxicology and Teratology.* 28, no. 5 (September–October 2006): 573–88.

74. Rahman, M. M., et al. "Early hippocampal volume loss as a marker of eventual memory deficits caused by repeated stress." *Scientific Reports.* 6 (July 4, 2016): 29127. doi: 10.1038/srep29127.

75. Lilleston, R. "For Surrogate Grandparents, the Ties Still Bind." AARP. Accessed November 11, 2019. https://www.aarp.org/home-family/friends-family/info-2017/ surrogate-grandparents-benefits-fd.html.

76. Gordon, E. "5 Pet Cafes in NYC: Eat, Sip, and Play With Your Furry Friends." *Untapped New York.* Last modified August 7, 2017. https://untappedcities.com/ 2017/08/07/the-top-5-pet-cafes-in-nyc-including-the-first-ever-dog-cafe/.

## CONCLUSION

1. "Take Control of your Cancer Risk: Nearly Fifty Percent of common Cancers are Preventable." American Institute for Cancer Research. Last modified February 1, 2018. https://www.aicr.org/press/press-releases/2018/nearly-fifty-percent-of -common-cancers-are-preventable.html.

2. Wu, J., and L. L. Lanier. "Natural killer cells and cancer." Advances in Cancer Research. 90 (2003): 127–56. doi: 10.1016/s0065-230x(03)90004-2.

# INDEX

Coley's toxins, 36–37, 38, 39
colorectal cancer
diet and, 180–182
healing stories, 29–30, 227–238
incidence of, 179
research studies, 6, 7, 8, 11, 180–182, 185, 187
community. *See* social support network
contentment. *See* positive emotions
control of health. *See* empowerment
Cousins, Norman, 85, 125–126, 127–128
*Crazy Sexy Cancer* (documentary), 184–185
Cromwell, Kristi, 80
Customized Oncology Nutrition, 169, 170
cytometric cancer profiling, 259–260

**D**

death. *See also* reasons for living
embracing, 91, 97–98
fear of, 145, 147, 162, 244
near-death experience (NDE), 150–151
Demartini, John, 87–88
depression
cancer diagnosis and, 75–76
cancer treatment and, 90–91
empowerment and, 55–56
exercise and, 5, 6, 22
positive emotions and, 91
detoxification (body), 217–219, 238, 240–241
detoxification, from technology, 106, 149, 174–175
Dietary Approaches to Stop Hypertension (the DASH diet), 182
dietary changes, 177–211
about, 177–178
action steps, 209–211
autoimmune issues and, 133–135
cancer prevention and, 181–183
cancer rates and, 178–181
cancer survival rates and, 183–184
gut health and microbiome, 193–197, 210–211. *See also* gut health and microbiome
healing stories, 16, 27–28, 37–40, 42, 64–65, 100, 128–131, 133–134, 166–168, 171–172, 184–185, 197–209, 232, 234–235, 260–261, 292
intermittent fasting and, 171–172, 190–193, 210, 292
intuition and, 130–131, 133–134
ketogenic diet, 167, 171–172, 177, 187–188, 190, 292, 297
Mediterranean diet, 177, 182–183
metabolic diseases and, 189–190
new trends, 178–197
personalization of, 104, 166–168, 169, 171–172, 234–235
plant-based diets, 177, 184–186, 188, 195
Di's healing story, 86–105
Dispenza, Joe, 143
doctor's expertise, questioning, 47–49, 59–61, 66, 128–129. *See also* empowerment

**E**

Eden, Donna, 117
Edison, Thomas, 213
EFT (emotional freedom technique)/tapping, 116, 119, 153–157, 173–174
EHE (epithelioid hemangioendothelioma), 184–185
Einstein, Albert, 109
EMDR (eye movement desensitization and reprocessing), 152–153
emotional baggage. *See* suppressed emotion release
emotional freedom technique (EFT)/tapping, 116, 119, 153–157, 173–174
empowerment, 47–73
about, 47–52
action steps, 71–73
healing stories, 36–37, 41, 50–52, 57–71, 88–90, 103–104, 128–129, 225–227, 287
new trends, 52–57
positive emotions and, 103–104
research studies, 55–57
endometrial cancer, 7
energy healing
about, 115–117
action steps, 44, 139–140
intuition and, 115–117
yoga as, 116, 130–131, 140
energy kinesiology (muscle testing), 117–119, 136
Environmental Working Group (EWG), 211
epigenetics, 30–31, 42, 135–136, 155
epithelioid hemangioendothelioma (EHE), 184–185
esophageal cancer, 195
exercise, 1–24
about, 1–4
action steps, 21–24
benefits for cancer patients, 5–7
benefits for everyone, 4–5
cancer survival and, 7–8
detoxification and, 240
healing stories, 2–3, 13–21, 23, 65, 100, 104, 130, 166, 170, 207, 236, 292, 297
positive emotions and, 81, 104
research studies, 3, 4–9
suppressed emotions and, 165–166, 170
as targeted medicine, 8–9
types of, 9–12
Exercise Medicine Research Institute, 9
extra-virgin olive oil (EVOO), 182
eye movement desensitization and reprocessing (EMDR), 152–153

**F**

fear, 145, 146–147, 151
fecal microbiota transplantation (FMT), 84
fight-or-flight mode
after cancer diagnosis, xi, 122
positive emotions versus, 76

Page, Ivelisse, 225–227
Palmer's healing story, 123–139
pancreatic cancer, 2–3, 181, 187
peace. *See* positive emotions
peritoneal cancer, 57–71, 158–159, 278
personalization
for Alzheimer patients, 287–288
cancer cure and, 48
of chemotherapy, 259–260, 261–262, 264
of dietary changes, 104, 166–168, 169, 171–172, 234–235
of herbs and supplements, 213–214, 216, 233–234, 235
Pew Research Center, 26
pharynx cancer, 181
*Physical Activity Guidelines for Americans* (2018), 4
physical activity. *See* exercise
plant-based diets, 177, 184–186, 188, 195
playfulness and purpose, 250–251, 267
Pollan, Michael, 177
positive emotions, 75–107
about, 75–78
action steps, 105–107
defined, 76
gratitude, 43, 79–81, 84, 96–97
happiness, as public policy, 79
healing stories, 17–19, 42, 61–62, 64, 66–68, 86–105, 291
laughter and, 80, 85, 105–107, 125–126
new trends, 78–86
oxytocin and, 76–77, 85–86, 105–106
psychobiotics, 84
psychoneuroimmunology, 83–84
tapping and, 155
technology addiction and, 81–82
post-traumatic stress disorder (PTSD), 148, 152–153, 154–155, 263
prostate cancer, 6, 7, 187, 196, 217, 260
psychobiotics, 84
psychoneuroimmunology (PNI), 83–84
psychosocial factors, 55
PubMed.gov, 53
purpose. *See* reasons for living

**Q**

qigong, 116
quality of life
cancer survival and, 55–56
coping skills and, 55–56
empowerment and, 55–57
energy healing and, 116–117
exercise's impact on, 6, 10
optimism and, 276–277
positive emotions and, 83
reasons for living and, 247

**R**

Radical Remission Foundation, xiv, 306–307
radical remissions

about, xvii, 304–305
author's personal story, xv–xvi
defined, xi–xii
docuseries and feature film on, xvi, 307
healing factors for, xii–xiii, xv, xviii. *See also* dietary changes; empowerment; exercise; herbs and supplements; intuition; positive emotions; reasons for living; social support network; spiritual connections; suppressed emotion release
as hope, xi, xviii
online database, xiv, 306
research studies, xiv, xvii–xviii, 303–304, 306–307
workshops and courses, xiii–xiv, 307–308
*Radical Remission: Surviving Cancer Against All Odds* (Turner)
about, xii–xiii
popularity of, xiii–xiv
radiofrequency radiation, 82
Rankin, Lissa, 146, 147
Rational Therapeutics, 259
reasons for living, 243–268
about, 243–245
action steps, 266–268
healing stories, 19, 36, 43, 69–70, 90, 103–104, 128, 137–138, 236–237, 248–250, 251, 252–265, 297
hope and, 21, 96–97, 137–138
new trends, 245–261
playfulness and purpose, 250–251, 267
positive emotions and, 103–104
research studies, 245–247
search for meaning, 247–250
rebounding, 12, 17
ReCODE (for Reversal of Cognitive Decline), 287–289, 296
Reiki, 116, 140
repressed emotions. *See* suppressed emotion release
rest and repair state, 76, 155–156, 191–192
RGCC (Research Genetic Cancer Centre), 63
Rust, Mary (healing story), 12, 13–21

**S**

salivary gland tumors, 82
Sally's healing story, 283–297
sarcomas, 184–185, 248–249, 252–265, 271–272
Sat Nam Rasayan, 116
Saupe, Henning, 83–84
Schneider, Jill Ayn, 27
self-love, 148–151, 173, 248
Sexton, Andrea, 275–276
shame, 32, 84, 159, 164, 281
Shoemaker, Ritchie, 293–294
Sielaff, Robin, 231
skin lymphoma, 197–209
sleep, 289–290
Slocum, Abdul Kadir, 246

# ACKNOWLEDGMENTS

## From Kelly Turner:

It took me 10 years to write my first book and six more to write this one. The only reason this one took less time was because of the many, many people who helped to make it possible. The main person to thank—without whom this book would have never happened—is my co-author Tracy White, who somehow convinced me that we should undertake the gargantuan effort of writing a second book. Her motivation, writing, and partnership throughout the entire process made it all so much more enjoyable than I could have ever imagined. Tracy, thank you for stepping into your destiny as an author to help bring *Radical Hope* into the world.

I am also exceedingly grateful to Lisa and Alexander Laing for stepping in right when I needed them with their superb writing and editing skills. This book would not have made it to the finish line without you two, and for that, I am forever grateful.

My heart goes out to my agent Ned Leavitt, for being up for another creative adventure with me, and also to Lisa Cheng, Patty Gift, Reid Tracy, and everyone else at Hay House who believed in this book and worked so hard to help make it the best it could be. Many thanks also to my editor at HarperOne, Gideon Weil, and my publicist there, Melinda Mullin, for their unwavering support of *Radical Remission*.

*Radical Hope* is not being launched in a vacuum because there are many new facets of the Radical Remission Project that have developed over the past six years. I am grateful to Cindy Handler, our Director of Trainings, and to all our certified Radical Remission teachers (I'm looking at you, Elders and Wild Ones!) for their patience and understanding when I was busy writing *Radical Hope*. Thank you also to everyone who submitted their healing story to our website, took our online course, or attended an in-person workshop over the past six years—our mission is to serve you, and we hope that this book is yet another way of achieving that mission.

Boundless thanks goes to Junaidah Barnett, Ph.D., Michelle Holmes, Ph.D., and George Wang, M.D., Ph.D., the principal investigators of our pilot study with Harvard University, for their interest in and commitment to taking my qualitative research to the quantitative level. Finally, by the time this book is published, our 10-part docuseries on radical remission will have aired, and I'm so grateful to my film crew—Jennifer, Ryan, Taylor, and Karli—for taking so many weeks out of their lives to help me bring radical remission stories to visual life.

I am so grateful to my sisters Lisa, Melissa, and Sarah for our weekly accountability calls, which helped keep my writing and editing on track. Mom, Dad, Chris, Carrie, Andy, and Patrick were also sending their support from afar, as were my adorable nieces and nephews, cousins, aunts, and uncles. I am truly so blessed to have the family I have.

This book certainly would not have happened without Tracy, but it equally would not have happened without the support of my amazing husband and partner in life, Aaron, whose emotional support knows no bounds. I would accomplish nothing without him to lean on. And words cannot express how much love I have in my heart for our two incredible children, who were always there to offer cuddles and hugs when I was tired of editing. And Lisa Malota, you are our very own Mary Poppins—our family would not function without you.

Finally, a huge thank-you goes to all the survivors of cancer and other diseases who agreed to be interviewed for this book. By allowing us to analyze, learn from, and share your experiences, you are helping the world to learn more about the human body and human potential. Thank you for being our teachers. And to all of the doctors, healers, and experts who lent their wisdom to this book, thank you for being guiding lights as we move collectively closer to health and wholeness. May we all continue learning and improving upon the human experience.

— *Kelly Turner, Ph.D.*

## From Tracy G. White—November 2019:

This book is not my cancer story. This book is about helping patients find the same hope I desperately needed when I was diagnosed with metastatic cervical cancer in 2016. I have many people to thank for the opportunity and privilege to work on this project. Writing *Radical Hope* has been the highlight of my life.

My contribution to this book would not have been possible without the trust and faith of Dr. Kelly Turner. I'm eternally grateful to Kelly for so many things. In 2016, the principles of *Radical Remission* unequivocally led to my miraculous remission. I was blissfully stable for three years. During that time, I became a Radical Remission teacher, coach, and advocate. I connected to the Radical Remission tribe, which was an essential support group, and I got the pleasure of knowing Kelly as a person and mentor.

I have deep gratitude to Kelly; our agent, Ned Leavitt; Patty Gift; Lisa Cheng; and the entire Hay House team for taking a chance on a first-time co-author. It's been an honor to write *Radical Hope* and I hope it will provide some of the same inspiration as reading *Radical Remission* did for me in 2016. Because there's always hope!

In January 2019, I experienced an aggressive cancer recurrence. Lest you think having a recurrence implies these principles don't work, remember that I'm still alive two and a half years after the "expiration date" given to me by my doctors. This proves to me there are tangible benefits and that the 10 factors strengthened my immune system to be stronger during my conventional treatments. Ultimately, though, we must surrender to the universe's big picture of our survival.

I'm deeply moved by my loving, loyal, and compassionate husband, Paul, who has been with me every step of the way. In addition, my gracious, charming, and compassionate son, Blake, has always been my biggest cheerleader. Blake, you're the best thing that's ever happened to me. I love you even when I can't see you.

I am humbled by the support and outreach from so many friends. The outpouring of love is overwhelming and deeply touching. Especially my dear friends and gorgeous souls: Stacey Staaterman,

Melissa Myers, Clare Hand, Hillary Periera, SMS tribe, and the West Palm Beach posse, who gave so much of themselves to help get me well.

I have been blessed to work with an amazing medical team of doctors and healers, including my traditional oncologist, Dr. Kevin Holcomb, who, unlike many doctors, remained open-minded about my integrative treatments and never discouraged me. There's also my talented naturopath, Dr. Mark Bricca, whose kindness, knowledge, and compassion make him a gift to cancer patients. Dr. Nasha Winters spent years getting my terrain better aligned for my health. I also want to thank Dr. Mark Rosenberg of Advanced Medical Therapeutics for providing research and cancer solutions with out-of-the-box thinking. May more doctors see his good results as an example of the mind-body-spirit connection.

Last, I wish to acknowledge the team of spiritual healers that have helped me find my soul's path and purpose: Carrie Severson, Gina Martin, and Janet O'Shea, specifically, as well as the other healers I have met along the way.

Finally, thank you, dear reader, for investing in *Radical Hope*. I wish it brings you encouragement when you most need it.

In light and love,

*Tracy*

# ABOUT THE AUTHORS

**KELLY TURNER, PH.D.**, is the *New York Times* best-selling author of *Radical Hope* and *Radical Remission,* now in 22 languages, which summarizes her research into radical remission—when someone heals from a serious illness without conventional medicine or after conventional medicine has failed. Over the past 15 years, she has conducted research in 10 different countries and analyzed over 1,500 cases of radical remission. She is a frequent guest on *The Dr. Oz Show* and holds a B.A. from Harvard University and a Ph.D. from the University of California, Berkeley. She is the founder of the Radical Remission Project at RadicalRemission .com, which provides courses, workshops, and a free database of healing stories for patients and their loved ones. She is the founder of the Radical Remission Foundation, a nonprofit whose mission is to further scientific research on radical remissions, as well as the director and producer of *Radical Remission,* a docuseries about radical remission. Also a screenwriter, Kelly has written a feature-length film script about radical remission entitled *Open-Ended Ticket.* You can learn more at Kelly-Turner.com.

**TRACY WHITE** is the co-author of *Radical Hope.* Prior to her diagnosis of recurrent cervical cancer in 2016 and being given 15 months to live by her doctors, Tracy enjoyed a successful career as a marketing executive for leading magazines and websites. She spent 20 years creating intricate advertising deals and partnerships for brands such as Travel + Leisure, Food & Wine, Traditional Home, Fortune, Inc., Seventeen, and Bankrate. As a writer, speaker, and teacher on the topic of wellness, Tracy was published on SheKnows, SurvivorNet, and Elephant Journal. She taught workshops and gave lectures at such places as the Omega Institute, T.E.A.L., and SHARE. Tracy defied the odds by living an additional two and a half high-quality years after her doctors predicted she would die, during which time she co-authored *Radical Hope* and cherished extra years spent with her son and husband.

# Hay House Titles of Related Interest

*YOU CAN HEAL YOUR LIFE, the movie,*
starring Louise Hay & Friends
(available as a 1-DVD program, an expanded 2-DVD set,
and an online streaming video)
Learn more at www.hayhouse.com/louise-movie

*THE SHIFT, the movie,*
starring Dr. Wayne W. Dyer
(available as a 1-DVD program, an expanded 2-DVD set,
and an online streaming video)
Learn more at www.hayhouse.com/the-shift-movie

*CANCER-FREE WITH FOOD: A Step-by-Step Plan with 100+ Recipes to Fight Disease, Nourish Your Body & Restore Your Health,* by Liana Werner-Gray

*CHRIS BEAT CANCER: A Comprehensive Plan for Healing Naturally,* by Chris Wark

*CRAZY SEXY JUICE: 100+ Simple Juice, Smoothie & Nut Milk Recipes to Supercharge Your Health,* by Kris Carr

*DYING TO BE ME: My Journey from Cancer, to Near Death, to True Healing,* by Anita Moorjani

*OUTSIDE THE BOX CANCER THERAPIES: Alternative Therapies That Treat and Prevent Cancer,* by Dr. Mark Stengler and Dr. Paul Anderson

*REGENERATE: Unlocking Your Body's Radical Resilience through the New Biology,* by Sayer Ji

All of the above are available at your local bookstore,
or may be ordered by contacting Hay House (see next page).

We hope you enjoyed this Hay House book. If you'd like to receive our online catalog featuring additional information on Hay House books and products, or if you'd like to find out more about the Hay Foundation, please contact:

Hay House, Inc., P.O. Box 5100, Carlsbad, CA 92018-5100
(760) 431-7695 or (800) 654-5126
(760) 431-6948 (fax) or (800) 650-5115 (fax)
www.hayhouse.com® • www.hayfoundation.org

———

*Published in Australia by:* Hay House Australia Pty. Ltd.,
18/36 Ralph St., Alexandria NSW 2015
*Phone:* 612-9669-4299 • *Fax:* 612-9669-4144
www.hayhouse.com.au

*Published in the United Kingdom by:* Hay House UK, Ltd.,
The Sixth Floor, Watson House, 54 Baker Street, London W1U 7BU
*Phone:* +44 (0)20 3927 7290 • *Fax:* +44 (0)20 3927 7291
www.hayhouse.co.uk

*Published in India by:* Hay House Publishers India,
Muskaan Complex, Plot No. 3, B-2, Vasant Kunj, New Delhi 110 070
*Phone:* 91-11-4176-1620 • *Fax:* 91-11-4176-1630
www.hayhouse.co.in

———

## Access New Knowledge.
## Anytime. Anywhere.

Learn and evolve at your own pace
with the world's leading experts.

www.hayhouseU.com

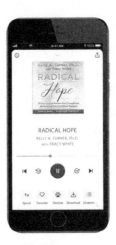